Handbook of Tumor Viruses

Handbook of Tumor Viruses

Editor: Park Wharton

AMERICAN
MEDICAL PUBLISHERS
www.americanmedicalpublishers.com

AMERICAN
MEDICAL PUBLISHERS
www.americanmedicalpublishers.com

Cataloging-in-Publication Data

Handbook of tumor viruses / edited by Park Wharton.
p. cm.
Includes bibliographical references and index.
ISBN 978-1-63927-688-2
1. Oncogenic viruses. 2. Viruses. 3. Viral carcinogenesis. I. Wharton, Park.
QR372.O6 H36 2023
616.994 019--dc23

American Medical Publishers,
41 Flatbush Avenue,
1st Floor, New York,
NY 11217, USA

ISBN 978-1-63927-688-2 (Hardback)

Contents

Preface

This book has been a concerted effort by a group of academicians, researchers and scientists, who have contributed their research works for the realization of the book. This book has materialized in the wake of emerging advancements and innovations in this field. Therefore, the need of the hour was to compile all the required researches and disseminate the knowledge to a broad spectrum of people comprising of students, researchers and specialists of the field.

Tumor viruses are members of six distinct families of animal viruses. They have the potential to cause cancer in animals and humans. Viruses which belong to five of the six families of tumor viruses have DNA genomes and are therefore called DNA tumor viruses. Retroviruses belong to the sixth family of tumor viruses that have RNA genomes in virus particles. These viruses replicate in infected cells through the synthesis of a DNA provirus. The viruses that cause cancers in humans are papillomaviruses, which causes anogenital and cervical cancers, Epstein-Barr virus which causes nasopharyngeal carcinoma and Burkitt's lymphoma, and Kaposi's sarcoma related herpesvirus. The genomes of tumor viruses are small in size, which facilitate identification of genes inducing cancer and enhance the understanding of cancer on the molecular level. This book is a compilation of chapters that discuss the most vital and emerging trends in the study of tumor viruses. It will serve as a reference to a broad spectrum of readers.

At the end of the preface, I would like to thank the authors for their brilliant chapters and the publisher for guiding us all-through the making of the book till its final stage. Also, I would like to thank my family for providing the support and encouragement throughout my academic career and research projects.

Editor

1

Merkel Cell Polyomavirus: Molecular Insights into the Most Recently Discovered Human Tumor Virus

Gabrielė Stakaitytė, Jennifer J. Wood, Laura M. Knight, Hussein Abdul-Sada, Noor Suhana Adzahar, Nnenna Nwogu, Andrew Macdonald and Adrian Whitehouse *

School of Molecular and Cellular Biology and Astbury Centre of Structural Molecular Biology, University of Leeds, Leeds, LS2 9JT, UK; E-Mails: bsgst@leeds.ac.uk (G.S.); bsjjw@leeds.ac.uk (J.J.W.); bslmk@leeds.ac.uk (L.M.K.); bshkas@leeds.ac.uk (H.A.-S.); bsnsba@leeds.ac.uk (N.S.A.); bsnoun@leeds.ac.uk (N.N.); A.Macdonald@leeds.ac.uk (A.M.)

* Author to whom correspondence should be addressed; E-Mail: A.Whitehouse@leeds.ac.uk;

Abstract: A fifth of worldwide cancer cases have an infectious origin, with viral infection being the foremost. One such cancer is Merkel cell carcinoma (MCC), a rare but aggressive skin malignancy. In 2008, Merkel cell polyomavirus (MCPyV) was discovered as the causative agent of MCC. It is found clonally integrated into the majority of MCC tumours, which require MCPyV oncoproteins to survive. Since its discovery, research has begun to reveal the molecular virology of MCPyV, as well as how it induces tumourigenesis. It is thought to be a common skin commensal, found at low levels in healthy individuals. Upon loss of immunosurveillance, MCPyV reactivates, and a heavy viral load is associated with MCC pathogenesis. Although MCPyV is in many ways similar to classical oncogenic polyomaviruses, such as SV40, subtle differences are beginning to emerge. These unique features highlight the singular position MCPyV has as the only human oncogenic polyomavirus, and open up new avenues for therapies against MCC.

Keywords: Merkel cell polyomavirus; Merkel cell carcinoma; large T antigen; small T antigen; tumourigenesis

---

1. Introduction

The causes of cancer are many and varied, but viruses and other infectious agents are being recognised as increasingly important. The International Agency for Research on Cancer estimates that around 20% of cancer cases worldwide are caused by infection, with most being viral in origin [1]. Today, seven human oncogenic viruses are thought to account for 10%–15% of human cancers.

Oncogenic viruses can cause cancer by interrupting the control of cell proliferation. Most express specific oncogenes that promote cell growth and proliferation, thus transforming cells. The first oncogenic virus, Rous sarcoma virus or RSV, was discovered by Peyton Rous in 1911, and causes cancer in chickens [2]. In the following decades, a series of mammalian oncogenic viruses were discovered, including murine polyomavirus (MPyV) and simian vacuolating virus 40 (SV40) [3–5]. The latter have served as an excellent model for both studying oncogenic viruses and fundamental oncogenic processes.

Human oncogenic viruses have been the focus of intensive study, ever since the discovery of Epstein-Barr virus (EBV) in 1964 [3]. They represent a variety of different types of viruses, from small DNA viruses to RNA viruses to retroviruses, representing the range of possible viral life cycles and modes of reproduction. Table 1 elaborates on these viruses and their links to cancers.

Table 1. The human oncogenic viruses. The seven human oncogenic viruses, their year of discovery, genome and various cancers they are associated with. ds-double-stranded, ss-single-stranded, (+)-positive-stranded.

VIRUS	YEAR	FAMILY	GENOME	ONCOGENES	CANCER ASSOCIATION
Epstein-Barr Virus (EBV)	1964	Herpesviridae	dsDNA	LMP1	Including Burkitt's lymphoma, nasopharyngeal carcinoma, and some other lymphoproliferative disorders
Hepatitis B virus (HBV)	1965	Hepadnaviridae	ssDNA and dsDNA	HBx	Some hepatocellular carcinomas
Human T-lymphotropic virus-I (HTLV-I)	1980	Retroviridae	ssRNA	Tax	Adult T cell leukaemia
Human papillomaviruses (HPV) 16 and 18	1983-1984	Papillomaviridae	dsDNA	E5, E6, E7	Most cervical cancer and penile cancers.
Hepatitis C virus (HCV)	1989	Hepaciviridae	(+)ssRNA	NS5A	Some hepatocellular carcinomas and lymphomas
Kaposi's sarcoma herpesvirus (KSHV)	1994	Herpesviridae	dsDNA	LANA, vflip, and vBcl-2, among others	Kaposi's sarcoma and primary effusion lymphoma
Merkel Cell Polyomavirus (MCPyV)	2008	Polyomaviridae	dsDNA	T antigens	Most Merkel cell carcinomas,

The newest addition to the human oncogenic virus classification is Merkel cell polyomavirus (MCPyV), discovered in 2008 [6]. It has been confirmed to be the causative agent behind the majority of cases of Merkel cell carcinoma (MCC), a rare and highly aggressive human malignancy.

2. Merkel Cell Carcinoma

Merkel cell carcinoma is a rare and highly malignant primary neuroendocrine carcinoma of the skin. Over 90% of cases arise in sun-exposed areas, with half around the head and neck. This suggests that sunlight, primarily as ultraviolet radiation, plays a role in the development of MCC. MCC can also be found on the trunk and genitals but at a significantly reduced frequency (<10%) [7]. Epidemiological studies highlight that older, lighter-skinned individuals and people who have been subjected to organ transplant or infected with HIV/AIDS are more vulnerable to infection [8,9].

MCC is thought to arise in Merkel cells, a type of mechanoreceptor cell located in the stratum basale in touch sensitive areas of the epidermis (Figure 1). Merkel cells were first described over a century ago by the leading German histopathologist Friedrich Sigmund Merkel [10]. These cells are oval and around 10–15 μm in diameter, resembling a hemisphere with spinous projections on their surfaces. They are found attached to the disk-like sensory terminal of nerve fibres, in a complex termed a Merkel or tactile disk [11]. The function of Merkel cells is still unclear. Studies indicate that the presence of neuropeptides, accumulated near the nerve fibre junction, signifies their action in the expression of voltage gated ion channels which are essential for synaptic transmission. However, conflicting evidence, using histochemical markers, suggests a paracrine function of Merkel cells [12].

Figure 1. Cross section of skin. Illustration of the six layers of skin, from the dermis to the stratum corneum. Examples of residents cells are included, among them a healthy Merkel cell and a cell that is part of a Merkel cell carcinoma tumour. Merkel cells are located in the stratum basale.

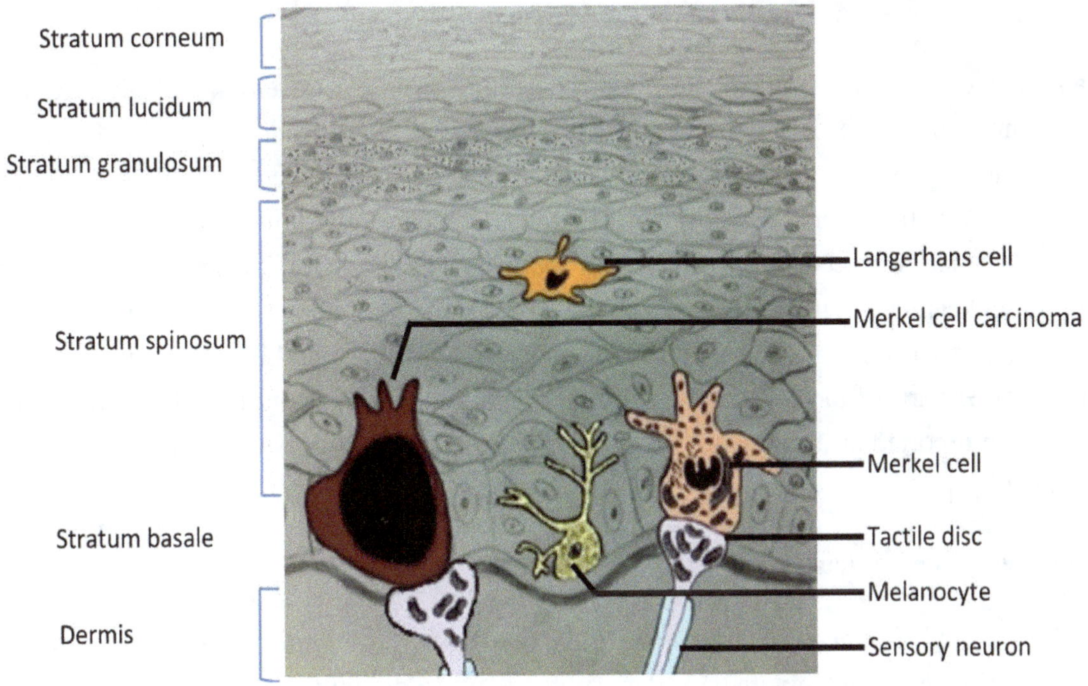

MCC was first described in 1972 by Cyril Toker [10], who noted a flesh-coloured or bluish-red glassy painless nodule (Figure 2) with solid trabeculae in five different areas (forearm, lip, face, leg and buttock) of two older men, who later died as a result of this tumour, and three older women. Toker used the name trabecular carcinoma of the skin to describe these tumours, assuming that they represented an endocrine, sweat gland-derived carcinoma.

Figure 2. Merkel cell carcinoma. A typical MCC nodule present on the leg of a patient. Image credit to Howard Peach, Leeds Teaching Hospitals NHS Trust, UK.

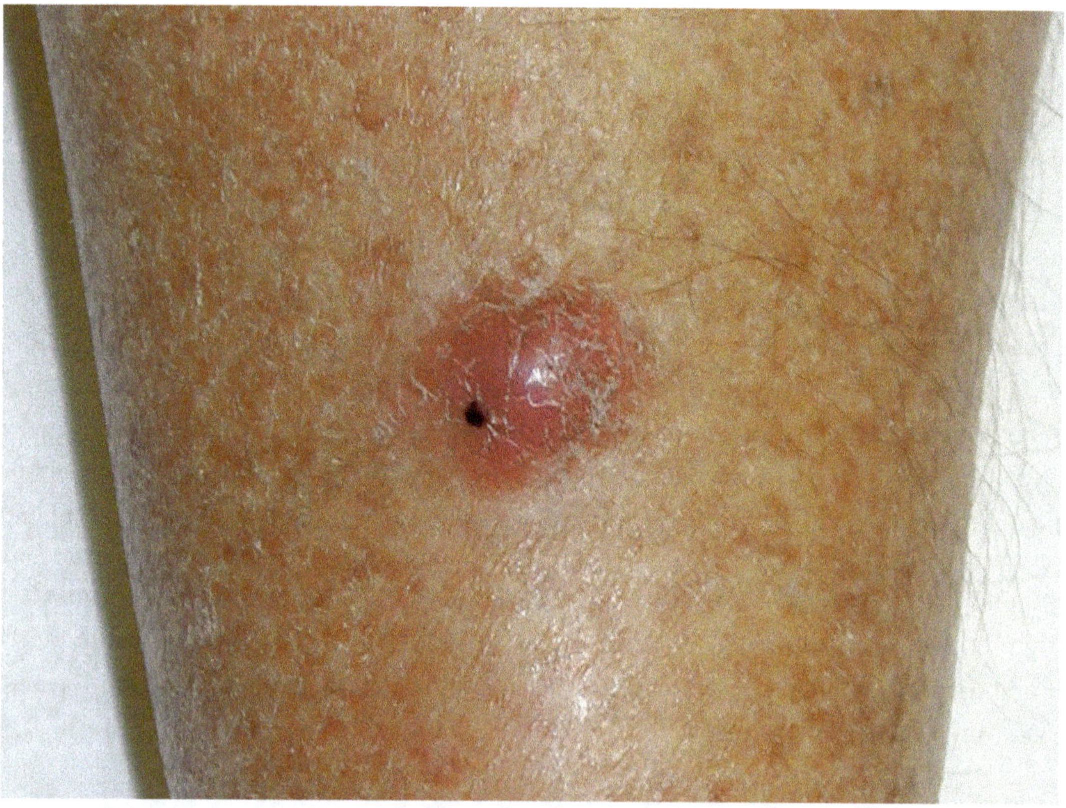

Advanced age (>65 years) and male gender correlate with the development of MCC [13]. The estimated annual incidence of MCC has increased during the last decade from 0.29 to 2.2 cases per million, and more than half of infected patients die within 5 years of diagnosis. Though the mortality rate of MCC is much higher than those for other skin cancers [14], this may in part be due to the increased incidence of secondary cancers in patients diagnosed with MCC, such as chronic lymphocytic leukaemia, multiple myeloma, malignancies of the biliary tract and salivary gland, and other skin malignancies, such as basal cell carcinoma [15]. MCC is a highly metastatic tumour and can transplant to other parts of the body by transiting through the lymphatic drainage [16]. MCC metastasis have often been reported at distant sites including the pancreas and breast [17], the heart [18], and the palatine tonsil [19].

3. Merkel Cell Polyomavirus

MCPyV is a double-stranded DNA virus of the *Polyomaviridae* family. It was discovered in 2008 by Moore and Chang at the University of Pennsylvania, using digital transcriptome subtraction (DTS), a novel method of detecting viruses in cancerous tissue. DTS involves extracting mRNA from tumor cells, converting it to cDNA, and then sequencing. The data obtained is then compared to known human sequences, and matching stretches of DNA are "subtracted", leaving the remainder as likely non-human. The remaining sequences are then compared against the pathogen sequence database. The analysis highlighted a sequence related to polyomaviruses, but distinct enough to be considered a novel virus [6].

Initially, the MCPyV genome was found integrated into the genome of MCC cells in a clonal pattern [6]. Moreover, based on the fact that MCPyV infection and genome integration happens before the clonal expansion of tumor cells suggests that MCPyV might be a contributing factor to MCC. The mechanism by which MCPyV causes tumorigenesis is still questionable. Following initial findings, several other reports confirmed clonal integration of the viral genome into the cellular genome in MCC tumors [20–22]. These reports support the theory that MCPyV is an etiological factor of MCC, rather than being a passenger virus. In addition, MCC tumour metastases were also found to be MCPyV-positive and possess the same integration patterns as the original tumour [20]. MCPyV is the only polyomavirus that has been conclusively associated with a human tumor, and has now been detected in 80%–97% of MCC tumors [6,23].

All MCC cells display membrane-bound cytoplasmic structures with a unique arrangement of cytokeratin 20 (CK20) filaments in a perinuclear distribution [24]. This feature is used to distinguish and diagnose MCC. The primary diagnostic panel of MCC also includes the thyroid transcription factor and leukocyte common antigen. Moreover, the presence of chromogranin and synoptophysin confirm the positive diagnostic results of MCC.

In addition, immunohistochemistry has been used to detect MCPyV viral antigens in MCC tumours, with antigen expression being limited to MCC cells [25]. More recent serological assays that detect MCPyV VP1 and VP2 proteins by enzyme-linked immunosorbent assay (ELISA) of blood sample have made the diagnosis of MCPyV easier [26]. These depend on the lack of similarity between the MCPyV VP1 and the capsid protein of other polyomaviruses. These assays have been used to determine the incidence of MCPyV in the general population, as well as giving clues about its epidemiology. MCPyV shows a worldwide distribution, and has been detected in samples from the United States [27], Europe [28], Japan [29], Cameroon in Africa [30] and Australia [31], among others. This highlights the startling fact that not only are the majority of MCC patients positive for the virus, but in the wider population, 50% of children under 15 and up to 80% of healthy adults are infected with MCPyV, as reflected by seroprevalence [27]. It is likely that MCPyV is acquired at some point during childhood, either by transmission between siblings or from mother to child, through close contact, involving skin and/or saliva [30]. In addition, recent evidence has suggested that there are geographical variations of MCPyV [32,33], with the possibility of as many as five different genotypes present across the globe [34]. The virus is considered a common skin commensal, and further work is bound to uncover more details of its epidemiology and genotypical variations.

4. MCPyV Genome

The MCPyV genome (Figure 3) comprises 5,387 base pairs, with a non-coding control region (NCRR), containing the bipartite origin of replication, separating the early and late gene coding regions.

Separation allows for temporal control of viral gene expression. This type of genome structure is closely related to that of all known polyomaviruses. While there is much shared homology between MCPyV and other well-studied human polyomaviruses, the MCPyV genome seems to be most closely related to the African Green Monkey lymphotropic polyomavirus [35]. Currently, MCPyV is classified in the Orthopolyomavirus genus of the *Polyomaviridae* family, which include mammalian polyomaviruses such as MPyV, SV40 and the human polyomaviruses JC (JCPyV) and BK (BKPyV) [36].

Figure 3. MCPyV genome organisation. Non-coding control region (NCCR): bipartite origin of replication. Early gene region: Large T antigen (LT), small T antigen (ST), 57kT antigen (57kT), alternative T antigen open reading frame (ALTO), microRNA (miRNA). Late gene region: capsid proteins (VP1-3).

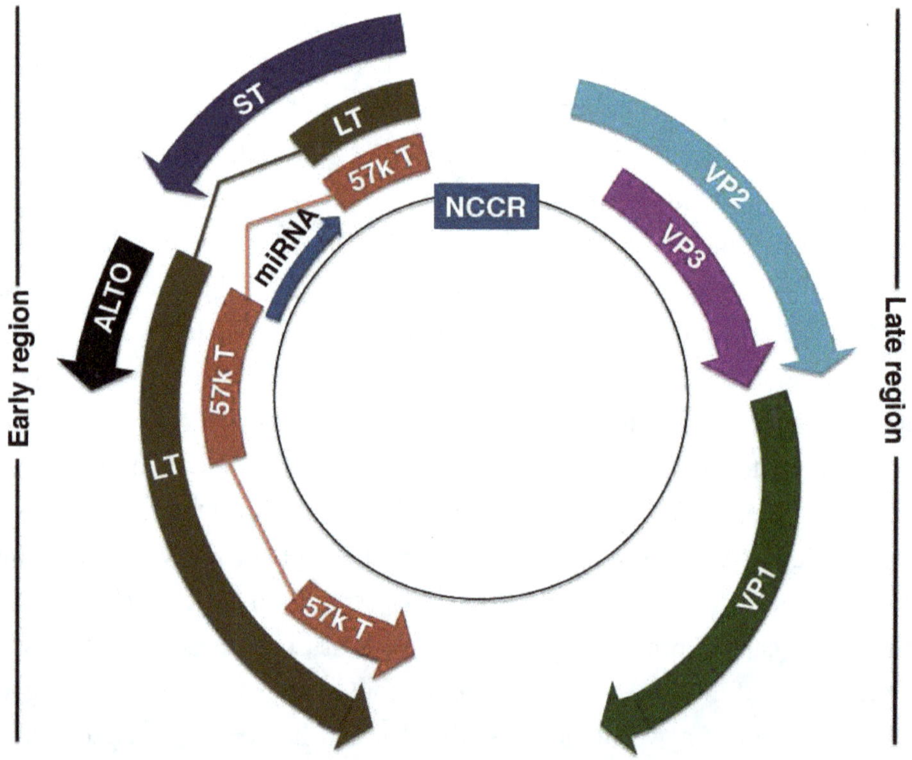

4.1. MCPyV Origin of Replication

The NCCR contains the 71 base pair long origin of replication. The origin of replication, like those of other polyomaviruses, has an AT rich region, an early enhancer domain and a binding site for the large T antigen. The binding site is composed of ten repeating guanine-rich pentanucleotide sequences: eight corresponding to the general polyomavirus consensus of 5'-GAGGG-3', while two are somewhat different: 5'-GGGGC-3' and 5'-GAGCC-3'. The number of sequences and their proximity to each other are unlike other polyomaviruses [37].

4.2. MCPyV T Antigen Locus

Polyomavirus early gene regions encode proteins that interfere in cell cycle regulation, and, in some cases, lead to tumour formation. For this reason, the polyomavirus early gene region is also known as the "tumour antigen" or T antigen locus (Figure 4). The MCPyV T antigen locus is about 3000 base pairs in length. After transcription as a single transcript, the T antigen is differentially spliced into the large T antigen (LT), the small T antigen (ST), and the 57 kD T antigen (57kT) [6]. LT, ST and 57kT all share the same short amino-terminal sequence, including the J domain. This contains the DnaJ (HPDKGG) domain, which is essential for binding the cellular heat shock protein, Hsc70, and a conserved Cr1 epitope (LXXLL) [6]. Alternative splicing produces a distinct carboxy-terminus, which determines the variability in the functions of the T antigen splice products.

Figure 4. Mapping of the multiply-spliced MCPyV T antigens. The three T antigens are LT, ST and 57kT. All three encode CR1 (yellow, LXXLL) and DnaJ (lilac, HPDKGG) domains. ST also contains two PP2A Aα binding sites (R7 and L142), a PP2A Aβ/PP4C binding site (amino acids 97–111) and an large T-stabilisation domain (LSD, amino acids 91–95). LT shares the pRb binding domain with 57kT; in addition, it has unique origin binding (OBD), zinc finger, leucine zipper, ATPase and helicase domains. The MCPyV-unique region (MUR) of LT contains the hVam6p binding site.

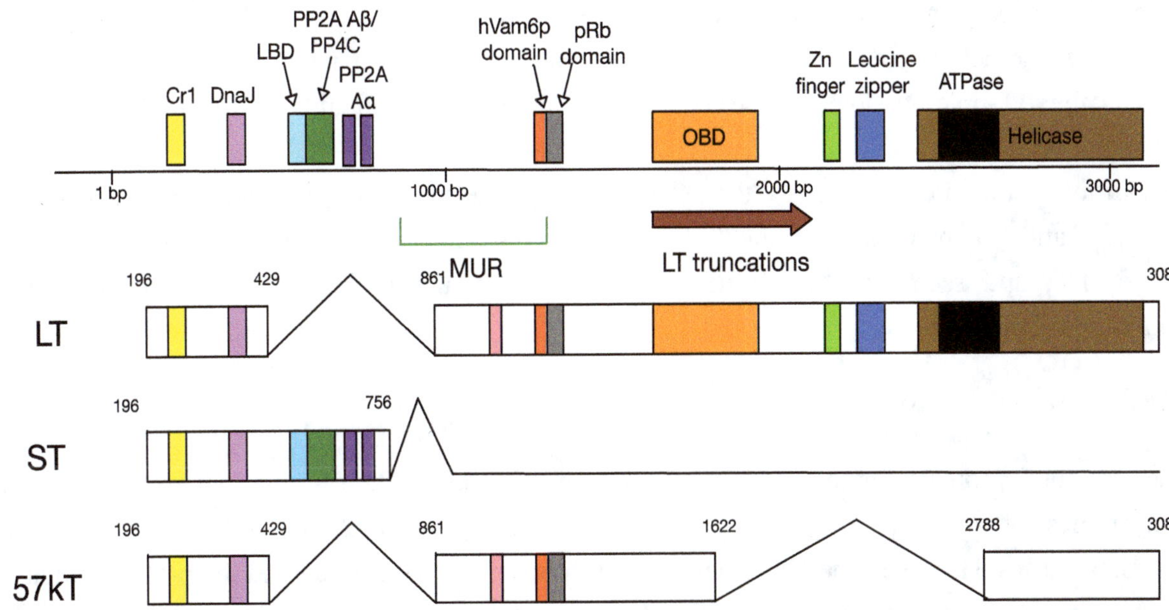

MCPyV LT, 816 amino acids in size, is composed of two exons. It has numerous functions in MCPyV infection, including the initiation of viral replication and manipulation of the host cell cycle. MCPyV LT contains several conserved domains found across polyomaviruses: the retinoblastoma protein (pRb) binding domain (LXCXE), a nuclear localisation signal (NLS) and the origin-binding domain (OBD). The carboxy-terminal half of the polyomavirus LT has viral DNA binding and helicase features [38–41]. The presence of a nuclear localisation signal (NLS) results in MCPyV LT localising to the nucleus when expressed in mammalian cells [42].

It may be possible to infer some interactions between MCPyV LT and cellular factors by considering SV40 LT. The DnaJ domain of SV40 LT interacts with the cellular chaperone Hsc70, and the LXCXE domain binds to pRb and pRb family members p107 and p130 [43,44]. The E3 ligase component Cullin 7 and the spindle checkpoint protein BUB1 are cellular factors which have been demonstrated to bind between these two regions [45,46]. The OBD and helicase region recruit numerous proteins required for viral replication, including p53, p300 and CBP [47,48]. However,

MCPyV LT shares only 34% sequence identity with SV40 LT [40]. MCPyV LT also contains the MCPyV unique region (MUR), consisting of a 200 amino acid sequence located between the first exon and the OBD [42]. This unique LT region binds the host cellular factor Vam6p and redistributes it to the nucleus, in addition to encoding a viral miRNA [42,49].

MCPyV 57kT, 432 amino acids in length, is the product of alternative splicing linking three exons. Little is known about this protein, although it shares the DnaJ domain and CR1 epitope with LT and sT, as well as containing the MUR region and the pRB-binding domain. In addition, 57kT is homologous with SV40 17kT [50], which plays a role in promoting host cell proliferation [51].

Finally, MCPyV ST is 186 amino acids long, and, like LT, has roles in viral replication and cellular transformation. The unique carboxy-terminal ST region is produced via transcriptional read-through of the exon splice site used by both LT and 57kT. ST localises both to the nucleus and the cytoplasm [52]. In addition, it contains the typical polyomavirus protein phosphatase 2A (PP2A) Aα subunit binding site [6], which is important for viral replication and virus-induced transformation in other polyomaviruses [53]. However, recently, a PP2A Aβ and/or protein phosphatase 4C (PP4C) binding site near its carboxy terminus has also been discovered, which may have a role to play in protecting MCPyV from the cellular immune response [54]. In addition, another newly-discovered MCPyV ST domain is the LT-binding domain (LBD), which stabilises LT and aids in the replication of the MCPyV genome [55].

In addition to the three T antigens, the MCPyV early gene locus also encodes a fourth protein, the alternative T antigen open reading frame (ALTO). ALTO is transcribed from the 200 amino acid MUR region of LT, and seems to be evolutionarily related to the middle T antigen of the murine polyomavirus [56].

4.3. MCPyV Late Proteins

The structural proteins for the virus capsid are encoded in the late region. There are three open reading frames for capsid proteins, viral proteins 1, 2, and 3 (VP1, VP2 and VP3), which is typical of all polyomaviruses. However, the VP3 open reading frame is not conserved and the protein is inactive, not part of the capsid, or not expressed at all [57].

MCPyV has an unenveloped, icosahedral capsid made up of 72 pentamers of the major capsid protein, VP1. VP2, the minor capsid protein, is important for infectivity, while the presence of VP3 has not been detected in native MPCyV virions [57]. Despite the apparent absence of VP3, the viral capsid is about 40–55 nm in size, which is comparable to other polyomaviruses. The ratio of VP1:VP2 seems to be about 5:2, which means there are two VP2 molecules for each VP1 pentamer [57].

The crystal structure of VP1 was determined as a symmetrical, ring-shaped homopentamer with the five monomers arranged around a central five-fold axis. Each VP1 monomer is composed of two antiparallel β sheets, which form a β-sandwich with jelly-roll topology. Variable loops create unique interaction surfaces on the outer surface of the pentamer [58]. VP1 has a nuclear-localisation signal (NLS) at its amino-terminus, and shows a diffuse nuclear pattern.

VP2 seems to be dispensable for most entry steps in some cell lines, as it does not affect trafficking, viral DNA packaging, or binding to cellular receptors. However, it is possible that myristoylation of VP2, which is required during entry, may help to disrupt cellular membranes. VP2 seems to lack a

NLS, and thus localises in the cytoplasm. However, presence of VP1 shifts the signature of VP2 to a similar, diffuse nuclear pattern [57].

4.4. MCPyV MicroRNA

Numerous polyomaviruses, including SV40, JCV and BKV, encode miRNAs which regulate early viral transcript levels [59,60]. It is therefore unsurprising, that in addition to the structural proteins, the late region also encodes a 22-nucleotide-long microRNA (miRNA), MCV-miR-M1-5p. The miRNA is encoded antisense to the LT coding region [49]. It is thought to regulate the expression of the early genes, reducing the levels of early gene transcripts, and has complementarity with a section of the LT transcript. Furthermore, it may have a role to play in cellular transformation, and its expression is preserved in at least half of MCPyV-positive MCC tumours [61].

Therefore, the MCPyV genome shares a many similarities in its organisation and gene products with other polyomaviruses. However, there are unique characteristics, and the reasons for these divergences are not yet fully understood.

5. The Lifecycle of MCPyV

The cellular tropism of MCPyV has not yet been established, as it was discovered within a malignancy, rather than its natural host cell. However, the origin of Merkel cell carcinoma as well as the findings that MCPyV is chronically shed from the skin [62], point to an epidermal source of host cells. MCPyV pseudovirions exhibit infectious entry into human skin-derived primary keratinocytes (HEKa) and transformed melanocytes, while primary transformed keratinocytes (HeCat) and primary melanocytes did not permit infection. In addition, none of the 60 human tumour cell lines investigated show tropism for MCPyV [63]. It is possible to propagate the virus in human embryonic kidney cell-derived cultures (HEK-293), when LT and ST are expressed *in trans* [64], and this is the presently used to study the life cycle of MCPyV.

5.1. MCPyV Attachment and Entry

As a rule, most polyomaviruses, such as MPyV, SV40, and BKPyV use sialic acid-containing glycolipids, or gangliosides, to attach to cells [65,66]. However, in the case of MCPyV, the initial attachment appears to involve glycosaminoglycans, in particular heparan sulfate. In addition, binding to gangliosides, specifically Gt1b, which carries three different sialic acids, is required for post-attachment entry [64].

Using X-ray crystallography, researchers have been able to determine that the MCPyV major capsid protein VP1 has a shallow binding site for cellular glycans containing sialic acid with a Neu5Ac moiety. Specifically, it interacts with carbohydrates bearing a linear Neu5Ac-α2,3-Gal motif. Mutating these binding sites has no effect on initial attachment [58]. Therefore, the current model of MCPyV entry (Figure 5) is a two-step attachment-and-entry process involving two separate types of host cell plasma membrane factors.

Figure 5. Two-step attachment and entry process of MCPyV. GAG—glycosaminoglycan, such as heparan sulfate. Neu5Ac—ganglioside with a linear Neu5Ac-α2,3-Gal motif.

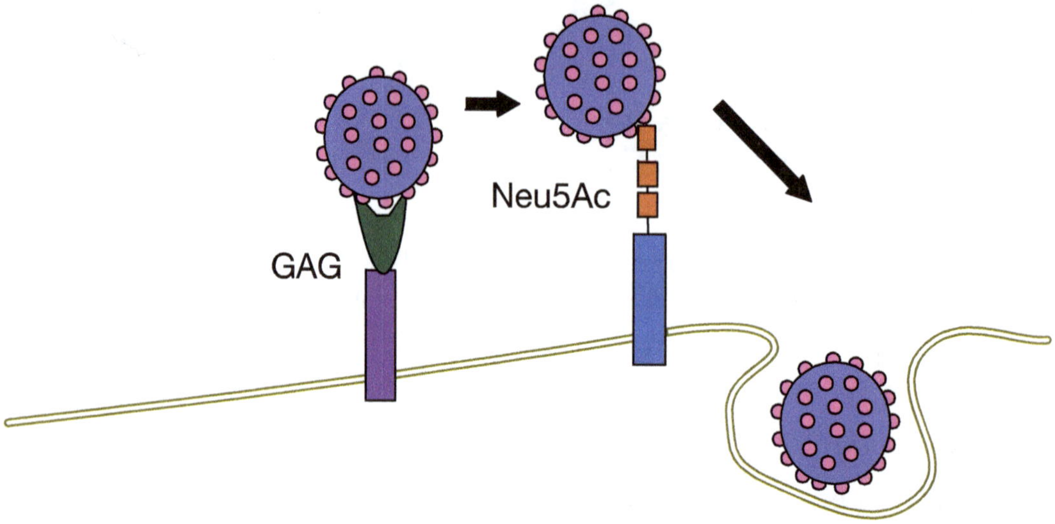

The utilisation of glycosaminoglycans by MCPyV for cellular attachment is reminiscent to the entry tactics of papillomaviruses, which are exclusively tropic for keratinocytes, a type of epithelial cell. This is a possible example of convergent evolution, and further suggests the epidermis as playing host to MCPyV.

5.2. MCPyV Replication

Under typical conditions, in permissive cells, MCPyV is able to complete its replication cycle in the cell nucleus and form virions, without inducing tumourigenesis. As a small double-stranded DNA virus, it relies heavily on host factors to transcribe its genome and replicate. However, as in other polyomaviruses, the T antigens are vital for this purpose, and are transcribed immediately upon entry into the nucleus of the host cell. These genes induce the cell to enter S-phase, altering the cellular environment to be hospitable to viral replication. Once sufficient levels of the T antigens are present, it is possible that the miRNA encoded by the MCPyV genome inhibits further early gene transcription, and thus shifts the focus to viral replication and the transcription of the late region capsid proteins [49].

Polyomaviruses require expression of the LT antigen for initiation of genome replication. Prior to SV40 replication, LT must oligomerise to form hexameric molecules, two of which bind to the origin of replication in a head to head orientation [67]. The LT helicase domain is then responsible for unwinding DNA and replication proceeds in a bidirectional manner, with hexamers moving in opposite directions. As mentioned, the MCPyV origin of replication maps to a 71 bp minimal core region composed of a poly(T) rich tract and eight GAGGC-like pentanucleotide sequences [37]. The LT OBD interacts with the origin region via recognition of these GAGGC-like motifs. A crystal structure of the origin revealed the requirement for three of these pentanucleotide sequences for initiation of replication [68]. The number and proximity of LT binding sites on the origin likely allows for intermolecular OBD-OBD interactions between molecules of LT [37].

Several viral and cellular factors have been demonstrated to affect LT mediated replication. The cellular vacuolar sorting protein, hVam6p, binds to LT through a domain adjacent to the Rb binding site in the MUR region of the protein [42]. hVam6p is involved in late endosome and lysosome fusion as part of the homotropic fusion and protein sorting (HOPS) complex. This interaction promotes translocation of hVam6p from the cytoplasm to the nucleus, disrupting lysosome clustering. Overexpression of hVam6p was shown to reduce MCPyV particle production by over 90%, whereas mutation of the LT hVam6p binding domain increased virion production by 4 to 6 fold [69]. This indicates an inhibitory role for hVam6p, the significance of which remains unclear, although it may have to do with diminishing viral replication and establishing a persistent infection.

Another cellular factor that plays a role in MCPyV replication is the chromatin-associated bromodomain containing protein 4 (Brd4), a member of the BET protein family. Brd4 interacts with LT, acting to recruit the cellular replication factor C (RFC) to MCPyV replication complexes. RFC is needed for the loading of the PCNA clamp and the tethering of the processive DNA polymerase δ to allow for the elongation of viral DNA [70]. Expression of a dominant negative inhibitor of Brd4 abrogates viral replication *in vitro* and *in vivo*, indicating a critical role for this interaction in the MCPV life cycle. Recently, it has been shown that host DNA damage response (DDR) factors are also involved in MCPyV replication, as they co-localise to the replication foci when LT is present and active. Both the ATM- and ATR-mediated pathways seem to be involved [71]. DDR factor [72] and Brd4 [73] activation and recruitment have been observed in HPV replication, suggesting a similar suite of host factors involved in MCPyV replication.

While LT is necessary for the replication of MCPyV DNA, on its own, it does not facilitate the process efficiently. ST is needed to enhance replication, with knockdown of ST leading to inhibition of replication [37]. One way ST could play a role is by promoting the hyperphosphorylation of the translation regulator eIF4E binding protein (4E-BP1) [74], which leads to an increase in the production of cellular proteins, including host factors necessary for viral replication. In addition, ST prevents the turnover of LT by targeting the cellular SCF^{Fbw7}E3 ligase. This cellular complex, of which Fbw7 is the recognition component [75], targets LT for proteasomal degradation. Fbw7 is important in cancer studies and it is deregulated in multiple cancers [76,77], with loss of Fbw7 resulting in tumourigenesis and genetic instability [78,79]. Degradation of LT can be reversed by adding the proteasome inhibitor MG132. However, binding of ST to SCF^{Fbw7} via its LT-stabilisation domain (LSD) inhibits LT degradation. In the absence of ST, the half-life of LT is 3–4 hours, while co-expression of the two proteins increases the half-life of LT to 24 hours [55]. The requirement of MCPyV ST in efficient viral replication is in stark contrast to SV40, as SV40 ST co-expression has minimal effect on SV40 LT mediated genome replication and SV40 ST is unable to cross-enhance MCPyV LT-induced viral replication despite having conserved PP2A and Hsc domains [55]. The shared DnaJ domain, which binds to the heat shock protein Hsc70, a feature important in polyomavirus replication is absolutely necessary for LT function, but is not essential for ST. Finally, neither ST nor the 57kT proteins are sufficient for replication on their own, and co-expression of 57kT with LT shows no increase in replication efficiency [37].

5.3. MCPyV and the Immune Response

Innate immunity is a critical intracellular barrier against invading microbes, thus it is unsurprising that pathogens commit a large proportion of their resources to evading it. Until very recently, little was known about how MCPyV responds to threats from its host cell. However, recent literature has highlighted an intriguing role of MCPyV T antigens in subverting the innate immune response to allow the establishment of early and persistent viral infection.

MCPyV ST has been found to play a role in downregulating the innate immune response through interference with the NF-κB family of transcription factors. NF-κB is crucial in regulating a number of genes important in both the inflammatory and antiviral response (Figure 6). NF-κB can be activated in response to numerous innate immunity signaling cascades, including tumour necrosis factor alpha (TNF-α) and pattern recognition receptors (PRRs). PRRs detect pathogen associated molecular patterns (PAMPs), such as foreign proteins or nucleic acids. This results in the activation of a coordinated signaling cascade, leading to the activation of the IKK complex. The phosphorylation and degradation of IκB allows the release and translocation of NF-κB to the nucleus, where it can activate gene transcription of proinflammatory cytokines and upregulation of late expression of type 1 interferons. The IKK complex is composed of two catalytic components (IKKα and IKKβ) and a non-catalytic regulator subunit, NF-κB essential modulator (NEMO). NEMO is a crucial component of the IKK complex, and acts as a molecular scaffold to recruit upstream signaling complexes [80].

Figure 6. NF-κB signaling. The IKK is activated after PAMP recognition by PRRs. This leads to the proteasomal degradation of IκB and release of NF-κB, which can then translocate into the nucleaus and activate the transcription of genes that have functions in the innate immunity.

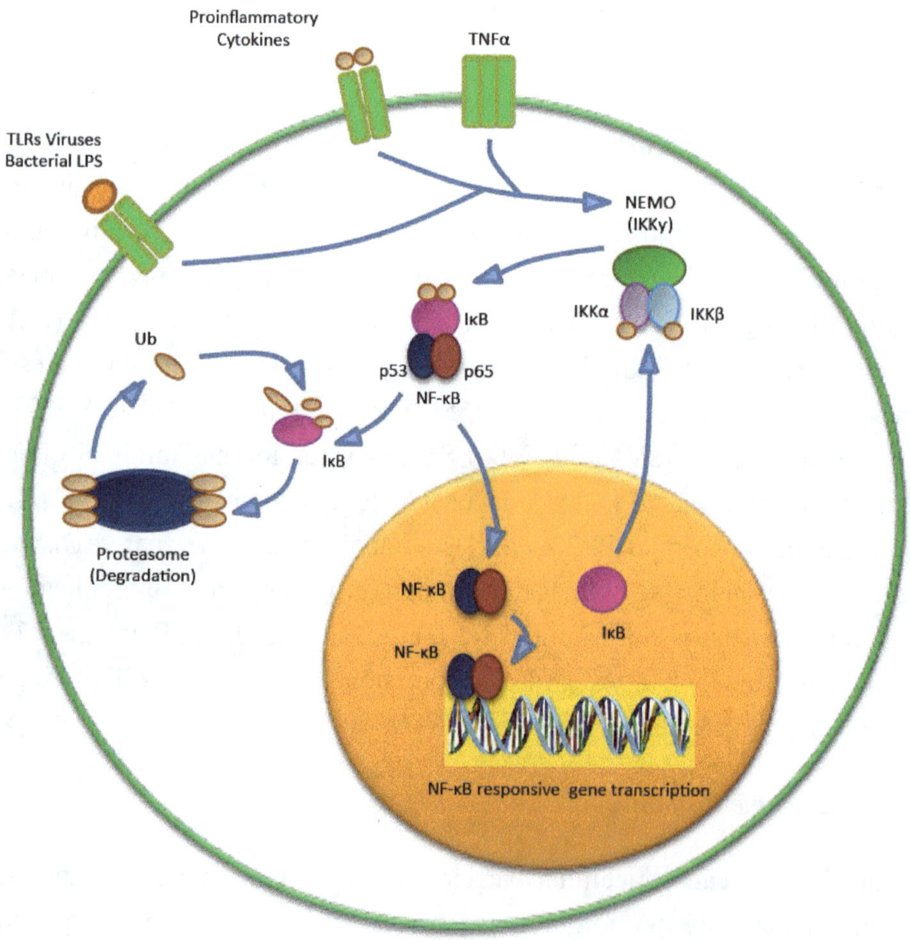

Multiple viral proteins have been shown to interfere with NF-κB signaling [81], including hepatitis C virus (HCV) core protein and HPV E7, both of which inhibit IKK activation preventing IκB degradation [82,83]. Other viruses, such as cytomegalovirus (CMV) and molluscum contagiosum poxvirus, directly target the NEMO scaffold protein, which disrupts IKK activation [84,85]. Interestingly, SV40 ST has been shown to upregulate NF-κB activation in a PP2A dependent manner, although specific inflammatory targets such as IL-8 are downregulated by expression of SV40 ST [86].

MCPyV ST expression results in a marked decrease in genes associated with the innate immune repose, such as CCL20, IL-8, TANK and CXCL-9 [54]. Many of the genes downregulated upon MCPyV ST expression are those associated with the NF-κB pathway. ST is able to negatively regulate NF-κB mediated transcriptional activation of NF-κB responsive genes, through a previously undescribed interaction of ST with NEMO. This interaction specifically inhibits phosphorylation of IKKα/IKKβ, thus rendering NF-κB unable to translocate to the nucleus [54].

The poylomavirus ST-PP2A Aα interaction is well known. However MCPyV ST has also been found to interact with PP4C and/or PP2A Aβ, and this is thought to regulate NF-κB activation [54]. To date, it is unclear whether ST directly interacts with PP4C to promote dephosphorylation of this complex or if PP4C is part of a complex with ST and PP2A Aβ. Despite this uncertainty, it is clear that the activity of cellular phosphatases and their association with MCPyV ST is important for IKK complex dephosphorylation and NF-κB-mediated transcription.

MCPyV LT expression has also been found to play a role in downregulating the innate immune response. It inhibits Toll-like receptor 9 (TLR9) expression in epithelial and MCC cells [87]. TLRs are a subset of PRRs, and are an indispensable part of the innate immune response. TLR activation by PAMPs produces molecules for clearing infection, such as antimicrobial peptides, cytokines, and chemokines [88]. In particular, TLR9 senses viral or bacterial double-stranded DNA, as these contain many nonmethylated CpG motifs [89]. Importantly, when TLR9 recognises pathogenic DNA, it activates NF-κB in immune cells, leading to increased production of inflammatory molecules [90]. A number of double-stranded DNA oncogenic viruses, including HPV, inhibit the expression of TLR9 [91–93]. MCPyV LT also inhibits TLR9 expression. It does so by decreasing the mRNA levels of the C/EBPβ transactivator, which is a positive regulator of the TLR9 promoter. This leads to a greatly reduced binding of C/EBPβ to its response element on the TLR9 promoter. ST may also play a role in this, as its expression also appears to inhibit TLR9, but the mechanism is unknown. As such, LT targeting of C/EBPβ may therefore be important in establishing viral persistence [87]. These findings show that MCPyV has a complex and multifaceted defence against innate immunity. This allows the virus to persist, and may contribute to eventual tumourigenesis.

5.4. MCPyV Assembly and Egress

MCPyV virions tend to localise to the nucleus and the nuclear periphery prior to egress [94]. Apart from this, very little is known about MCPyV assembly and egress. It may be that LT-mediated sequestration of hVam6p to the cell nucleus might contribute to egress through lysosomal processing during virus replication [42]. Unlike other polyomaviruses, such as SV40, JCPyV and BKPyV, MCPyV does not encode an agnoprotein, which is known to be important in virus particle assembly and maturation [95]. In addition, it does not seem to encode an equivalent of the SV40 VP4, which has been shown to trigger lytic virion release [96]. Therefore, it must employ an alternative pathway.

In general, cell lysis is thought to be the primary mechanism of polyomavirus virion release, but accumulation of viral particles in SV40-infected cells, which subsequently shed, has also been observed [97]. One possibility is that, if the natural host of MCPyV is a type of skin cell, it may not require lysis for release, as the natural process of keratinocyte desquamation may serve this purpose. Polyomavirus assembly and egress is still poorly understood, and until a permissive cell culture model is developed for MCPyV, questions about the stages of the viral lifecycle cannot be fully addressed.

6. MCPyV and Tumourigenesis

MCPyV infection is common in the general population, and the virus is considered a component of normal skin flora. However, in a limited number of cases, MCPyV clonally integrates into a Merkel cell, which may initiate tumourigenesis (Figure 7). As a tumour virus, MCPyV is considered to be a direct carcinogen, as it expresses oncogenes that directly contribute to cell transformation. However, MCPyV-induced oncogenesis often requires the virus to become replication-defective, allowing cellular proliferation [3].

Figure 7. Models of MCPyV-induced MCC tumourigenesis. MCPyV infection is thought to occur early in childhood of most people. Before tumourigenesis can occur, loss immunosurveillance must lead to proliferation of the virus. At least two mutations are needed before MCPyV can transform cells. In model A, the first mutation is thought to be the integration of the full-length viral genome into host DNA, while the second mutation is the truncation of LT. In model B, truncation of LT is thought to occur before integration. Either way, these changes in the virus lead to cellular transformation and tumour proliferation.

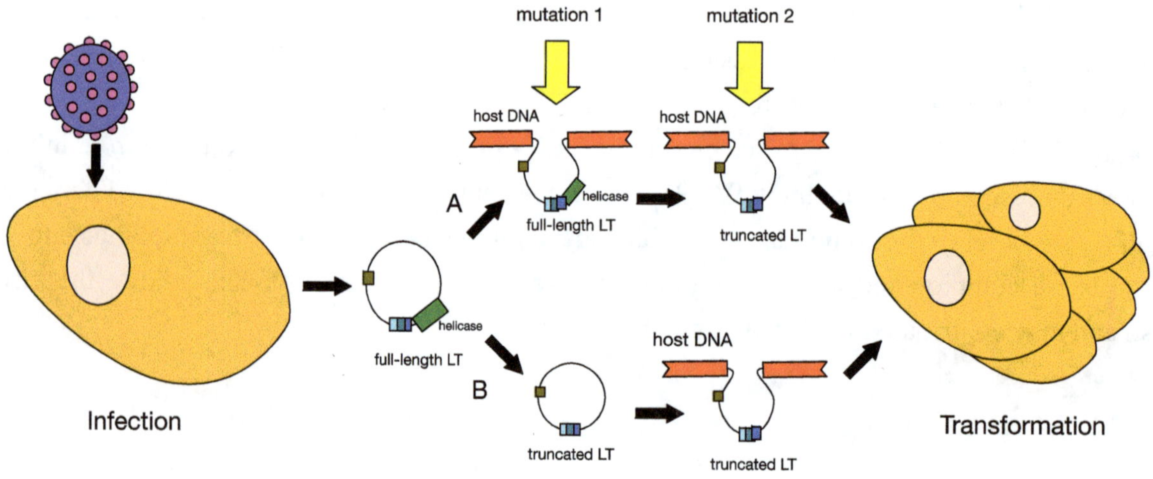

Old age and immunosuppression are both risk factors for MCC. This may in part be due to the loss of immunosurveillance against MCPyV, allowing the normally low levels of virus to rise. The presence of antibodies against the capsid proteins of MCPyV in patients with MCPyV-positive MCC suggests viraemia prior to tumour formation.

Upon MCPyV discovery, understanding of its oncogenic mode of action was initially drawn from established animal polyomavirus studies into the tumourigenic mechanisms associated with polyomavirus T antigens. However, recent years have seen an increase in the knowledge of MCPyV involvement in cellular transformation and the role that the MCPyV T antigens play in the viral life cycle.

The vast majority of polyomavirus literature asserts that polyomavirus LT, rather than ST is the major oncogene. For example, SV40 LT has been shown to be the major transforming protein, with ST playing an accessory role in tumourigensis [98,99]. In the case of MCPyV, however, the tumourigenesis mechanism appears to be more complicated. MCC cells appear to be reliant upon T antigen expression as pan-T antigen knockdown in MCPyV positive cell lines triggered growth arrest and cell death [100]. This presents the question as to whether LT or ST has a dominant effect upon cellular transformation.

6.1. Truncation of MCPyV Large T Antigen

The signature feature of MCPyV-positive MCC is the presence of mutations in LT. These mutations prematurely truncate the LT protein at its carboxy-terminus, which leads to the loss of the domains associated with viral replication [20,101–103]. The sites of mutations are randomly distributed in the LT from different tumours, but the pRB binding site is consistently preserved. Thus, LT proteins expressed in different tumours vary in size, depending on the site of their mutations [104]. The truncated LT lack the OBD and helicase domains required for viral replication but retains the capacity to trigger host cell proliferation. This indicates a strong selective pressure within the MCC tumours to eliminate the viral replication capabilities, and retain only replication-deficient copies of MCPyV. Besides the mutations in LT, several groups have also reported mutations in the origin of replication and the VP1 gene in MCC-derived MCPyV genomic sequences that prevent efficient replication and progeny virion production, respectively [37,69,94,104]. Therefore, a two-step mutation process towards tumourigenesis has been suggested.

Upon MCPyV integration, the viral genome retains the full-length LT, capable of initiating host DNA replication. This unlicensed replication will result in replication fork collision and DNA breakage, which will lead to cytopathic cell death [103]. Thus a second mutation is needed to eliminate LT-initiated DNA replication for the cell to survive once MCPyV has integrated, and only a cell with both mutations is likely to develop into a tumour. The requirement for two separate events prior to tumourigenesis may help to explain why MCC is so rare [3]. It is also possible, however, that LT may first become truncated, with MCPyV going through rolling circle replication prior to integration [105]. There is some evidence for this alternative hypothesis. It has been shown that, upon exposure to UV radiation, expression of truncated LT leads to defective DNA repair and cell cycle arrest [106], and this increase in genomic instability may promote integration of the viral genome.

6.2. MCPyV Large T Antigen as an Oncogene

The MCPyV genome has been demonstrated to be clonally integrated in up to 97% of MCC samples [23,107]. Expression of MCV T antigens from the integrated genome contributes to transformation of host cells. LT DNA is present at an average of 5.2 copies per tumour cell and LT protein expression can be detected in the nuclei of these cells [108].

In other oncogenic polyomaviruses, such as SV40, LT has been shown to be the major oncoprotein, with sT playing a lesser role. Overexpression of the SV40 LT is sufficient to transform mouse fibroblasts [109]. This transforming ability of LT is dependent upon manipulation of the key tumour suppressor proteins, p53 and Rb. The cell cycle checkpoint protein p53 is activated by cellular stress and blocks genome replication under conditions that could perpetuate DNA damage induced errors [110]. This is achieved by p53 promoting the expression of genes that induce DNA repair, cell-cycle arrest and apoptosis. Binding of SV40 LT to p53 inhibits this transcriptional activity and therefore permits inappropriate cellular proliferation [47]. The Rb protein controls entry into S-phase of the cell cycle. In resting cells pRb is bound to E2F, however upon activation of cyclin-dependent kinases pRb is phosphorylated, disrupting this complex. This permits E2F to activate the transcription of genes required for cell cycle progression. The LXCXE motif within LT mediates binding to Rb (Figure 8), which inhibits the interaction with E2F, thus bypassing this S-phase checkpoint. The DnaJ domain of LT also plays a role in this interaction, bringing together Hsp70 and Rb family members to facilitate the release of E2F in an ATP dependent fashion [111].

Figure 8. Effect of LT on cell proliferation. Upon MCPyV infection and T antigen expression, LT binds the regulatory protein pRb, thus inactivating it. This allows E2F to activate the transcription of cell cycle progression-associated genes, which switches the cell into S-phase and leads to cell proliferation.

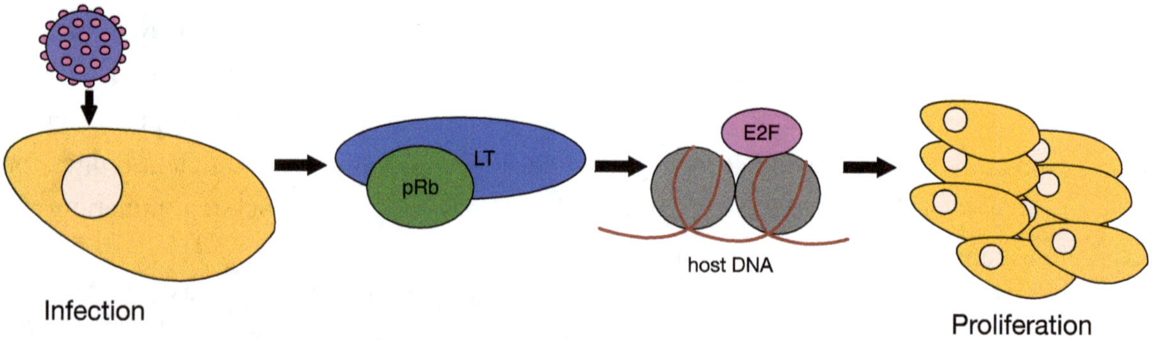

MCPyV LT is truncated in tumour cells, and one reason, as mentioned above, is to prevent unlicensed gene replication. However, the majority of reported LT mutations involve truncation of the entire C-terminal domain, as opposed to more subtle inactivating mutations. This suggests that there is an additional selective pressure upon transforming cells for removal of this region of LT. Consequently it has been shown that truncated LT is more efficient at inducing cellular proliferation than full length LT [112]. Moreover, overexpression of the LT carboxy-terminal 100 amino acids had an inhibitory effect upon the growth of certain cells types. Subsequent investigations have revealed that MCV infection activates the cellular DNA damage response in a manner dependent upon the LT carboxy-terminus [113]. Activation of DNA damage kinases was found to promote cell cycle arrest in a p53 dependent manner. Comparable to this, SV40 infection activates the ATM DNA damage pathway [114]. However, as the SV40 LT inhibits downstream activities of p53, cellular proliferation is not inhibited. Therefore LT truncations are likely selected to avoid activation of the DDR in the absence of p53 inactivation. In addition, LT has also been shown to increase levels of the cellular oncoprotein, survivin, which is dependent upon its Rb binding capacity [115]. Survivin is a member of the inhibitor-of-apoptosis proteins family, the overexpression of which is associated with numerous cancers [116].

With SV40 as the model, MCPyV LT would be expected to be the main viral oncoprotein driving cellular transformation. However, in contrast to SV40, neither full length, nor truncated MCPyV LT can initiate cellular transformation [74]. Some evidence suggests that MCPyV differs from other polyomaviruses in this respect, with ST the major oncogenic factor, which will be discussed below. One contributing factor to this diminished transformation ability of LT is that it does not appear to interact with p53, unlike the SV40 homologue [112]. This does not imply that LT does not play a role in MCPyV tumourigenesis, as it binds to both pRb and Hsc70, which are known to play a role in cell proliferation [37,103]. In addition, MCPyV LT does interfere with pRb-E2F binding, and is therefore capable of effecting cellular proliferation. In addition, recent data appear to support the role of LT as the major oncogenic factor, demonstrating that ectopic expression of LT alone could rescue pan-T antigen knockdown [117]. The relative importance of the small and large T antigens in MCC therefore requires further investigation.

6.3. MCPyV Small T Antigen as an Oncogene

There is new evidence that, unlike in other oncogenic polyomaviruses, MCPyV ST is as important for tumourigenesis, if not more so, than MCPyV LT. For example, it has been demonstrated that ST is more commonly expressed in MCC tumour samples than LT, indicating a significant role of ST in tumourigensis and tumour cell maintenance. In fact, 92% of MCC tumour samples are positive for ST expression, while only 75% are positive for LT. In addition, knockdown of ST in MCPyV-positive MCC cells inhibits growth [74]. Furthermore, expression of ST is sufficient to induce rodent fibroblast transformation, loss of contact inhibition, anchorage-independent and serum independent growth, while expression of LT does not lead to these changes [74]. These are key hallmarks of an oncogenic viral protein and confirm the important role that MCPyV ST plays in MCC tumourigenesis and pathology.

SV40 ST, being only an accessory oncogene, primarily contributes to cell transformation by targeting PP2A (Figure 9). This ability to bind PP2A is a common feature of polyomaviruses, as both SV40 ST and MPyV ST/MT bind PP2A [37]. Both MCPyV and SV40 ST bind the PP2A structural Aα subunit and the catalytic subunit thereby altering the substrate specificity of the PP2A holoenzyme [53,118]. SV40 is able to subvert the normal host phosphatase systems, as its ST binds to PP2A Aα in such a way that it overlaps the B subunit-binding domain [54,119]. This allows SV40 ST to compete with B subunit binding thereby inhibiting PP2A targeting and subsequent dephosphorylation of target substrates [98,120,121]. Alternatively, ST could act in a positive manner by redirecting PP2A phosphatase activity to alternative proteins [120].

Although MCPyV is related to SV40 and shares similar gene structure, it is becoming apparent that these two polyomaviruses differ drastically in their carcinogenic mechanisms. While the SV40 ST-PP2A Aα interaction is critical for SV40 induced transformation and cell proliferation, this may not be the case for MCPyV ST. MCPyV ST mutants with disrupted ST-PP2A Aα interaction were fully capable of inducing both rodent cell transformation and anchorage-independent colony formation [74]. This clearly indicates that while these viruses may contain similar protein structure and binding domains, their mode of action is distinct. If MCPyV ST oncogenicity does not depend upon its ability to bind PP2A Aα, another mechanism must be in place, perhaps through binding to PP2A Aβ and/or PP4C. It has been demonstrated that SV40 ST activates the Akt pathway by preventing PP2A Aα mediated dephosphorylation of Akt [122,123]. However, MCPyV ST has little effect at that point in the AkT-mTOR pathway, instead acting downstream of mTOR [74].

Figure 9. Interaction of ST with PP2A. Polyomavirus ST competes with the B subunit of PP2A for binding to the structural A subunit and the catalytic C subunit. In SV40, this interaction between ST and PP2A Aα leads to cell transformation. Although the interaction of MCPyV ST with PP2A Aα may not be necessary for transformation, interaction with PP2A Aβ or the related PP4C may play a role.

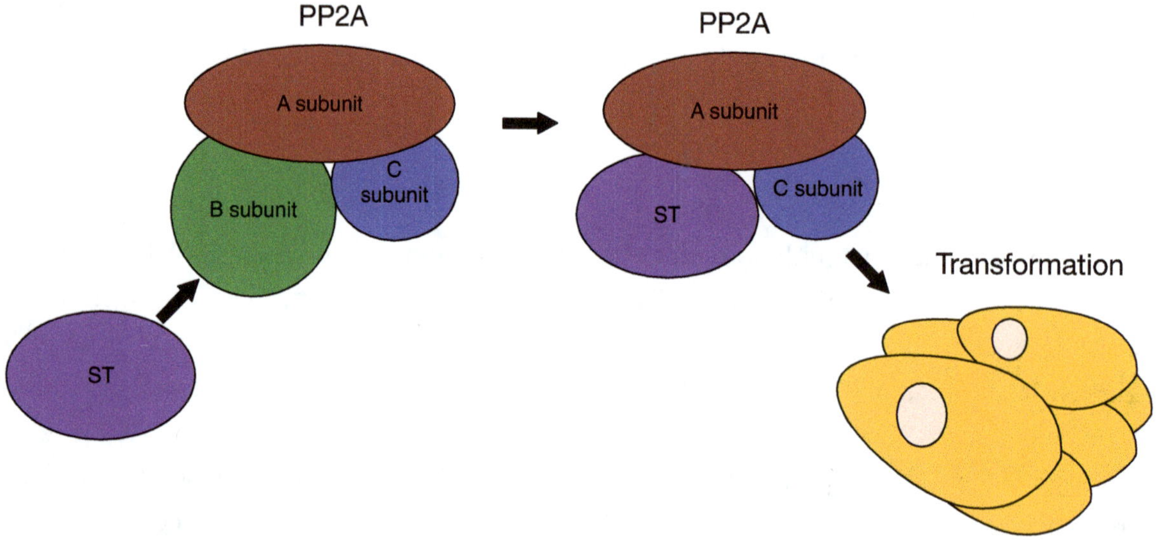

The PI3K-AkT-mTOR signalling pathway plays a significant role in the regulation of cap-dependent translation in tumourigenesis [124–126]. An important step in cap-dependent translation is the binding of the eukaryotic translation initiation factor 4E (eIF4E) to specific mRNA molecules [127]. Assembly of eIF4E at the mRNA cap as part of the multisubunit eIF4F complex initiates ribosome recruitment. A major regulator of this pathway is the eukaryotic translation initiation factor 4E-binding protein 1 (4E-BP1), which sequesters eIF4F to prevent eIF4F complex formation [128]. Interference with this pathway is important for tumour cell growth, as overexpression of eIF4F can induce rodent cell transformation [129,130]. Upon 4E-BP1 phosphorylation by mammalian target of rapamycin (mTOR) 4E-BP1 releases eIF4F, allowing cap assembly and cap-dependent translation [131].

MCPyV ST acts by reducing the turnover of hyperphosphorylated 4E-BP1, which increases eIF4F activity, and, in turn, cap-dependent translation. Moreover, expression of a constitutively active mutant 4E-BP1 protein reverses ST induced cell transformation and is independent of PP2A Aα and Hsc70 binding [74]. This demonstrates the importance of ST in regulating cap dependent translation, and that through this mechanism ST is able to contribute to MCC tumourigenesis. In contrast, it has been demonstrated that SV40 ST diminishes 4E-BP1 phosphorylation [132], which is another interesting difference to the established view that polyomavirus ST tumorigenic ability is intrinsically linked to PP2A Aα binding.

Interestingly, the newly-discovered LSD domain of MCPyV ST is not only important for stabilising LT and viral genome replication, but may be required for rodent cell transformation. A mutation within the LSD region ablates ST ability to induce transformation [55]. This mutation does not affect ST ability to bind PP2A, once again confirming that the ability of ST to induce transformation is independent of PP2A, and is distinct from other polyomaviruses in this respect.

However, at present there seems to be conflicting view points as to the tumorigenic nature of MCPyV ST. While expression levels of ST in MCC cell lines and MCC tissues appear to be low [117], ST is more commonly detected in MCC tissues than LT in immunohistochemistry analysis, and knocking out ST in MCPyV-positive MCC inhibits cell growth [74]. Furthermore, as discussed above, there is some controversy as to which of the two proteins is most important for cancer cell growth and proliferation. It may be that ST is essential for initial transformation, while LT is necessary for subsequent survival and proliferation.

It is clear that there is a degree of uncertainty that needs to be addressed. Regardless, there is a large robust body of evidence that indicates that MCPyV ST is crucial to tumourigensis and maintenance of the tumour state. Indeed, the fact that MCPyV is the only human polyomavirus associated with tumourigenesis indicates that there are some aspects of this virus that do not follow the normal polyomavirus stereotype, and that there likely are novel mechanisms that set it apart from its relatives.

7. Therapies for MCC

Conventional treatment of MCC depends on the disease stage. The standard therapy for localised tumours is surgical excision with 2–3 cm margins. If regional lymph nodes are thought to be involved, dissection is undertaken. In most cases, adjuvant radiotherapy to the tumour site and, if necessary, regional lymph node site, is given. This has been associated with decreased risk of regional relapse [133]. If a tumour cannot be excised, radiation on its own can be performed, as MCC is a relatively radiosensitive tumour [134]. If MCC has metastasised, various regimens of broad-spectrum chemotherapy have been used, such as anthracyclines, cyclophosphamide, etoposide, and platinum derivatives, alone or in combination. Over half of MCC patients respond to chemotherapy, but prognosis is poor, and the median survival is 21.5 months [135].

Previous to the discovery of MCPyV as the causative agent of the majority of MCC cases, the molecular basis of the cancer was not well researched. Therefore, only generic therapies are available for treatment. However, this is likely to change as more is uncovered about MCPyV tumourigenesis and drug targets are identified. MCPyV T antigen expression is necessary for survival of MCPyV-positive MCC cells, therefore LT and ST are considered to be potential therapeutic targets.

Some preliminary drugs inhibiting MCPyV-positive MCC have been identified *in vitro*. For example, type I interferon (IFN) reduces LT expression and inhibits cell viability in MpyV-positive MCC cell lines [136]. However, IFN treatment failed to induce a clinical response in two patients with late-stage MCC [137]. On the other hand, YM155, a drug inhibiting surivin expression, which is upregulated by LT and is important for the surivival of MCPyV-positive MCC cell lines, is cytotoxic in the nanomolar range and shows a cytostatic effect in MCC xenograft tumours in mice [115,138]. The most promising drug at the moment, however, is the small-molecule tyrosine kinase inhibitor, pazopanib [139], currently in a phase II clinical trial. The field remains open for novel drugs, especially those that target the newly-discovered effects MCPyV T antigens have on the innate immune response. In addition, inhibiting cap-dependent translation and mTOR signalling may also be beneficial in treating MCC.

MCC, like other virus-induced cancers, has viral antigens in its cells, and is thus immunologically responsive. In fact, improved immunosurveillance is likely behind the occasional spontaneous regression of disseminated MCC tumours [140]. Immunity-based approaches to treating MCPyV-positive MCC are promising, and work in this area is ongoing. Specific T lymphocytes that recognise various MCPyV epitopes have been identified, both within tumour cells and in the blood of both MCC patients and healthy test subjects [141]. 58 CD8+ T lymphocytes against 35 MCPyV T antigen epitopes have been identified, and these responses are present only in MCC patients [142]. Despite these specific T lymphocyte responses, MCC tumours persist and grow. This suggests that MCC tumours inhibit T lymphocyte cytotoxicity or otherwise evade the immune response. Nevertheless, DNA vaccines are a possibility, and preliminary work using murine tumour models to create vaccines has shown that it is possible to that target both ST and LT and elicit both CD4+ and CD8+ T lymphocyte response [143,144]. In addition, MCPyV-specific CD8+ T lymphocytes exhibit targetable exhaustion markers PD-1 and Tim-3 [145]. These markers are associated with reversible T-lymphocyte dysfunction, thus investigating antagonists of the PD-1 and Tim-3 pathways may yield additional MCC treatment measures.

Merkel cell carcinoma is highly metastatic, and designing drugs to inhibit this property would limit the mortality rate of late-stage disease. Uncovering the mechanism of what drives MCC metastasis is therefore of paramount importance. Determining if and how one or both of the oncoproteins of MCPyV induces cell motility and invasion will allow for the rational design of inhibitors to interfere with this mechanism.

8. Conclusions

From our understanding of MCPyV, a broad model of tumourigenesis can be presented. The virus is acquired by the advent of adulthood. The route of transmission is not yet known, as the virus is part of the microflora of the skin, it is likely that infection is cutaneous. Immunosupression, whether in the form of aging, HIV-AIDS, drugs, or UV damage, leads to loss of immunosurveillance and MCPyV reactivation. It is at that time that the mutations associated with MCPyV tumourigenesis can occur. It may be that UV or other types of external stimuli contribute to the likelihood of mutagenesis.

Regardless of the order of the two mutations, cells which have an integrated copy of replication-defective MCPyV display viral oncogene expression, which leads to clonal expansion, neoplastic progression, and, ultimately, development of MCC.

Each year, more studies shed light on the lifecycle and the tumourigenic potential of MCPyV. There is a mechanism for tumourigenesis, although it is not yet fully determined. In addition, details about the natural lifecycle of the virus are coming into light, such as attachment steps and the mechanism of replication. However, until a fully permissive cell culture model is developed, it will not be possible to fully elucidate the entry, replication, and egress of MCPyV.

There is some evidence that MCC might not be the only cancer MCPyV plays a role in, although the findings are, as yet, inconclusive. Chronic lymphocytic leukaemia (CLL) is one cancer where replication-deficient MCPyV has been isolated from a subset of tumours [146]. In addition, patients with

MCPyV-positive MCC have a greater risk of developing CLL than patients with MCPyV-negative MCC [147]. CLL tumours in general do not reveal a pattern of MCPyV presence [25,148], although this does not preclude the virus from playing a role in a fraction of CLL cases. Another cancer where MCPyV might play a role is squamous cell carcinoma (SCC). Although some reports find no significant association [145,149], others stress that MCPyV DNA is present in 40% of cutaneous SCCs, which significantly correlates with MCPyV seropositivty [150]. In addition, nearly all MCPyV-positive SCCs have mutations within exon 2 that could produce a truncated version of LT [151]. Finally, a full-length MCPyV genome has been isolated from a Kaposi's sarcoma, and this genome expresses a truncated LT [152]. Thus MCPyV could have a role to play in the development of a number of cancers.

MCC is a highly invasive and metastatic cancer. The reason behind these features has not been elucidated, but it may be that the T antigens are involved in promoting the characteristic, aggressive metastasis of MCPyV-transformed cells. Furthermore, the T antigens could have functions in such areas as lipid metabolism, the cell cycle, and DNA damage and repair. At the moment, knowledge of how LT and ST influence the multitude of cancer pathways is limited, and drawn mainly from work with SV40, despite mounting evidence that many mechanisms MCPyV LT and ST employ are divergent. A growing number of interactions between LT, ST, and host factors are being uncovered, but, undoubtedly, there is still much more left to find.

In order to understand both MCPyV as a virus and how it causes cellular transformation, and ultimately cancer, much more work needs to be done on the molecular virology of the virus, on the cellular biology of MCPyV-transformed cells and on the immunology of MCC. It has come to light that MCPyV has many unique features, and detailing further its molecular virology may uncover more important mechanisms of transformation, carcinogenesis, and cancer spread.

Acknowledgements

The authors would like to thank all members of the Whitehouse and Macdonald laboratories for useful discussions. This work was supported in parts by the British Skin Foundation, Rosetrees Trust, BBSRC DTG and DTP studentships, BBSRC Research Development Fellowship, Cancer Research UK, Yorkshire Cancer Research, University of Basrah, Ministry of Higher Education and Scientific Research Iraq scholarship and Ministry of Higher Education Scholarship, Malaysia.

References

1. Parkin, D.M. The global health burden of infection-associated cancers in the year 2002. *Int. J. Cancer* **2006**, *118*, 3030–3044.
2. Javier, R.T.; Butel, J.S. The History of tumor virology. *Cancer Res.* **2008**, *68*, 7693–7706.
3. Moore, P.S.; Chang, Y. Why do viruses cause cancer? Highlights of the first century of human tumour virology. *Nat. Rev. Cancer* **2010**, *10*, 878–889.
4. Stewart, S.E.; Eddy, B.E.; Borgese, N. Neoplasms in mice inoculated with a tumor agent carried in tissue culture. *J. Natl. Cancer Inst.* **1958**, *20*, 1223–1243.
5. Sweet, B.H.; Hilleman, M.R. The Vacuolating Virus, SV40. *Exp. Biol. Med.* **1960** *105*, 420–427.

6. Feng, H.; Shuda, M.; Chang, Y.; Moore, P.S. Clonal integration of a polyomavirus in human merkel cell carcinoma. *Science* **2008**, *319*, 1096–1100.
7. Kaae, J.; Hansen, A.V.; Biggar, R.J.; Boyd, H.A.; Moore, P.S.; Wohlfahrt, J.; Melbye, M. Merkel cell carcinoma: Incidence, mortality, and risk of other cancers. *J. Natl. Cancer Inst.* **2010**, *102*, 793–801.
8. Lanoy, E.; Costagliola, D.; Engels, E.A. Skin cancers associated with HIV infection and solid-organ transplantation among elderly adults. *Int. J. Cancer* **2010**, *126*, 1724–1731.
9. Toker, C. Trabecular Carcinoma of the Skin. *Arch. Dermatol.* **1972**, *105*, 107–110.
10. Merkel, F. Tastzellen and Tastkoerperchenbei den Hausthieren und beim Menschen. *Arch. Mikr. Anat.* **1875**, *11*, 636–652.
11. Lacour, J.P.; Dubois, D.; Pisani, A.; Ortonne, J.P. Anatomical mapping of Merkel cells in normal human adult epidermis. *Br. J. Dermatol.* **1991**, *125*, 535–542.
12. May, C.A.; Osterland, I. Merkel cell distribution in the human eyelid. *Eur. J. Histochem.* **2013**, *57*, 224–226.
13. Koljonen, V.; Kluger, N.; Sihto, H.; Bohling, T. Lateral distribution of merkel cell carcinoma in a nationwide cohort. *J. Eur. Acad. Dermatol. Venereol.* **2013**, *27*, 884–888.
14. Hodgson, N.C. Merkel Cell Carcinoma: Changing Incidence Trends. *J. Surg. Oncol.* **2005**, *89*, 1–4.
15. Bzhalava, D.; Bray, F.; Storm, H.; Dillner, J. Risk of second cancers after the diagnosis of Merkel cell carcinoma in Scandinavia. *Br. J. Cancer* **2011**, *104*, 178–180.
16. Gupta, S.G.; Wang, L.C.; Penas, P.F.; Gellenthin, M.; Lee, S.J.; Nghiem, P. Sentinel lymph node biopsy for evaluation and treatment of patients with Merkel cell carcinoma: The dana-farber experience and meta-analysis of the literature. *Arch. Dermatol.* **2006**, *142*, 685–690.
17. Vernadakis, S.; Moris, D.; Bankfalvi, A.; Makris, N.; Sotiropoulos, G.C. Metastatic Merkel cell carcinoma (MCC) of pancreas and breast: A unique case. *World J. Surg. Oncol.* **2013**, *11*, 261.
18. Suttie, C.F.; Hruby, G.; Horvath, L.; Thompson, J. Cardiac metastasis in Merkel cell carcinoma. *J. Clin. Oncol.* **2014**, *32*, 1–2.
19. Vasileiadis, I.; Sofopoulos, M.; Arnogiannaki, N.; Georgopoulos, S. A Merkel cell carcinoma metastatic to the tonsil: A case report and review of the literature. *J. Oral Maxillofac. Surg.* **2013**, *71*, 1812.
20. Laude, H.C.; Jonchère, B.; Maubec, E.; Carlotti, A.; Marinho, E.; Couturaud, B.; Peter, M.; Sastre-Garau, X.; Avril, M.-F.; Dupin, N.; *et al.* Distinct Merkel cell polyomavirus molecular features in tumour and non tumour specimens from patients with merkel cell carcinoma. *PLoS Pathog.* **2010**, *6*, e1001076.
21. Martel-Jantin, C.; Filippone, C.; Cassar, O.; Peter, M.; Tomasic, G.; Vielh, P.; Briere, J.; Petrella, T.; Aubriot-Lorton, M.H.; Mortier, L.; *et al.* Genetic Variability and integration of Merkel cell polyomavirus in Merkel cell carcinoma. *Virology* **2012**, *426*, 134–142.
22. Sastre-Garau, X.; Peter, M.; Avril, M.-F.; Laude, H.; Couturier, J.; Rozenberg, F.; Almeida, A.; Boitier, F.; Carlotti, A.; Couturaud, B.; *et al.* Merkel cell carcinoma of the skin: Pathological and molecular evidence for a causative role of MCV in oncogenesis. *J. Pathol.* **2009**, *218*, 48–56.
23. Rodig, S.J.; Cheng, J.; Wardzala, J.; DoRosario, A.; Scanlon, J.J.; Laga, A.C.; Martinez-Fernandez, A.; Barletta, J.A.; Bellizzi, A.M.; Sadasivam, S.; *et al.* Improved detection suggests all Merkel cell carcinomas harbor merkel polyomavirus. *J. Clin. Invest.* **2012** *122*, 4645 4653.

24. Donepudi, S.; DeConti, R.C.; Samlowski, W.E. Recent Advances in the understanding of the genetics, etiology, and treatment of Merkel cell carcinoma. *Semin. Oncol.* **2012**, *39*, 163–172.
25. Shuda, M.; Arora, R.; Kwun, H.J.; Feng, H.; Sarid, R.; Fernandez-Figueras, M.-T.; Tolstov, Y.; Gjoerup, O.; Mansukhani, M.M.; Swerdlow, S.H.; *et al.* Human Merkel cell polyomavirus infection I. MCV T antigen expression in Merkel cell carcinoma, lymphoid tissues and lymphoid tumors. *Int. J. Cancer* **2009**, *125*, 1243–1249.
26. Viscidi, R.P.; Rollison, D.E.; Sondak, V.K.; Silver, B.; Messina, J.L.; Giuliano, A.R.; Fulp, W.; Ajidahun, A.; Rivanera, D. Age-specific seroprevalence of Merkel cell polyomavirus, BK virus, and JC virus. *Clin. Vaccine Immunol.* **2011**, *18*, 1737–1743.
27. Tolstov, Y.L.; Pastrana, D.V.; Feng, H.; Becker, J.C.; Jenkins, J.J.; Moschos, S.; Chang, Y.; Buck, C.B.; Moore, P.S. Human Merkel cell polyomavirus infection II. MCV is a common human infection that can be detected by conformational capsid epitope immunoassays. *Int. J. Cancer* **2009**, *125*, 1250–1256.
28. Becker, J.C.; Houben, R.; Ugurel, S.; Trefzer, U.; Pfohler, C.; Schrama, D. MC polyomavirus is frequently present in Merkel cell carcinoma of European patients. *J. Invest. Dermatol.* **2009**, *129*, 248–250.
29. Matsushita, M.; Kuwamoto, S.; Iwasaki, T.; Higaki-Mori, H.; Yashima, S.; Kato, M.; Murakami, I.; Horie, Y.; Kitamura, Y.; Hayashi, K. Detection of Merkel cell polyomavirus in the human tissues from 41 japanese autopsy cases using polymerase chain reaction. *Intervirology* **2013**, *56*, 1–5.
30. Martel-Jantin, C.; Pedergnana, V.; Nicol, J.T.J.; Leblond, V.; Trégouët, D.-A.; Tortevoye, P.; Plancoulaine, S.; Coursaget, P.; Touzé, A.; Abel, L.; *et al.* Merkel Cell polyomavirus infection occurs during early childhood and is transmitted between siblings. *J. Clin. Virol.* **2013**, *58*, 288–291.
31. van der Meijden, E.; Bialasiewicz, S.; Rockett, R.J.; Tozer, S.J.; Sloots, T.P.; Feltkamp, M.C.W. Different serologic behavior of MCPyV, TSPyV, HPyV6, HPyV7 and HPyV9 polyomaviruses found on the skin. *PLoS One* **2013**, *8*, e81078:1–e81078:9.
32. Hashida, Y.; Imajoh, M.; Kamioka, M.; Taniguchi, A.; Kuroda, N.; Hayashi, K.; Nakajima, H.; Sano, S.; Daibata, M. Phylogenetic analysis of Merkel cell polyomavirus based on full-length LT and VP1 gene sequences derived from neoplastic tumours in Japanese patients. *J. Gen. Virol.* **2014**, *95*, 135–141.
33. Matsushita, M.; Iwasaki, T.; Kuwamoto, S.; Kato, M.; Nagata, K.; Murakami, I.; Kitamura, Y.; Hayashi, K. Merkel cell polyomavirus (MCPyV) strains in Japanese Merkel cell carcinomas (MCC) are distinct from caucasian type MCPyVs: Genetic variability and phylogeny of MCPyV genomes obtained from Japanese MCPyV-infected MCCs. *Virus Genes* **2014**, *48*, 233–242.
34. Martel-Jantin, C.; Filippone, C.; Tortevoye, P.; Afonso, P.V.; Betsem, E.; Descorps-Declere, S.; Nicol, J.T.J.; Touzé, A.; Coursaget, P.; Crouzat, M.; *et al.* Molecular epidemiology of Merkel cell polyomavirus: Evidence for geographically related variant genotypes. *J. Clin. Microbiol.* **2014**, *52*, 1687–1690.
35. Dalianis, T.; Ramqvist, T.; Andreasson, K.; Kean, J.M.; Garcea, R.L. KI, WU and Merkel cell polyomaviruses: A new era for human polyomavirus research. *Semin. Cancer Biol.* **2009**, *19*, 270–275.

36. Johne, R.; Buck, C.B.; Allander, T.; Atwood, W.J.; Garcea, R.L.; Imperiale, M.J.; Major, E.O.; Ramqvist, T.; Norkin, L.C. Taxonomical developments in the family polyomaviridae. *Arch. Virol.* **2011**, *156*, 1627–1634.
37. Kwun, H.J.; Guastafierro, A.; Shuda, M.; Meinke, G.; Bohm, A.; Moore, P.S.; Chang, Y. The minimum replication origin of Merkel cell polyomavirus has a unique large T-antigen loading architecture and requires small T-antigen expression for optimal replication. *J. Virol.* **2009**, *83*, 12118–12128.
38. Peden, K.W.C.; Srinivasan, A.; Farber, J.M.; Pipas, J.M. Mutants with changes within or near a hydrophobic region of simian virus-40 Large Tumor Antigen are Defective for Binding Cellular Protein p53. *Virology* **1989**, *168*, 13–21.
39. Kierstead, T.D.; Tevethia, M.J. Association of p53 binding and immortalization of primary C57bl/6 mouse embryo fibroblasts by using simian-virus 40 T-antigen mutants bearing internal overlapping deletion mutations. *J. Virol.* **1993**, *67*, 1817–1829.
40. Topalis, D.; Andrei, G.; Snoeck, R. The large tumor antigen: A "Swiss Army Knife" protein possessing the functions required for the polyomavirus life cycle. *Antiviral Res.* **2013**, *97*, 122–136.
41. Nakamura, T.; Sato, Y.; Watanabe, D.; Ito, H.; Shimonohara, N.; Tsuji, T.; Nakajima, N.; Suzuki, Y.; Matsuo, K.; Nakagawa, H.; *et al.* Nuclear localization of Merkel cell polyomavirus large T antigen in Merkel cell carcinoma. *Virology* **2010**, *398*, 273–279.
42. Liu, X.; Hein, J.; Richardson, S.C.W.; Basse, P.H.; Toptan, T.; Moore, P.S.; Gjoerup, O.V.; Chang, Y. Merkel cell polyomavirus large T antigen disrupts lysosome clustering by translocating human vam6p from the cytoplasm to the nucleus. *J. Biol. Chem.* **2011**, *286*, 17079–17090.
43. DeCaprio, J.A.; Ludlow, J.W.; Figge, J.; Shew, J.Y.; Huang, C.M.; Lee, W.H.; Marsilio, E.; Paucha, E.; Livingston, D.M. SV40 large tumor-antigen forms a specific complex with the product of the retinoblastoma susceptibility gene. *Cell* **1988**, *54*, 275–283.
44. Srinivasan, A.; McClellan, A.J.; Vartikar, J.; Marks, I.; Cantalupo, P.; Li, Y.; Whyte, P.; Rundell, K.; Brodsky, J.L.; Pipas, J.M. The amino-terminal transforming region of simian virus 40 large T and small T antigens functions as a J domain. *Mol. Cell. Biol.* **1997**, *17*, 4761–4773.
45. Ali, S.H.; Kasper, J.S.; Arai, T.; DeCaprio, J.A. Cul7/p185/p193 binding to simian virus 40 large T antigen has a role in cellular transformation. *J. Virol.* **2004**, *78*, 2749–2757.
46. Cotsiki, M.; Lock, R.L.; Cheng, Y.; Williams, G.L.; Zhao, J.; Perera, D.; Freire, R.; Entwistle, A.; Golemis, E.A.; Roberts, T.M.; *et al.* Simian virus 40 large T antigen targets the spindle assembly checkpoint protein Bub1. *Proc. Natl. Acad. Sci. USA* **2004**, *101*, 947–952.
47. Lane, D.P.; Crawford, L.V. T-antigen is bound to a host protein in SV40-transformed cells. *Nature* **1979**, *278*, 261–263.
48. Poulin, D.L.; Kung, A.L.; DeCaprio, J.A. p53 Targets Simian virus 40 large T antigen for acetylation by CBP. *J. Virol.* **2004**, *78*, 8245–8253.
49. Seo, G.J.; Chen, C.J.; Sullivan, C.S. Merkel cell polyomavirus encodes a MicroRNA with the ability to autoregulate viral gene expression. *Virology* **2009**, *383*, 183–187.
50. Zerrahn, J.; Knippschild, U.; Winkler, T.; Deppert, W. Independent expression of the transforming amino-terminal domain of SV40 large T-antigen from an alternatively spliced 3rd

SV40 early messenger-RNA. *EMBO J.* **1993**, *12*, 4739–4746.

51. Comerford, S.A.; Schultz, N.; Hinnant, E.A.; Klapproth, S.; Hammer, R.E. Comparative analysis of SV40 17kT and LT function *in vivo* demonstrates that it's C-terminus reprograms hepatic gene expression and is necessary for tumorigenesis in the liver. *Oncogenesis* **2012**, *1*, e28.
52. Moens, U.; van Ghelue, M.; Johannessen, M. Oncogenic potentials of the human polyomavirus regulatory proteins. *Cell. Mol. Life. Sci.* **2007**, *64*, 1656–1678.
53. Pallas, D.C.; Shahrik, L.K.; Martin, B.L.; Jaspers, S.; Miller, T.B.; Brautigan, D.L.; Roberts, T.M. Polyoma small and middle T-antigens and SV40 small T-antigen form stable complexes with protein phosphatase-2A. *Cell* **1990**, *60*, 167–176.
54. Griffiths, D.A.; Abdul-Sada, H.; Knight, L.M.; Jackson, B.R.; Richards, K.; Prescott, E.L.; Peach, A.H.; Blair, G.E.; Macdonald, A.; Whitehouse, A. Merkel cell polyomavirus small T antigen targets the NEMO adaptor protein to disrupt inflammatory signaling. *J. Virol.* **2013**, *87*, 13853–13867.
55. Kwun, H.J.; Shuda, M.; Feng, H.; Camacho, C.J.; Moore, P.S.; Chang, Y. Merkel cell polyomavirus small T antigen controls viral replication and oncoprotein expression by Targeting the cellular ubiquitin ligase SCFFbw7. *Cell Host Microbe* **2013**, *14*, 125–135.
56. Carter, J.J.; Daugherty, M.D.; Qi, X.; Bheda-Malge, A.; Wipf, G.C.; Robinson, K.; Roman, A.; Malik, H.S.; Galloway, D.A. Identification of an overprinting gene in Merkel cell polyomavirus provides evolutionary insight into the birth of viral genes. *Proc. Natl. Acad. Sci. USA* **2013**, *110*, 12744–12749.
57. Schowalter, R.M.; Buck, C.B. The Merkel cell polyomavirus minor capsid protein. *PLoS Pathog.* **2013**, *9*, e1003558.
58. Neu, U.; Hengel, H.; Blaum, B.S.; Schowalter, R.M.; Macejak, D.; Gilbert, M.; Wakarchuk, W.W.; Imamura, A.; Ando, H.; Kiso, M.; *et al.* Structures of Merkel cell polyomavirus VP1 complexes define a sialic acid binding site required for infection. *PLoS Pathog.* **2012**, *8*, e1002738.
59. Sullivan, C.S.; Grundhoff, A.T.; Tevethia, S.; Pipas, J.M.; Ganem, D. SV40-encoded MicroRNAs regulate viral gene expression and reduce susceptibility to cytotoxic T cells. *Nature* **2005**, *435*, 682–686.
60. Seo, G.J.; Fink, L.H.L.; O'Hara, B.; Atwood, W.J.; Sullivan, C.S. Evolutionarily conserved function of a viral microRNA. *J. Virol.* **2008**, *82*, 9823–9828.
61. Lee, S.; Paulson, K.G.; Murchison, E.P.; Afanasiev, O.K.; Alkan, C.; Leonard, J.H.; Byrd, D.R.; Hannon, G.J.; Nghiem, P. Identification and validation of a novel mature microRNA encoded by the Merkel cell polyomavirus in human Merkel cell carcinomas. *J. Clin. Virol.* **2011**, *52*, 272–275.
62. Schowalter, R.M.; Pastrana, D.V.; Pumphrey, K.A.; Moyer, A.L.; Buck, C.B. Merkel cell polyomavirus and two previously unknown polyomaviruses are chronically shed from human skin. *Cell Host Microbe* **2010**, *7*, 509–515.
63. Schowalter, R.M.; Reinhold, W.C.; Buck, C.B. Entry tropism of BK and Merkel cell polyomaviruses in cell culture. *PLoS One* **2012**, *7*, e42181.
64. Schowalter, R.M.; Pastrana, D.V.; Buck, C.B. Glycosaminoglycans and sialylated glycans sequentially facilitate Merkel cell polyomavirus infectious entry *PLoS Pathog.* **2011** *7*, e1002161.

65. Bauer, P.H.; Cui, C.; Stehle, T.; Harrison, S.C.; DeCaprio, J.A.; Benjamin, T.L. Discrimination between sialic acid-containing receptors and pseudoreceptors regulates polyomavirus spread in the mouse. *J. Virol.* **1999**, *7*, 5826–5832.
66. Sapp, M.; Day, P.M. Structure, attachment and entry of polyoma- and papillomaviruses. *Virology* **2009**, *384*, 400–409.
67. Wessel, R.; Schweizer, J.; Stahl, H. Simian virus-40 T-antigen DNA helicase is a hexamer which forms a binary complex during bidirectional unwinding from the viral origin of DNA-replication. *J. Virol.* **1992**, *66*, 804–815.
68. Harrison, C.J.; Meinke, G.; Kwun, H.J.; Rogalin, H.; Phelan, P.J.; Bullock, P.A.; Chang, Y.; Moore, P.S.; Bohm, A. Asymmetric assembly of Merkel cell polyomavirus large T-antigen origin binding domains at the viral origin. *J. Molec. Biol.* **2011**, *409*, 529–542.
69. Feng, H.; Kwun, H.J.; Liu, X.; Gjoerup, O.; Stolz, D.B.; Chang, Y.; Moore, P.S. Cellular and viral factors regulating Merkel cell polyomavirus replication. *PLoS One* **2011**, *6*, e22468.
70. Wang, X.; Li, J.; Schowalter, R.M.; Jiao, J.; Buck, C.B.; You, J. Bromodomain protein Brd4 plays a key role in Merkel cell polyomavirus DNA replication. *PLoS Pathog.* **2012**, *8*, e1003021.
71. Tsang, S.H.; Wang, X.; Li, J.; Buck, C.B.; You, J. Host DNA damage response factors localize to Merkel cell polyomavirus DNA replication sites to support efficient viral DNA replication. *J. Virol.* **2014**, *88*, 3285–3297.
72. Gillespie, K.A.; Mehta, K.P.; Laimins, L.A.; Moody, C.A. Human papillomaviruses recruit cellular DNA repair and homologous recombination factors to viral replication centers. *J. Virol.* **2012**, *86*, 9520–9526.
73. Wang, X.; Helfer, C.M.; Pancholi, N.; Bradner, J.E.; You, J. Recruitment of Brd4 to the human papillomavirus type 16 DNA replication complex is essential for replication of viral DNA. *J. Virol.* **2013**, *87*, 3871–3884.
74. Shuda, M.; Kwun, H.J.; Feng, H.; Chang, Y.; Moore, P.S. Human Merkel cell polyomavirus small T antigen is an oncoprotein targeting the 4E-BP1 translation regulator. *J. Clin. Invest.* **2011**, *121*, 3623–3634.
75. Welcker, M.; Clurman, B.E. FBW7 ubiquitin ligase: A tumour suppressor at the crossroads of cell division, growth and differentiation. *Nat. Rev. Cancer* **2008**, *8*, 83–93.
76. Maser, R.S.; Choudhury, B.; Campbell, P.J.; Feng, B.; Wong, K.K.; Protopopov, A.; O'Neil, J.; Gutierrez, A.; Ivanova, E.; Perna, I.; *et al.* Chromosomally Unstable mouse tumours have genomic alterations similar to diverse human cancers. *Nature* **2007**, *447*, 966–971.
77. Wood, L.D.; Parsons, D.W.; Jones, S.; Lin, J.; Sjöblom, T.; Leary, R.J.; Shen, D.; Boca, S.M.; Barber, T.; Ptak, J.; *et al.* The genomic landscapes of human breast and colorectal cancers. *Science* **2007**, *318*, 1108–1113.
78. Mao, J.H.; Perez-Losada, J.; Wu, D.; Delrosario, R.; Tsunematsu, R.; Nakayama, K.I.; Brown, K.; Bryson, S.; Balmain, A. Fbxw7/Cdc4 Is a p53-dependent, haploinsufficient tumour suppressor gene. *Nature* **2004**, *432*, 775–779.
79. Rajagopalan, H.; Jallepalli, P.V.; Rago, C.; Velculescu, V.E.; Kinzler, K.W.; Vogelstein, B.; Lengauer, C. Inactivation of hCDC4 can cause chromosomal instability. *Nature* **2004**, *428*, 77–81.
80. Hayden, M.S.; Ghosh, S. Signaling to NF-kappa B. *Genes Dev.* **2004**, *18*, 2195–2224.

81. Le Negrate, G. Viral interference with innate immunity by preventing NF-kappa B activity. *Cell. Microbiol.* **2012**, *14*, 168–181.

82. Joo, M.S.; Hahn, Y.S.; Kwon, M.; Sadikot, R.T.; Blackwell, T.S.; Christman, J.W. Hepatitis C virus core protein suppresses NF-kappa B activation and cyclooxygenase-2 expression by direct interaction with I kappa B kinase beta. *J. Virol.* **2005**, *79*, 7648–7657.

83. Spitkovsky, D.; Hehner, S.P.; Hofmann, T.G.; Moller, A.; Schmitz, M.L. The Human papillomavirus oncoprotein E7 attenuates NF-kappa B activation by targeting the I kappa B kinase complex. *J. Biol. Chem.* **2002**, *277*, 25576–25582.

84. Randall, C.M.H.; Jokela, J.A.; Shisler, J.L. The MC159 Protein from the molluscum contagiosum poxvirus inhibits NF-kappa B activation by interacting with the I kappa B kinase complex. *J. Immunol.* **2012**, *188*, 2371–2379.

85. Fliss, P.M.; Jowers, T.P.; Brinkmann, M.M.; Holstermann, B.; Mack, C.; Dickinson, P.; Hohenberg, H.; Ghazal, P.; Brune, W. Viral mediated redirection of NEMO/IKK gamma to autophagosomes curtails the inflammatory cascade. *PLoS Pathog.* **2012**, *8*, e1002517.

86. Moreno, C.S.; Ramachandran, S.; Ashby, D.G.; Laycock, N.; Plattner, C.A.; Chen, W.; Hahn, W.C.; Pallas, D.C. Signaling and transcriptional changes critical for transformation of human cells by simian virus 40 small tumor antigen or protein phosphatase 2A B56 gamma knockdown. *Cancer Res.* **2004**, *64*, 6978–6988.

87. Shahzad, N.; Shuda, M.; Gheit, T.; Kwun, H.J.; Cornet, I.; Saidj, D.; Zannetti, C.; Hasan, U.; Chang, Y.; Moore, P.S.; *et al.* The T antigen locus of Merkel Cell polyomavirus downregulates human toll-like receptor 9 expression. *J. Virol.* **2013**, *87*, 13009–13019.

88. Takeda, K.; Akira, S. Toll-like receptors in innate immunity. *Int. Immunol.* **2005**, *17*, 1–14.

89. Beutler, B. Inferences, questions and possibilities in toll-like receptor signalling. *Nature* **2004**, *430*, 257–263.

90. Tsujimura, H.; Tamura, T.; Kong, H.J.; Nishiyama, A.; Ishii, K.J.; Klinman, D.M.; Ozato, K. Toll-like receptor 9 signaling activates NF-κB through IFN regulatory factor-8/IFN consensus sequence binding protein in dendritic cells. *J. Immunol.* **2004**, *172*, 6820–6827.

91. Fathallah, I.; Parroche, P.; Gruffat, H.; Zannetti, C.; Johansson, H.; Yue, J.; Manet, E.; Tommasino, M.; Sylla, B.S.; Hasan, U.A. EBV latent membrane protein 1 is a negative regulator of TLR9. *J. Immunol.* **2010**, *185*, 6439–6447.

92. Hasan, U.A.; Bates, E.; Takeshita, F.; Biliato, A.; Accardi, R.; Bouvard, V.; Mansour, M.; Vincent, I.; Gissmann, L.; Iftner, T.; *et al.* TLR9 Expression and Function is abolished by the cervical cancer-associated human papillomavirus type 16. *J. Immunol.* **2007**, *178*, 3186–3197.

93. Vincent, I.E.; Zannetti, C.; Lucifora, J.; Norder, H.; Protzer, U.; Hainaut, P.; Zoulim, F.; Tommasino, M.; Trépo, C.; Hasan, U.; *et al.* Hepatitis B virus impairs TLR9 expression and function in plasmacytoid dendritic cells. *PLoS One* **2011**, *6*, e26315.

94. Neumann, F.; Borchert, S.; Schmidt, C.; Reimer, R.; Hohenberg, H.; Fischer, N.; Grundhoff, A. Replication, gene expression and particle production by a consensus Merkel cell polyomavirus (MCPyV) genome. *PLoS One* **2011**, *6*, e29112.

95. Khalili, K.; White, M.K.; Sawa, H.; Nagashima, K.; Safak, M. The agnoprotein of polyomaviruses: A multifunctional auxiliary protein. *J. Cell Physiol.* **2005**, *204*, 1–7.

96. Daniels, R.; Sadowicz, D.; Hebert, D.N. A Very late viral protein triggers the lytic release of SV40. *PLoS Pathog.* **2007**, *3*, 0929–0938.
97. Clayson, E.T.; Brando, L.V.; Compans, R.W. Release of simian virus 40 virions from epithelial cells is polarized and occurs without cell lysis. *J. Virol.* **1989**, *63*, 2278–2288.
98. Hahn, W.C.; Dessain, S.K.; Brooks, M.W.; King, J.E.; Elenbaas, B.; Sabatini, D.M.; DeCaprio, J.A.; Weinberg, R.A. Enumeration of the simian virus 40 early region elements necessary for human cell transformation. *Mol. Cell. Biol.* **2002**, *22*, 2111–2123.
99. Bikel, I.; Montano, X.; Agha, M.E.; Brown, M.; McCormack, M.; Boltax, J.; Livingston, D.M. SV40 small T-antigen enhances the transformation activity of limiting concentrations of SV40 Large T-antigen. *Cell* **1987**, *48*, 321–330.
100. Houben, R.; Shuda, M.; Weinkam, R.; Schrama, D.; Feng, H.; Chang, Y.; Moore, P.S.; Becker, J.C. Merkel cell polyomavirus-infected merkel cell carcinoma cells require expression of viral T antigens. *J. Virol.* **2010**, *84*, 7064–7072.
101. Fischer, N.; Brandner, J.; Fuchs, F.; Moll, I.; Grundhoff, A. Detection of merkel cell polyomavirus (MCPyV) in Merkel cell carcinoma cell lines: Cell morphology and growth phenotype do not reflect presence of the virus. *Int. J. Cancer* **2010**, *126*, 2133–2142.
102. Katano, H.; Ito, H.; Suzuki, Y.; Nakamura, T.; Sato, Y.; Tsuji, T.; Matsuo, K.; Nakagawa, H.; Sata, T. Detection of Merkel cell polyomavirus in Merkel cell carcinoma and Kaposi's sarcoma. *J. Med. Virol.* **2009**, *81*, 1951–1958.
103. Shuda, M.; Feng, H.; Kwun, H.J.; Rosen, S.T.; Gjoerup, O.; Moore, P.S.; Chang, Y. T antigen mutations are a human tumor-specific signature for Merkel cell polyomavirus. *Proc. Natl. Acad. Sci. USA* **2008**, *105*, 16272–16277.
104. Kassem, A.; Schopflin, A.; Diaz, C.; Weyers, W.; Stickeler, E.; Werner, M.; Zur Hausen, A. Frequent detection of Merkel cell polyomavirus in human Merkel cell carcinomas and identification of a unique deletion in the VP1 gene. *Cancer Res.* **2008**, *68*, 5009–5013.
105. DeCaprio, J.A.; Garcea, R.L. A cornucopia of human polyomaviruses. *Nat. Rev. Microbiol.* **2013**, *11*, 264–276.
106. Demetriou, S.K.; Ona-Vu, K.; Sullivan, E.M.; Dong, T.K.; Hsu, S.-W.; Oh, D.H. Defective DNA repair and cell cycle arrest in cells expressing Merkel cell polyomavirus T antigen. *Int. J. Cancer* **2012**, *131*, 1818–1827.
107. Busam, K.J.; Jungbluth, A.A.; Rekthman, N.; Coit, D.; Pulitzer, M.; Bini, J.; Arora, R.; Hanson, N.C.; Tassello, J.A.; Frosina, D.; *et al*. Merkel cell polyomavirus expression in Merkel cell carcinomas and its absence in combined tumors and pulmonary neuroendocrine carcinomas. *Am. J. Surg. Pathol.* **2009**, *33*, 1378–1385.
108. Shuda, M.; Arora, R.; Kwun, H.J.; Feng, H.; Sarid, R.; Fernandez-Figueras, M.-T.; Tolstov, Y.; Gjoerup, O.; Mansukhani, M.M.; Swerdlow, S.H.; *et al*. Human Merkel cell polyomavirus infection I. MCV T antigen expression in Merkel cell carcinoma, lymphoid tissues and lymphoid tumors. *Int. J. Cancer* **2009**, *125*, 1243–1249.
109. Brown, M.; McCormack, M.; Zinn, K.G.; Farrell, M.P.; Bikel, I.; Livingston, D.M. A recombinant murine retrovirus for simian virus-40 large T-cDNA transforms mouse fibroblasts to anchorage-independent growth. *J. Virol.* **1986**, *60*, 290–293.
110. Vousden, K.H.; Lane, D.P. p53 in health and disease. *Nat. Rev. Mol. Cell. Biol.* **2007**, *8*, 275–283.

111. Sullivan, C.S.; Cantalupo, P.; Pipas, J.M. The molecular chaperone activity of simian virus 40 large T antigen is required to Disrupt Rb-E2F family complexes by an ATP-dependent mechanism. *Mol. Cell. Biol.* **2000**, *20*, 6233–6243.
112. Cheng, J.; Rozenblatt-Rosen, O.; Paulson, K.G.; Nghiem, P.; DeCaprio, J.A. Merkel cell polyomavirus large T antigen has growth-promoting and inhibitory activities. *J. Virol.* **2013**, *87*, 6118–6126.
113. Li, J.; Wang, X.; Diaz, J.; Tsang, S.H.; Buck, C.B.; You, J. Merkel cell polyomavirus large T antigen disrupts host genomic integrity and inhibits cellular proliferation. *J. Virol.* **2013**, *87*, 9173–9188.
114. Shi, Y.L.; Dodson, G.E., Rundell, K.; Tibbetts, R.S. Ataxia-telangiectasia-mutated (ATM) Is a T-antigen kinase that controls SV40 viral replication *in vivo*. *J. Biol. Chem.* **2005**, *280*, 40195–40200.
115. Arora, R.; Shuda, M.; Guastafierro, A.; Feng, H.; Toptan, T., Tolstov, Y.; Normolle, D.; Vollmer, L.L.; Vogt, A.; Doemling, A.; *et al.* Survivin is a therapeutic target in Merkel cell carcinoma. *Sci. Transl. Med.* **2012**, *4*, 133ra56.
116. Coumar, M.S.; Tsai, F.Y.; Kanwar, J.R.; Sarvagalla, S.; Cheung, C.H.A. Treat cancers by targeting survivin: Just a dream or future reality? *Cancer Treat. Rev.* **2013**, *39*, 802–811.
117. Angermeyer, S.; Hesbacher, S.; Becker, J.C.; Schrama, D.; Houben, R. Merkel cell polyomavirus-positive Merkel cell carcinoma cells do not require expression of the viral small T antigen. *J. Invest. Dermatol.* **2013**, *133*, 2059–2064.
118. Sontag, E.; Fedorov, S.; Kamibayashi, C.; Robbins, D.; Cobb, M.; Mumby, M. The interaction of SV40 small tumor-antigen with protein phosphatase-2a stimulates the MAP kinase pathway and induces cell-proliferation. *Cell* **1993**, *75*, 887–897.
119. Ruediger, R.; Hentz, M.; Fait, J.; Mumby, M.; Walter, G. Molecular Model of the a subunit of protein phosphatase 2A: Interaction with other subunits and tumor antigens. *J. Virol.* **1994**, *68*, 123–129.
120. Yang, S.I.; Lickteig, R.L.; Estes, R.; Rundell, K.; Walter, G.; Mumby, M.C. Control of protein phosphatase-2A by simian virus-40 small-T antigen. *Mol. Cell. Biol.* **1991**, *11*, 1988–1995.
121. Yu, J.; Boyapati, A.; Rundell, K. Critical role for SV40 small-T antigen in human cell transformation. *Virology* **2001**, *290*, 192–198.
122. Zhao, J.J.; Gjoerup, O.V.; Subramanian, R.R.; Cheng, Y.; Chen, W.; Roberts, T.M.; Hahn, W.C. Human Mammary epithelial cell transformation through the activation of phosphatidylinositol 3-kinase. *Cancer Cell* **2003**, *3*, 483–495.
123. Rodriguez-Viciana, P.; Collins, C.; Fried, M. Polyoma and SV40 proteins differentially regulate PP2A to activate distinct cellular signaling pathways involved in growth control. *Proc. Natl. Acad. Sci. USA* **2006**, *103*, 19290–19295.
124. Buchkovich, N.J.; Yu, Y.; Zampieri, C.A.; Alwine, J.C. The TORrid affairs of viruses: Effects of mammalian DNA viruses on the PI3K-Akt-mTOR signalling pathway. *Nat. Rev. Microbiol.* **2008**, *6*, 266–275.
125. Dowling, R.J.O.; Topisirovic, I.; Alain, T.; Bidinosti, M.; Fonseca, B.D.; Petroulakis, E.; Wang, X.; Larsson, O.; Selvaraj, A.; Liu, Y.; *et al.* mTORC1-mediated cell proliferation, but not cell growth, controlled by the 4E-BPs. *Science* **2010**, *328*, 1172–1176.

126. She, Q.-B.; Halilovic, E.; Ye, Q.; Zhen, W.; Shirasawa, S.; Sasazuki, T.; Solit, D.B.; Rosen, N. 4E-BP1 is a key effector of the oncogenic activation of the AKT and ERK signaling pathways that integrates their function in tumors. *Cancer Cell* **2010**, *18*, 39–51.
127. Richter, J.D.; Sonenberg, N. Regulation of cap-dependent translation by eIF4E inhibitory proteins. *Nature* **2005**, *433*, 477–480.
128. Pause, A.; Belsham, G.J.; Gingras, A.C.; Donzé, O.; Lin, T.A.; Lawrence, J.C., Jr.; Sonenberg, N. Insulin-dependent stimulation of protein-synthesis by phosphorylation of a regulator of 5'-Cap function. *Nature* **1994**, *371*, 762–767.
129. Lazariskaratzas, A.; Montine, K.S.; Sonenberg, N. Malignant transformation by a eukaryotic initiation-factor subunit that binds to messenger-RNA 5' cap. *Nature* **1990**, *345*, 544–547.
130. Avdulov, S.; Li, S.; Michalek, V.; Burrichter, D.; Peterson, M.; Perlman, D.M.; Manivel, J.C.; Sonenberg, N.; Yee, D.; Bitterman, P.B.; *et al.* Activation of translation complex eIF4F is essential for the genesis and maintenance of the malignant phenotype in human mammary epithelial cells. *Cancer Cell* **2004**, *5*, 553–563.
131. Beretta, L.; Gingras, A.C.; Svitkin, Y.V.; Hall, M.N.; Sonenberg, N. Rapamycin blocks the phosphorylation of 4E-BP1 and inhibits cap-dependent initiation of translation. *EMBO J.* **1996**, *15*, 658–664.
132. Yu, J.; Boyapati, A.; Rundell, K. Critical role for SV40 small-T antigen in human cell transformation. *Virology* **2001**, *290*, 192–198.
133. Jouary, T.; Leyral, C.; Dreno, B.; Doussau, A.; Sassolas, B.; Beylot-Barry, M.; Renaud-Vilmer, C.; Guillot, B.; Bernard, P.; Lok, C.; *et al.* Adjuvant prophylactic regional radiotherapy *versus* observation in stage I Merkel cell carcinoma: A multicentric prospective randomized study. *Ann. Oncol.* **2012**, *23* 1074–1080.
134. Pape, E.; Rezvoy, N.; Penel, N.; Salleron, J.; Martinot, V.; Guerreschi, P.; Dziwniel, V.; Darras, S.; Mirabel, X.; Mortier, L. Radiotherapy alone for Merkel cell carcinoma: A comparative and retrospective study of 25 patients. *J. Am. Acad. Dermatol.* **2011**, *65*, 983–990.
135. Tai, P.T.; Yu, E.; Winquist, E.; Hammond, A.; Stitt, L.; Tonita, J.; Gilchrist, J. Chemotherapy in neuroendocrine/Merkel cell carcinoma of the skin: Case series and review of 204 cases. *J. Clin. Oncol.* **2000**, *18*, 2493–2499.
136. Willmes, C.; Adam, C.; Alb, M.; Völkert, L.; Houben, R.; Becker, J.C.; Schrama, D. Type I and II IFNs inhibit Merkel cell carcinoma via modulation of the Merkel Cell polyomavirus T antigens. *Cancer Res.* **2012**, *72*, 2120–2128.
137. Biver-Dalle, C.; Nguyen, T.; Touzé, A.; Saccomani, C.; Penz, S.; Cunat-Peultier, S.; Riou-Gotta, M.-O.; Humbert, P.; Coursaget, P.; Aubin, F. Use of interferon-alpha in two patients with Merkel cell carcinoma positive for Merkel cell polyomavirus. *Acta Oncol.* **2010**, *50*, 479–480.
138. Dresang, L.R.; Guastafierro, A.; Arora, R.; Normolle, D.; Chang, Y.; Moore, P.S. Response of Merkel cell polyomavirus-positive Merkel cell carcinoma xenografts to a survivin inhibitor. *PLoS One* **2013**, *11*, e80543.
139. Davids, M.; Charlton, A.; Ng, S.S.; Chong, M.L.; Laubscher, K.; Dar, M.; Hodge, J.; Soong, R.; Goh, B.C. Response to a novel multitargeted tyrosine kinase inhibitor pazopanib in metastatic Merkel cell carcinoma. *J. Clin. Oncol.* **2009**, *27*, e97–e100.

140. Sugamata, A.; Goya, K.; Yoshizawa, N. A Case of complete spontaneous regression of extremely advanced Merkel cell carcinoma. *J. Surg. Case Rep.* **2011**, *10*, 7.

141. Iyer, J.G.; Afanasiev, O.K.; McClurkan, C.; Paulson, K.; Nagase, K.; Jing, L.; Marshak, J.O.; Dong, L.; Carter, J.; Lai, I.; *et al.* Merkel cell polyomavirus-specific CD8+ and CD4+ T-cell responses identified in Merkel cell carcinomas and blood. *Clin. Cancer Res.* **2011**, *17*, 6671–6680.

142. Lyngaa, R.; Pedersen, N.W.; Schrama, D.; Thrue, C.A.; Ibrani, D.; Met, Ö.; Thor Straten, P.; Nghiem, P.; Becker, J.C.; Hadrup, S.R. T-cell responses to oncogenic Merkel cell polyomavirus proteins distinguish Merkel cell carcinoma patients from healthy donors. *Clin. Cancer Res.* **2014**, *20*, 1768–1778.

143. Gomez, B.; He, L.; Tsai, Y.C.; Wu, T.-C.; Viscidi, R.P.; Hung, C.-F. Creation of a Merkel cell polyomavirus small T antigen-expressing murine tumor model and a DNA vaccine targeting small T antigen. *Cell Biosci.* **2013**, *3*, 29.

144. Zeng, Q.; Gomez, B.P.; Viscidi, R.P.; Peng, S.; He, L.; Ma, B.; Wu, T.-C.; Hung, C.-F. Development of a DNA vaccine targeting Merkel cell polyomavirus. *Vaccine* **2012**, *30*, 1322–1329.

145. Afanasiev, O.K.; Yelistratova, L.; Miller, N.; Nagase, K.; Paulson, K.; Iyer, J.G.; Ibrani, D.; Koelle, D.M.; Nghiem, P. Merkel polyomavirus-specific T cells fluctuate with Merkel cell carcinoma burden and express therapeutically targetable PD-1 and Tim-3 exhaustion markers. *Clin. Cancer Res.* **2013**, *19*, 5351–5360.

146. Pantulu, N.D.; Pallasch, C.P.; Kurz, A.K.; Kassem, A.; Frenzel, L.; Sodenkamp, S.; Kvasnicka, H.M.; Wendtner, C.M.; Zur Hausen, A. Detection of a novel truncating Merkel cell polyomavirus large T antigen deletion in chronic lymphocytic leukemia cells. *Blood* **2010**, *116*, 5280–5284.

147. Koljonen, V.; Kukko, H.; Pukkala, E.; Sankila, R.; Bohling, T.; Tukiainen, E.; Sihto, H.; Joensuu, H. Chronic lymphocytic leukaemia patients have a high risk of Merkel-Cell polyomavirus DNA-positive Merkel cell carcinoma. *Br. J. Cancer* **2009**, *101*, 1444–1447.

148. Teman, C.J.; Tripp, S.R.; Perkins, S.L.; Duncavage, E.J. Merkel cell polyomavirus (MCPyV) in chronic lymphocytic leukemia/small lymphocytic lymphoma. *Leuk Res.* **2011**, *35*, 689–692.

149. Andres, C.; Belloni, B.; Puchta, U.; Sander, C.A.; Flaig, M.J. Prevalence of MCPyV in Merkel cell carcinoma and non-MCC tumors. *J. Cutan. Pathol.* **2010**, *37*, 28–34.

150. Reisinger, D.M.; Shiffer, J.D.; Cognetta, A.B., Jr.; Chang, Y.; Moore, P.S. Lack of evidence for basal or squamous cell carcinoma infection with Merkel cell polyomavirus in immunocompetent patients with Merkel cell carcinoma. *J. Am. Acad. Dermatol.* **2010**, *63*, 400–403.

151. Rollison, D.E.; Giuliano, A.R.; Messina, J.L.; Fenske, N.A.; Cherpelis, B.S.; Sondak, V.K.; Roetzheim, R.G.; Iannacone, M.R.; Michael, K.M.; Gheit, T.; *et al.* Case-control study of Merkel cell polyomavirus infection and cutaneous squamous cell carcinoma. *Cancer Epidemiol. Biomarkers Prev.* **2012**, *21*, 74–81.

152. Dworkin, A.M.; Tseng, S.Y.; Allain, D.C.; Iwenofu, O.H.; Peters, S.B.; Toland, A.E. Merkel cell polyomavirus in cutaneous squamous cell carcinoma of immunocompetent individuals. *J. Invest. Dermatol.* **2009**, *129*, 2868–2874.

2

How Human Tumor Viruses Make Use of Autophagy

Zachary L. Pratt [1] **and Bill Sugden** [2,*]

[1] Department of Bacteriology and Food Research Institute, Microbial Sciences Building, University of Wisconsin-Madison, Madison, WI 53706, USA; E-Mail: zpratt@wisc.edu

[2] Department of Oncology, McArdle Laboratory for Cancer Research, Madison, WI 53706, USA

* Author to whom correspondence should be addressed; E-Mail: sugden@oncology.wisc.edu;

Abstract: Viruses commandeer regulatory pathways of their hosts to optimize their success as cellular parasites. The human tumor viruses, Epstein-Barr Virus (EBV), Kaposi's Sarcoma Herpesvirus (KSHV), Hepatitis B Virus (HBV), and Hepatitis C Virus (HCV) all affect autophagy for their own ends. EBV and KSHV regulate it during latent infections, a phase when no progeny virus is produced, while HBV and HCV use autophagy to promote their productive infections. Here we shall compare and contrast how these human tumor viruses regulate autophagy and what they gain by the appropriation of this cellular pathway.

Keywords: Epstein-Barr Virus; Kaposi's Sarcoma Herpesvirus; Hepatitis B Virus; Hepatitis C Virus; human tumor virus; autophagy; cancer

---

1. Introduction

Autophagy is a cellular program that can be initiated by several stimuli, is carried out by multiple regulatory molecules and enzymes, and culminates in the formation of double-membrane bound vesicles, termed autophagosomes, containing macromolecules which are catabolized in autophagolysosomes upon fusion of autophagosomes with lysosomes [1,2]. To initiate autophagy, the phosphatidylinositol 3-phosphate kinase, Vps34 (abbreviations can be found in Table 1), must be activated and generate phosphatidylinositol 3-phosphate for the growing phagophore, a precursor structure to the autophagosome. The stimuli for autophagy range from nutrient starvation to acute exercise [3]. The autophagic program is controlled by regulators as diverse as mammalian target of rapamycin (mTOR) and B-cell chronic lymphocytic leukemia/lymphoma 2 (Bcl2) [1] and the participants in it include kinases, ubiquitin-like conjugating molecules, phosphatidylinositol 3-kinases, and transmembrane proteins [4].

Table 1. Full names of abbreviations used in this review.

Abbreviation	Full Name
3-MA	3-methyl adenine
6TM	6-transmembrane-spanning domain of LMP1
AIDS	acute immunodeficiency syndrome
ATF	activated transcription factor
ATG	autophagy-related
BALF1	*Bam*HI A leftward fragment 1
Bcl2	B-cell chronic lymphocytic leukemia/lymphoma 2
BHRF1	*Bam*HI H rightward fragment 1
CD	cluster of differentiation
CRE	cAMP responsive element
EBNA1	Epstein-Barr nuclear antigen 1
EBV	Epstein-Barr Virus
eIF2α	eukaryotic initiation factor 2 alpha
HBs	Hepatitis B small surface protein
HBV	Hepatitis B Virus
HBx	Hepatitis B X protein
HCC	hepatocellular carcinoma
HCV	Hepatitis C Virus
HFFs	human foreskin fibroblasts
IFN	interferon
IRGM	immunity related GTPase M
ISG56	interferon-stimulated gene 56
KSHV	Kaposi's Sarcoma Herpesvirus
LC3	light chain 3
LMP1	latent membrane protein 1
MAVS	mitochondrial antiviral signaling protein
MHC	major histocompatibility complex
mTOR	mammalian target of rapamycin
NAF1	nutrient-deprivation autophagy factor 1
NFκB	nuclear factor kappa B
NS4B	non-structural protein 4B
PE	phosphatidylethanolamine
PEL	primary effusion lymphoma
PERK	protein kinase RNA-like endoplasmic reticulum kinase
RIG-I	retinoic acid inducible gene I protein
RTA	replication and transcription activator
siRNA	small interfering RNA
TNFα	tumor necrosis factor alpha
UPR	Unfolded Protein Response
v-FLIP	FADD-like interleukin-1 beta-converting enzyme inhibitory protein
Vps34	vesicle-mediated vacuolar protein sorting 34

Viruses are obligate cellular parasites and human tumor viruses, in particular, are obligate cellular parasites that can affect their host cells oncogenically. Viruses need to amplify their numbers to survive and spread. They use the synthetic machinery of their host cells to make more of themselves and these productive cycles often end in cell death and pathology. Human tumor viruses must produce more of themselves, too, but can drive the infected cells both to survive and proliferate aberrantly. Several human tumor viruses make use of autophagy either during their productive cycles, or during non-productive infections, or both (Table 2). Here we review how four human tumor viruses involve autophagy in their life-cycles to foster their own parasitic ends and to induce their pathologies.

Table 2. Multiple roles for autophagy in the life-cycles of human tumor viruses.

Virus	Role of Autophagy in Viral Life-cycle	References
EBV	Autophagy contributes to the generation of epitopes of EBNA1, a pivotal viral protein, presented on MHC II	[5,6]
	Along with the UPR, autophagy regulates expression of LMP1, a viral oncogene	[7,8]
KSHV	Autophagy inhibits survival and proliferation of latently-infected cells	[9,10]
	Supports viral replication and productive life-cycle	[11]
HCV	Autophagy blocks an interferon response during the early stages of infection allowing HCV to establish its infection	[12]
HBV	Autophagy supports infection and may provide a scaffold for reverse transcription or viral envelopment during the productive life-cycle	[13,14]

2. Epstein-Barr Virus

Epstein-Barr Virus (EBV) is a Herpesvirus, and as with other members of this family, its viral particle is enveloped and contains a double-stranded DNA genome of 165 kbp. EBV infects the vast majority of people in the world without causing disease, but does cause a variety of cancers in a minority of infected people including Burkitt's lymphoma, Hodgkin's lymphomas, B-cell post-transplant lymphoproliferative disorder, Nasopharygeal carcinoma, and gastric carcinoma [15]. Once people are infected, the virus is latently maintained in memory B-cells for the life of the person [16]. There are at least two apparently unrelated ways in which EBV has evolved to use autophagy in its host cell. EBV DNA is maintained as an extrachromosomal plasmid in latently infected cells, including all tumor cells. The virus contributes only one protein, Epstein-Barr nuclear antigen 1 (EBNA1), to the synthesis and maintenance of its plasmid; all other *trans*-acting factors are provided by the host cell [17]. EBNA1, though, is essential for EBV to be maintained in proliferating cells [18,19].

Surprisingly, the expression of EBNA1 in infected cells does not lead to those cells being recognized efficiently by cluster of differentiation 8 (CD8)-positive cytotoxic T-cells. A stretch of glycine-alanine repeats in this viral protein limits its presentation as an antigen on major histocompatibility complex (MHC) class I molecules [20]. Rather, EBNA1 stimulates CD4-positive T-cells when presented on infected B-cells by MHC class II molecules [5,21,22]. Some of these epitopes are generated via autophagy, and EBNA1 can be found in double membrane vesicles, consistent with its localization to autophagosomes (Table 2) [6,23,24]. Stimulation of CD4-positive T-cells after their exposure to EBV-positive cells is inhibited when autophagy is suppressed with small interfering RNAs (siRNAs) that target mediators of autophagy, ATG12 or ATG7 (ATG refers to "autophagy related") [6,23]. Similarly, CD4-positive T-cells remain unstimulated when the acidification of autophagolysosomes in infected cells is inhibited [23]. Despite its immunogenicity, EBNA1 is poorly presented on MHC II molecules, perhaps because it spends little time in the cytoplasm [5,6,25,26]. By disrupting its nuclear localization signal and rendering it cytosolic, Leung and colleagues were able to enhance EBNA1's degradation in autophagolysosomes and increase the stimulation of CD4-positive T-cell clones by 15-fold [6]. How the presentation of EBNA1 to CD4-positive T-cells contributes to EBV's life-cycle is unclear. However, its poor presentation by MHC class II molecules surely contributes to some EBV-positive tumors, such as canonical Burkitt's lymphomas, in which EBNA1 is the only viral protein expressed, escaping the hosts' immune response.

There is potentially a mechanism by which EBV regulates autophagy to affect the host's immune response. EBV encodes two proteins, *Bam*HI rightward fragment 1 (BHRF1) and *Bam*HI A leftward fragment 1 (BALF1), which are orthologs of the cellular antiapoptotic protein, Bcl2. These proteins can each inhibit apoptosis and at least one or the other needs to be expressed in newly infected B-lymphocytes for EBV to infect the cells successfully [27]. BHRF1 is expressed in a subset of Burkitt's lymphomas and helps to block apoptosis in these latently infected tumor cells, too [28]. Bcl2 and its ortholog encoded by KSHV bind Beclin1 and thereby inhibit autophagy [29]. If the EBV-encoded orthologs of Bcl2, BHRF1 and BALF1, bind Beclin1 too, which appears likely, then these EBV proteins will also inhibit autophagy. Their potential inhibition of autophagy would limit further the presentation of EBNA1-derived peptides by MHC class II molecules and simultaneously limit any other contributions to innate immunity mediated through autophagy.

EBV uses autophagy to regulate expression of one of its oncogenes, the latent membrane protein 1 (LMP1), which drives proliferation of infected B-cells (Table 1). LMP1 is expressed in a subset of latent infections and contains two domains that perform independent functions [30]. Its carboxy-terminal domain is a viral mimic of the human CD40 receptor, and activates signaling pathways, such as nuclear factor kappa B (NFκB), to drive cellular proliferation and inhibit apoptosis [7,30–32]. This carboxy-terminal signaling requires LMP1 to self-oligomerize, which is accomplished by a second domain, its six-transmembrane spanning domains (6TM) [8]. Recently, it has been shown that a single amino acid within transmembrane domain 5 is necessary for LMP1's oligomerization [33]. The 6TM of LMP1 dose-dependently induces autophagy via the Unfolded Protein Response (UPR) (Table 3) [34,35]. This induction is mediated at least in part by LMP1's activating protein kinase RNA-like endoplasmic reticulum kinase (PERK), a kinase that can phosphorylate eukaryotic initiation factor 2 alpha (eIF2α). These cellular mechanisms are used to regulate LMP1's own synthesis and degradation, thereby modulating its expression and signaling during infection (Table 2). When levels of LMP1 within B-cells are low, LMP1 promotes its own transcription by activating PERK to phosphorylate eIF2α [34,36]. An activated transcription factor/ cAMP responsive element (ATF/CRE) element in LMP1's promoter is activated during the UPR, likely via ATF4 whose translation is enhanced by phospho-eIF2α [35]. Translation of LMP1 is mediated by unphosphorylated eIF2α, which makes up the majority of the total eIF2α in these cells [35]. However, as the levels of LMP1 increase, the fraction of eIF2α phosphorylated increases and translation of LMP1 is limited [35].

Table 3. Viral proteins that affect autophagy.

Virus	Viral Protein	Autophagic Protein	Effect of Viral Proteins on Autophagy	References
EBV	LMP1	Unknown	Activates autophagy via the UPR	[7,8]
KSHV	v-FLIP	ATG3	Competes with LC3 for binding to ATG3, thereby inhibits the conjugation of LC3 to PE	[10]
	v-Bcl2	Beclin 1	Binds Beclin 1 and inhibits its activation of autophagy	[29,37,38]
	RTA	Unknown	Induces autophagy	[11]
HCV	NS4B	Vps34	Induces autophagy by stimulating the enzymatic activity of Vps34	[39]
	NS5B	ATG5	Stimulates conjugation of LC3 to PE	[40]
HBV	HBs	Unknown	Activates autophagy via UPR	[41]
	HBx	Vps34	Initiates autophagy, possibly by the generation of phosphatidylinositol 3-phosphate by Vps34	[14]

To induce its degradation, LMP1 stimulates autophagy via the UPR [34]. LMP1's activation of PERK likely contributes to the activation of autophagy via PERK's phosphorylation of eIF2α. The transcription factor, ATF4, which is translated by phospho-eIF2α, can stimulate transcription of genes encoding the autophagic proteins, light chain 3 (LC3) and autophagy-related 5 homolog (ATG5) [42]. LC3 is an ubiquitin-like protein that is conjugated to phosphatidylethanolamine (PE) [4]. LC3 is translated as an inactive protein (Pro-LC3), which is cleaved by the protease, ATG4, to generate cytosolic LC3-I. LC3-I is conjugated to PE (LC3-II) in a reaction requiring the E2-like enzyme, ATG3, and the E3-like complex, ATG16L complex [4]. The lipid-conjugation of LC3 allows LC3's insertion into the phagophore. Inhibiting autophagy or the acidification of lysosomes blocks LMP1's degradation, thus increasing its expression in EBV-positive cells [10,34]. Disrupting this complex regulation of expression is deleterious to the cell and inhibits cellular survival and/or proliferation. The levels of LMP1 vary in otherwise genetically identical cells; those expressing intermediate levels of LMP1 proliferate optimally, while those with low or high levels grow more slowly and likely will avoid immune detection [9,36]. A weak immune response will be elicited if too little antigen is expressed. When expressed at high levels, LMP1's 6TM inhibits proliferation, thereby rendering B-cells resistant to external apoptotic stimuli, such as tumor necrosis factor alpha (TNFα) [9]. This complex regulation of the LMP1 oncogene contributes to EBV's driving proliferation of both normal and some tumor cells.

3. Kaposi's Sarcoma Herpesvirus

Kaposi's Sarcoma Herpes Virus (KSHV) is also a Herpesvirus having an enveloped virus particle encapsidating a double-stranded DNA genome. The prevalence of infection by KSHV varies dramatically in different populations. Between 5%–10% of adult North Americans are infected on average, while up to 65% of isolated groups of indigenous people in Brazil are infected [43]. KSHV causes Kaposi's Sarcoma, an endothelial cancer associated often with acute immunodeficiency syndrome (AIDS), and primary effusion lymphomas (PELs), a lymphoma of B-cell origin [43]. Most

PEL cells are infected both with KSHV and EBV [43]. PEL cells do not usually express LMP1, and therefore autophagy does not affect expression of this viral oncogene.

KSHV appears to have a love/hate relationship with autophagy. It blocks autophagy during the latent phase of its life-cycle and depends on it during the productive phase of its life-cycle. KSHV encodes FADD-like interleukin-1 beta-converting enzyme inhibitory protein (v-FLIP), which inhibits autophagy [44]. v-FLIP does so by competing with LC3 for binding to ATG3, thereby inhibiting LC3's conjugation to PE and its insertion into phagophores (Table 3) [4,44]. The effect of v-FLIP on autophagy is at least two-fold (Table 2). First, v-FLIP inhibits autophagic cellular death [44]. Lee and colleagues examined how inhibiting v-FLIP's binding to ATG3 would affect tumor development by PEL cells grown as xenografts. They developed peptide mimics of the α-2 and α-4 domains of v-FLIP, which compete specifically for v-FLIP's binding to ATG3, and injected them into mice receiving KSHV-positive xenografts. By competing with v-FLIP, but not LC3, for binding to ATG3, the peptide mimics effectively reduced the size of the tumors [44]. Secondly, v-FLIP's suppression of autophagy inhibits v-cyclin-induced cellular senescence during viral infection [45]. KSHV's v-cyclin protein is an oncogenic mimic of the human cyclins that drives the proliferation of infected endothelial cells. When expressed alone in human foreskin fibroblasts (HFFs), v-cyclin induces senescence, but senescence is rarely observed during infection with KSHV [45]. Autophagy appears to contribute to cellular senescence in human fibroblasts, and its inhibition delays senescence in fibroblasts following the induction of the oncogene, Ras [11]. v-FLIP's suppression of autophagy is both necessary and sufficient to inhibit senescence of KSHV-infected HFFs [45]. Thus, it appears that KSHV inhibits autophagy via v-FLIP and this inhibition contributes to the infected cells' survival and potentially to its oncogenic progression.

Another means by which KSHV can inhibit autophagy is through its ortholog of Bcl2 which binds Beclin 1 [29,37]. Bcl2 itself binds Beclin 1 only at the endoplasmic reticulum where the nutrient-deprivation autophagy factor 1 (NAF1) is localized [29,46]. NAF1 is a member of the inositol-1,4,5 triphosphate receptor complex and is required for Bcl2 to bind Beclin 1 [29]. In comparison to the human Bcl2, KSHV's v-Bcl2 binds more strongly to Beclin 1, likely indicating a selection for this interaction in the life-cycle of KSHV [12]. KSHV's v-Bcl2 is expressed during the productive phase of the viral life cycle and it is not clear what advantage this inhibition provides the virus. Inhibiting autophagy could limit the presentation of antigens on MHC class II molecules and thereby protect infected cells from their immune recognition [21,22]. It is all reasonable to speculate that KSHV's v-Bcl2 is expressed soon after infection of B-cells or endothelial cells and blocks apoptosis as do the v-Bcl2 orthologs of EBV [27]. All of these viral orthologs may contribute to successful infections by their respective viruses by binding Beclin 1 to regulate autophagy, too.

One reason the role of KSHV's v-Bcl2 in inhibiting autophagy is uncertain is because the immediate-early transcription factor of KSHV, replication and transcription activator (RTA) stimulates autophagy, which in turn supports the productive phase of viral infection (Tables 2, 3). The expression of RTA is necessary to induce the productive cycle of KSHV. For example, sodium butyrate stimulates the expression of RTA in latently infected cells and activates a transcriptional cascade of viral genes required for producing infectious virions [38,47]. Independently of KSHV, RTA can induce autophagy in endothelial cells and B-cells by an unknown mechanism [40]. Treating PEL cells with 3-methyl adenine (3-MA), an inhibitor of autophagy, represses expression of viral genes needed for viral replication [40]. KSHV's productive cycle therefore benefits from autophagy. It is possible, given its inhibition of autophagy, that v-FLIP maintains viral latency, that is, blocks the transition from latent to productive infection via its inhibiting autophagy. KSHV uses autophagy to promote its productive cycle and inhibits it probably to foster its latent infections. Both activities would potentially contribute to the pathogenesis by KSHV.

4. Hepatitis C Virus

Hepatitis C Virus (HCV) causes a large fraction of cases of primary hepatocellular carcinoma (HCC) in the world today with about 200 million people currently being infected [38]. The virus is a member of the Flavivirus family with its particle containing a single, positive-sense RNA genome of close to 10 kb in length [38]. The RNA is translated during infection into a single polypeptide that is subsequently cleaved by cellular and viral proteases into four structural and six non-structural proteins [38]. By "structural" proteins is meant those that make up the virus particle; non-structural proteins are usually enzymes that regulate the viral life-cycle.

HCV infection initiated either by treatment of cells with infectious particles or transfection of viral RNAs into them induces autophagy (Table 2) [48,49]. It has also been found that HCV's non-structural protein 4B, NS4B, when expressed alone in cells induces autophagy (Table 3) [39]. Multiple studies indicate that the inhibition of this induced autophagy inhibits HCV infection. The inhibition of Beclin 1 and ATG4B with siRNAs in infected Huh7 cells decreases the levels of synthesized viral RNA by 100-fold [48]. Beclin 1 is a major regulator of autophagy and ATG4B cleaves pro-LC3, generating the cytosolic LC3-I protein prior to its conjugation to PE [1,13]. NS5B has been found to bind ATG5 in yeast two-hybrid assays; inhibition of ATG5 with siRNAs in infected Huh7 cells inhibits viral RNA synthesis 10-fold (Table 3) [50]. ATG5 forms a complex with ATG12 and then with ATG16L, which together determine where in phagophores LC3 is conjugated to PE [4,51]. ATG5 interacts with immunity related GTPase M (IRGM) and the inhibition of IRGM with siRNA inhibits HCV infection, too [14].

The mechanism by which inhibiting autophagy inhibits HCV infection is being elucidated in order to understand what this virus gains by its inducing autophagy. Inhibiting the induction of autophagy prior to infection inhibits viral RNA synthesis, but it does not do so after HCV replication has been initiated [48]. This timing of the importance of autophagy in the HCV life-cycle is consistent with observations indicating that autophagy inhibits an innate immune response to HCV early in the viral life-cycle [49]. These authors found that the inhibition of ATG5 (or of participants in the UPR which foster autophagy) with siRNAs enhanced both transcription of the interferon beta (IFNβ) promoter and of downstream response elements, such as interferon-stimulated gene 56 (ISG56). Their findings are consistent with HCV-induced autophagy limiting the innate immune response of retinoic acid inducible gene I protein (RIG-I) recognizing sequences in HCV's RNA genome [41]. This inhibition would be required by the virus only early during the course of infection because later in infection a viral protease, NS3/4A, cleaves the cellular protein, mitochondrial antiviral signaling protein (MAVS), which is required downstream of RIG-I to induce IFNα and β [52]. It now appears that HCV induces autophagy to block an interferon response and allow the early stages of its infection. HCV uses an independent mechanism to block this innate immune response later in its life-cycle. Inhibiting autophagy late in HCV's life-cycle when it has established a persistent infection is detrimental to the virus because it induces death [53]. It therefore appears that even in persistently infected cells, HCV's induction of autophagy is advantageous to the virus.

5. Hepatitis B Virus

Three hundred and fifty million people worldwide are infected with Hepatitis B Virus (HBV) despite the availability of a vaccine that prevents infection. HBV causes a large fraction of cases of HCC, as does HCV. HBV is a member of the Hepadnavirus family and its linear, partially double-stranded DNA molecule of 3.2 kb is found in a protein core, which itself is enveloped [54]. The DNA is transcribed into a 3.4 kb pregenomic mRNA during infection, which is encapsidated by the viral core protein and serves as a template for reverse transcription [54]. This large mRNA, as well as smaller ones with the same poly-adenylation site, encodes three envelope surface proteins, a core protein, reverse transcriptase, and the X protein (HBx) [54]. The surface proteins have an identical, four-spanning transmembrane domain and the small surface protein, HBs can self-oligomerize.

Two groups have found that HBV induces autophagy in cells transfected *in vitro* and in mice transgenic for HBV (Table 2) [55–57]. Their combined data support this induction by HBV persuasively [55–57]. For example, transfection of cells derived from human liver tumors with HBV DNA induces increased levels of PE-conjugated LC3 [55] and the formation of autophagosomes [57]. These combined studies also show that autophagy fosters HBV's life-cycle. Inhibiting autophagy with siRNAs to ATG7 inhibits formation of the products of HBV's reverse transcription [55] and siRNAs to Beclin 1 inhibit the appearance of viral DNA in extracellular medium [57]. These findings are also supported by an analysis in mice engineered to be null for ATG5 in their livers [51]. The null mice when transgenic for HBV have greatly reduced levels of viral DNA in their sera when compared to their ATG5-positive counterparts [56]. These studies support the ability of HBV to induce autophagy and for the viral life-cycle to be fostered by autophagy. Where they differ is in their notions of the mechanisms of induction and the benefits that subsequently accrue to HBV. One set of experiments indicates that the viral HBx gene is essential for the induction of autophagy (Table 2) [55]; the other indicates that the HBs gene is sufficient for this induction (Table 2) [57]. One finds that the inhibition of autophagy inhibits reverse transcription within the viral core [55]; the other that the inhibition of autophagy inhibits viral envelopment [57]. These varied findings cannot be straightforwardly reconciled. It is apparent that expression of HBs in cells does induce the UPR and that the UPR leads to autophagy in these cells [57]. Inhibiting key mediators of the UPR such as PERK or ATF6 with siRNAs does block autophagy in cells transfected with HBs, for example [51]. Perhaps some of the differences noted in the studies reflect differences in the authors' emphasis more than in their science. HBV likely induces and benefits from autophagy; the specifics of how it does so need elaboration.

6. Discussion

Some viruses that interact with the autophagic machinery repress it, thus ensuring their success in infected cells. The four human tumor viruses reviewed here all use—and even stimulate—autophagy for their own benefits (Figure 1). Each virus encodes one or more proteins that regulate the autophagic machinery either directly or indirectly.

Figure 1. Autophagy is initiated by stimuli that activate the phosphatidylinositol 3-phosphate kinase, Vps34. Vps34 generates phosphatidylinositol 3-phosphate, a substrate for the forming autophagosome, and its enzymatic activity is dependent on Beclin 1. For its localization in the phagophore, the unclosed double-membrane precursor to the autophagosome, the light chain 3 (LC3) is conjugated to phosphatidylethanolamine (PE) via an ubiquitin-like conjugation pathway. LC3 is cleaved from its inactive precursor form by ATG4B to render it cytosolic, and subsequently conjugated to PE via its binding the E2-like ligase, autophagy related 3 homolog (ATG3), and its transfer to the E3-like ATG16L complex (ATG16L, ATG5, and ATG12). Autophagy can be stimulated via the Unfolded Protein Response (UPR) via the phosphorylation and activation of protein kinase RNA-like endoplasmic reticulum kinase (PERK). Active PERK phosphorylates the eukaryotic initiation factor 2 alpha (eIF2α). Phospho-eIF2α cannot translate capped mRNAs, but can translate mRNAs with internal ribosome entry sites (IRES), such as activated transcription factor 4 (ATF4). ATF4 activates the transcription of LC3 and Beclin 1 to induce autophagy. Human tumor viruses can regulate autophagy at several steps of the pathway. Both latent membrane protein 1 (LMP1) and the small surface protein of HBV (HBs) stimulate the UPR and induce autophagy. LMP1's induction of autophagy regulates its degradation in autophagolysosomes. The Epstein-Barr nuclear antigen 1 (EBNA1) also can localize to autophagosomes and is degraded in autophagolysosomes, where epitopes of EBNA1 are generated for their presentation on MHC class II molecules. Autophagy fosters HBV's productive infection. In addition to HBs, the Hepatitis B X protein (HBx) can stimulate autophagy via its interaction with Vps34. Autophagy can support HBV's envelopment or reverse transcription. The non-structural proteins of HCV, NS4B and NS5B induce autophagy; the former appears to interact with Vps34, while the latter promotes LC3's conjugation to PE by binding ATG5. Autophagy inhibits the cellular interferon response during the early stages of HCV's infection. In contrast to NS5B, the KSHV viral FADD-like interleukin-1 beta-converting enzyme inhibitory protein (v-FLIP) inhibits LC3's lipid-conjugation by competing with it for ATG3. v-FLIP inhibits autophagy-induced apoptosis and senescence of KSHV-positive cells. Autophagy is induced by replication and transactivator (RTA) to support KSHV's replication, and v-FLIP may inhibit the productive life-cycle of the virus by repressing autophagy.

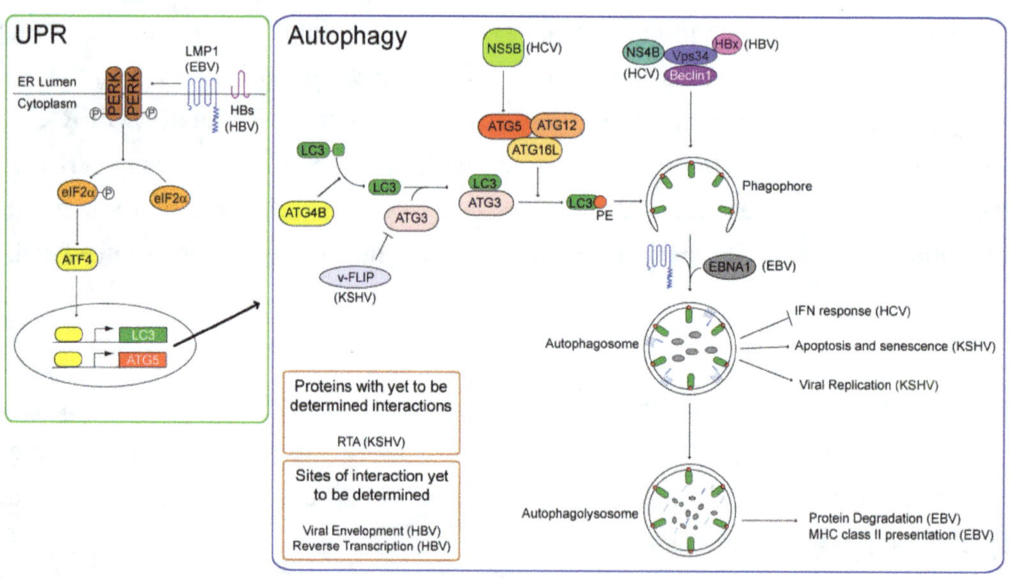

All four human tumor viruses induce autophagy, and KSHV also inhibits it. Two of these viruses, HBV and EBV, encode transmembrane proteins—HBs and LMP1, respectively—that localize to the endoplasmic reticulum and induce autophagy via the UPR [35,57]. In its induction of autophagy in EBV-positive B-cells, the viral protein LMP1 autocatalyzes its degradation, thereby likely avoiding immune detection and relieving the cytostasis it causes [34]. How LMP1 and HBs activate the UPR is not known. It is possible that their complex membrane structures are easily misfolded. It is also possible that via their self-oligomerization they are recognized as protein aggregates that require degradation. Evidence consistent with the latter idea comes from models of Parkinson's disease [58].

Whereas LMP1's induction of autophagy may contribute to EBV's avoidance of immune detection, the EBNA1 protein encoded by EBV can be presented on MHC class II molecules in part by autophagy [6,23]. HCV also uses autophagy to avoid immune detection. During the early stages of infection, NS5B of HCV interacts with ATG5 and stimulates the conjugation of LC3 to PE [50]. Autophagy inhibits the IFN response stimulated by RIG-I when liver cells are infected with HCV [49,53]. Though autophagy's inhibition of innate immunity is required only for early infection, autophagy appears also to inhibit cellular death during the late stages of HCV's infection.

Autophagy fosters the productive life-cycles of KSHV, HBV, and HCV; more virions are produced when autophagy is induced by viral proteins [40,48,55–57,59]. KSHV can also inhibit autophagy. Its v-FLIP, which is expressed during viral latency, competes with LC3 for binding to ATG3, thereby inhibiting LC3's lipid-conjugation [44]. In doing so, v-FLIP inhibits cellular death of KSHV-infected PEL cells and HFFs [44]. KSHV's v-Bcl2 can also inhibit autophagy by binding Beclin1 but the role this inhibition plays in the viral life-cycle is now unknown.

Given its role in the life-cycle of HCV, HBV, KSHV, and EBV, autophagy could be a potential target for anti-viral or tumor therapy. For example, suppressing autophagy would block the production of HBV and HCV virions; it could cause cellular death in EBV- and HCV-positive cells. In contrast, cellular death of KSHV-positive PELs and Kaposi's Sarcomas could occur when autophagy is induced. Elucidating the roles of autophagy in the life-cycles of human tumor viruses may lead to the identification of targets for new treatments of the many cancers these viruses cause.

Acknowledgements

This work was supported by grants from the United States National Institutes of Health (NIH, CA70723, CA133027, and CA22443) awarded to B.S. B.S. is an American Cancer Society Research Professor.

References

1. Kroemer, G.; Marino, G.; Levine, B. Autophagy and the integrated stress response. *Mol. Cell* **2010**, *40*, 280–293.
2. He, C.; Klionsky, D.J. Regulation mechanisms and signaling pathways of autophagy. *Annu. Rev. Genet.* **2009**, *43*, 67–93.
3. He, C.; Bassik, M.C.; Moresi, V.; Sun, K.; Wei, Y.; Zou, Z.; An, Z.; Loh, J.; Fisher, J.; Sun, Q.;

et al. Exercise-induced BCL2-regulated autophagy is required for muscle glucose homeostasis. *Nature* **2012**, *481*, 511–515.

4. Yang, Z.; Klionsky, D.J. Mammalian autophagy: Core molecular machinery and signaling regulation. *Curr. Opin. Cell Biol.* **2010**, *22*, 124–131.
5. Long, H.M.; Haigh, T.A.; Gudgeon, N.H.; Leen, A.M.; Tsang, C.W.; Brooks, J.; Landais, E.; Houssaint, E.; Lee, S.P.; Rickinson, A.B.; *et al.* CD4+ T-Cell responses to Epstein-Barr Virus (EBV) latent-cycle antigens and the recognition of EBV-transformed lymphoblastoid cell lines. *J. Virol.* **2005**, *79*, 4896–4907.
6. Leung, C.S.; Haigh, T.A.; Mackay, L.K.; Rickinson, A.B.; Taylor, G.S. Nuclear location of an endogenously expressed antigen, EBNA1, restricts access to macroautophagy and the range of CD4 Epitope display. *Proc. Natl. Acad. Sci. USA* **2010**, *107*, 2165–2170.
7. Dirmeier, U.; Hoffmann, R.; Kilger, E.; Schultheiss, U.; Briseno, C.; Gires, O.; Kieser, A.; Eick, D.; Sugden, B.; Hammerschmidt, W. Latent Membrane Protein 1 of Epstein-Barr Virus coordinately regulates proliferation with control of apoptosis. *Oncogene* **2005**, *24*, 1711–1717.
8. Lee, J.; Sugden, B. A membrane leucine heptad contributes to trafficking, signaling, and transformation by Latent Membrane Protein 1. *J. Virol.* **2007**, *81*, 9121–9130.
9. Kaykas, A.; Sugden, B. The amino-terminus and membrane-spanning domains of LMP-1 inhibit cell proliferation. *Oncogene* **2000**, *19*, 1400–1410.
10. Lee, D.Y.; Lee, J.; Sugden, B. The unfolded protein response and autophagy: Herpesviruses rule! *J. Virol.* **2009**, *83*, 1168–1172.
11. Young, A.R.; Narita, M.; Ferreira, M.; Kirschner, K.; Sadaie, M.; Darot, J.F.; Tavare, S.; Arakawa, S.; Shimizu, S.; Watt, F.M.; *et al.* Autophagy mediates the mitotic senescence transition. *Genes Dev.* **2009**, *23*, 798–803.
12. Sinha, S.; Colbert, C.L.; Becker, N.; Wei, Y.; Levine, B. Molecular basis of the regulation of Beclin 1-Dependent autophagy by the Gamma-Herpesvirus 68 Bcl-2 homolog M11. *Autophagy* **2008**, *4*, 989–997.
13. Kabeya, Y.; Mizushima, N.; Yamamoto, A.; Oshitani-Okamoto, S.; Ohsumi, Y.; Yoshimori, T. LC3, GABARAP and GATE16 localize to autophagosomal membrane depending on form-II formation. *J. Cell Sci.* **2004**, *117*, 2805–2812.
14. Gregoire, I.P.; Richetta, C.; Meyniel-Schicklin, L.; Borel, S.; Pradezynski, F.; Diaz, O.; Deloire, A.; Azocar, O.; Baguet, J.; Le Breton, M.; *et al.* IRGM is a common target of RNA viruses that subvert the autophagy network. *PLoS Pathog.* **2011**, *7*, e1002422.
15. Dar, W.A.; Sugden, B. Epstein-Barr Virus as a Pathogen. In *Viral Oncology: Basic Science and Clinical Applications*; Khalili, K., Jeang, K.T., Eds.; John Wiley & Sons, Inc.: Hoboken, NJ, USA, 2010; pp. 425–451.
16. Babcock, G.J.; Decker, L.L.; Volk, M.; Thorley-Lawson, D.A. EBV persistence in memory B cells *in vivo*. *Immunity* **1998**, *9*, 395–404.
17. Nanbo, A.; Sugden, A.; Sugden, B. The Coupling of Synthesis and partitioning of EBV's plasmid replicon is revealed in live cells. *EMBO J.* **2007**, *26*, 4252–4262.
18. Vereide, D.; Sugden, B. Proof for EBV's sustaining role in Burkitt's lymphomas. *Semin. Cancer Biol.* **2009** *19*, 389–393.

19. Vereide, D.; Sugden, B. Lymphomas depend on EBV in proportion to their expression of viral genes. *Blood* **2011**, *117*, 1977–1985.
20. Levitskaya, J.; Coram, M.; Levitsky, V.; Imreh, S.; Steigerwald-Mullen, P.M.; Klein, G.; Kurilla, M.G.; Masucci, M.G. Inhibition of antigen processing by the internal repeat region of the Epstein-Barr Virus nuclear Antigen-1. *Nature* **1995**, *375*, 685–688.
21. Leen, A.; Meij, P.; Redchenko, I.; Middeldorp, J.; Bloemena, E.; Rickinson, A.; Blake, N. Differential immunogenicity of Epstein-Barr Virus latent-cycle proteins for human CD4(+) T-Helper 1 responses. *J. Virol.* **2001**, *75*, 8649–8659.
22. Munz, C.; Bickham, K.L.; Subklewe, M.; Tsang, M.L.; Chahroudi, A.; Kurilla, M.G.; Zhang, D.; O'Donnell, M.; Steinman, R.M. Human CD4(+) T lymphocytes consistently respond to the latent Epstein-Barr Virus nuclear Antigen EBNA1. *J. Exp. Med.* **2000**, *191*, 1649–1660.
23. Paludan, C.; Schmid, D.; Landthaler, M.; Vockerodt, M.; Kube, D.; Tuschl, T.; Munz, C. Endogenous MHC class II processing of a viral nuclear antigen after autophagy. *Science* **2005**, *307*, 593–596.
24. Nimmerjahn, F.; Milosevic, S.; Behrends, U.; Jaffee, E.M.; Pardoll, D.M.; Bornkamm, G.W.; Mautner, J. Major histocompatibility complex class II-restricted presentation of a cytosolic antigen by autophagy. *Eur. J. Immunol.* **2003**, *33*, 1250–1259.
25. Mautner, J.; Pich, D.; Nimmerjahn, F.; Milosevic, S.; Adhikary, D.; Christoph, H.; Witter, K.; Bornkamm, G.W.; Hammerschmidt, W.; Behrends, U. Epstein-Barr Virus nuclear Antigen 1 evades direct immune recognition by CD4+ T helper cells. *Eur. J. Immunol.* **2004**, *34*, 2500–2509.
26. Paludan, C.; Bickham, K.; Nikiforow, S.; Tsang, M.L.; Goodman, K.; Hanekom, W.A.; Fonteneau, J.F.; Stevanovic, S.; Munz, C. Epstein-Barr nuclear Antigen 1-Specific CD4(+) Th1 cells kill Burkitt's lymphoma cells. *J. Immunol.* **2002**, *169*, 1593–1603.
27. Altmann, M.; Hammerschmidt, W. Epstein-Barr Virus provides a new paradigm: A requirement for the immediate inhibition of apoptosis. *PLoS Biol.* **2005**, *3*, e404.
28. Kelly, G.L.; Long, H.M.; Stylianou, J.; Thomas, W.A.; Leese, A.; Bell, A.I.; Bornkamm, G.W.; Mautner, J.; Rickinson, A.B.; Rowe, M. An Epstein-Barr Virus anti-apoptotic protein constitutively expressed in transformed cells and implicated in burkitt lymphomagenesis: The Wp/BHRF1 link. *PLoS Pathog.* **2009**, *5*, e1000341.
29. Pattingre, S.; Tassa, A.; Qu, X.; Garuti, R.; Liang, X.H.; Mizushima, N.; Packer, M.; Schneider, M.D.; Levine, B. Bcl-2 antiapoptotic proteins inhibit beclin 1-Dependent autophagy. *Cell* **2005**, *122*, 927–939.
30. Graham, J.P.; Arcipowski, K.M.; Bishop, G.A. Differential B-Lymphocyte regulation by CD40 and its viral mimic, Latent Membrane Protein 1. *Immunol. Rev.* **2010**, *237*, 226–248.
31. Zimber-Strobl, U.; Kempkes, B.; Marschall, G.; Zeidler, R.; van Kooten, C.; Banchereau, J.; Bornkamm, G.W.; Hammerschmidt, W. Epstein-Barr Virus Latent Membrane Protein (LMP1) is not sufficient to maintain proliferation of B cells but both it and activated CD40 can prolong their survival. *EMBO J.* **1996**, *15*, 7070–7078.
32. Rastelli, J.; Homig-Holzel, C.; Seagal, J.; Muller, W.; Hermann, A.C.; Rajewsky, K.; Zimber-Strobl, U. LMP1 signaling can replace CD40 signaling in B cells *in vivo* and has unique features of inducing class-switch recombination to IgG1. *Blood* **2008**, *111*, 1448–1455.

33. Sammond, D.W.; Joce, C.; Takeshita, R.; McQuate, S.E.; Ghosh, N.; Martin, J.M.; Yin, H. Transmembrane peptides used to investigate the homo-oligomeric interface and binding hotspot of Latent Membrane Protein 1. *Biopolymers* **2011**, *95*, 772–784.
34. Lee, D.Y.; Sugden, B. The Latent Membrane Protein 1 oncogene modifies B-Cell physiology by regulating autophagy. *Oncogene* **2008**, *27*, 2833–2842.
35. Lee, D.Y.; Sugden, B. The LMP1 oncogene of EBV activates PERK and the unfolded protein response to drive its own synthesis. *Blood* **2008**, *111*, 2280–2289.
36. Lam, N.; Sandberg, M.L.; Sugden, B. High physiological levels of LMP1 result in phosphorylation of eIF2 Alpha in Epstein-Barr Virus-infected cells. *J. Virol.* **2004**, *78*, 1657–1664.
37. Liang, C.Y.; E, X.F.; Jung, J.U. Downregulation of autophagy by herpesvirus Bcl-2 homologs. *Autophagy* **2008**, *4*, 268–272.
38. Sun, R.; Lin, S.F.; Gradoville, L.; Yuan, Y.; Zhu, F.; Miller, G. A viral gene that activates lytic cycle expression of Kaposi's Sarcoma-associated herpesvirus. *Proc. Natl. Acad. Sci. USA* **1998**, *95*, 10866–10871.
39. Su, W.C.; Chao, T.C.; Huang, Y.L.; Weng, S.C.; Jeng, K.S.; Lai, M.M. Rab5 and class III phosphoinositide 3-Kinase Vps34 are involved in Hepatitis C Virus NS4B-induced autophagy. *J. Virol.* **2011**, *85*, 10561–10571.
40. Wen, H.J.; Yang, Z.; Zhou, Y.; Wood, C. Enhancement of autophagy during lytic replication by the Kaposi's Sarcoma-associated herpesvirus replication and transcription activator. *J. Virol.* **2010**, *84*, 7448–7458.
41. Saito, T.; Owen, D.M.; Jiang, F.; Marcotrigiano, J.; Gale, M., Jr. Innate immunity induced by composition-dependent RIG-I recognition of Hepatitis C Virus RNA. *Nature* **2008**, *454*, 523–527.
42. Rouschop, K.M.; van den Beucken, T.; Dubois, L.; Niessen, H.; Bussink, J.; Savelkouls, K.; Keulers, T.; Mujcic, H.; Landuyt, W.; Voncken, J.W.; *et al.* The unfolded protein response protects human tumor cells during hypoxia through regulation of the autophagy genes MAP1LC3B and ATG5. *J. Clin. Invest.* **2010**, *120*, 127–141.
43. Martin, J.N. The Epidemiology of KSHV and its Association with Malignant Disease. In *Human Herpesviruses: Biology, Therapy, and Immunoprophylaxis*; Arvin, A., Campadelli-Fiume, G., Mocarski, E., Moore, P.S., Roizman, B., Whitley, R., Yamanishi, K., Eds.: Cambridge University Press: Cambridge, UK, 2007.
44. Lee, J.S.; Li, Q.; Lee, J.Y.; Lee, S.H.; Jeong, J.H.; Lee, H.R.; Chang, H.; Zhou, F.C.; Gao, S.J.; Liang, C.; *et al.* FLIP-mediated autophagy regulation in cell death control. *Nat. Cell Biol.* **2009**, *11*, 1355–1362.
45. Leidal, A.M.; Cyr, D.P.; Hill, R.J.; Lee, P.W.; McCormick, C. Subversion of autophagy by kaposi's sarcoma-associated herpesvirus impairs oncogene-induced senescence. *Cell. Host Microbe* **2012**, *11*, 167–180.
46. Chang, N.C.; Nguyen, M.; Germain, M.; Shore, G.C. Antagonism of Beclin 1-dependent autophagy by BCL-2 at the endoplasmic reticulum requires NAF-1. *EMBO J.* **2010**, *29*, 606–618.
47. Guito, J.; Lukac, D.M. KSHV Rta promoter specification and viral reactivation. *Front. Microbiol.* **2012**, *3*, 30.
48. Dreux, M.; Gastaminza, P.; Wieland, S.F.; Chisari, F.V. The autophagy machinery is required to

initiate Hepatitis C virus replication. *Proc. Natl. Acad. Sci. USA* **2009**, *106*, 14046–14051.

49. Ke, P.Y.; Chen, S.S. Activation of the unfolded protein response and autophagy after Hepatitis C virus infection suppresses innate antiviral immunity *in vitro*. *J. Clin. Invest.* **2011**, *121*, 37–56.
50. Guevin, C.; Manna, D.; Belanger, C.; Konan, K.V.; Mak, P.; Labonte, P. Autophagy protein ATG5 interacts transiently with the Hepatitis C Virus RNA Polymerase (NS5B) early during infection. *Virology* **2010**, *405*, 1–7.
51. Fujita, N.; Itoh, T.; Omori, H.; Fukuda, M.; Noda, T.; Yoshimori, T. The Atg16L complex specifies the site of LC3 lipidation for membrane biogenesis in autophagy. *Mol. Biol. Cell* **2008**, *19*, 2092–2100.
52. Li, X.D.; Chiu, Y.H.; Ismail, A.S.; Behrendt, C.L.; Wight-Carter, M.; Hooper, L.V.; Chen, Z.J. Mitochondrial antiviral signaling protein (MAVS) monitors commensal bacteria and induces an immune response that prevents experimental colitis. *Proc. Natl. Acad. Sci. USA* **2011**, *108*, 17390–17395.
53. Taguwa, S.; Kambara, H.; Fujita, N.; Noda, T.; Yoshimori, T.; Koike, K.; Moriishi, K.; Matsuura, Y. Dysfunction of autophagy participates in vacuole formation and cell death in cells replicating Hepatitis C Virus. *J. Virol.* **2011**, *85*, 13185–13194.
54. Schadler, S.; Hildt, E. HBV life cycle: Entry and morphogenesis. *Viruses* **2009**, *1*, 185–209.
55. Sir, D.; Tian, Y.; Chen, W.L.; Ann, D.K.; Yen, T.S.; Ou, J.H. The early autophagic pathway is activated by Hepatitis B Virus and required for viral DNA replication. *Proc. Natl. Acad. Sci. USA* **2010**, *107*, 4383–4388.
56. Tian, Y.; Sir, D.; Kuo, C.F.; Ann, D.K.; Ou, J.H. Autophagy required for Hepatitis B Virus replication in transgenic mice. *J. Virol.* **2011**, *85*, 13453–13456.
57. Li, J.; Liu, Y.; Wang, Z.; Liu, K.; Wang, Y.; Liu, J.; Ding, H.; Yuan, Z. Subversion of cellular autophagy machinery by Hepatitis B Virus for viral envelopment. *J. Virol.* **2011**, *85*, 6319–6333.
58. Doyle, K.M.; Kennedy, D.; Gorman, A.M.; Gupta, S.; Healy, S.J.; Samali, A. Unfolded proteins and endoplasmic reticulum stress in neurodegenerative disorders. *J. Cell. Mol. Med.* **2011**, *15*, 2025–2039.
59. Dreux, M.; Chisari, F.V. Impact of the autophagy machinery on Hepatitis C Virus infection. *Viruses* **2011**, *3*, 1342–1357.

3

Human Papillomaviruses: Epithelial Tropisms and the Development of Neoplasia

Nagayasu Egawa [1,2], Kiyofumi Egawa [3,4], Heather Griffin [1,2] and John Doorbar [1,2,*]

[1] Division of Virology, Department of Pathology, University of Cambridge, Tennis Court Road, Cambridge CB2 1QP, UK; E-Mails: ne259@cam.ac.uk (N.E.); hmg36@cam.ac.uk (H.G.)

[2] The Francis Crick Institute Mill Hill Laboratory, the Ridgeway, Mill Hill, London NW7 1AA, UK

[3] Department of Dermatology, The Jikei University School of Medicine, 3-25-8 Nishi-shinbashi, Minato-ku, Tokyo 105-0003, Japan; E-Mail: amamino.kuroibo@gmail.com

[4] Department of Microbiology, Kitasato University School of Allied Health and Sciences, 1-15-1 Kitasato, Sagamihara, Kanagawa 252-0373, Japan

* Author to whom correspondence should be addressed; E-Mail: jd121@cam.ac.uk;

Academic Editor: Joanna Parish

Abstract: Papillomaviruses have evolved over many millions of years to propagate themselves at specific epithelial niches in a range of different host species. This has led to the great diversity of papillomaviruses that now exist, and to the appearance of distinct strategies for epithelial persistence. Many papillomaviruses minimise the risk of immune clearance by causing chronic asymptomatic infections, accompanied by long-term virion-production with only limited viral gene expression. Such lesions are typical of those caused by Beta HPV types in the general population, with viral activity being suppressed by host immunity. A second strategy requires the evolution of sophisticated immune evasion mechanisms, and allows some HPV types to cause prominent and persistent papillomas, even in immune competent individuals. Some Alphapapillomavirus types have evolved this strategy, including those that cause genital warts in young adults or common warts in children. These strategies reflect broad differences in virus protein function as well as differences in patterns of viral gene expression, with genotype-specific associations underlying the recent introduction of DNA testing, and also the introduction of vaccines to protect against cervical cancer. Interestingly, it appears that cellular environment and the site of infection affect viral pathogenicity by modulating viral gene expression. With the high-risk HPV gene products, changes in E6 and E7 expression are thought to account for the development of neoplasias at the endocervix, the anal and cervical transformation zones, and the tonsilar crypts and other oropharyngeal sites. A detailed analysis of site-specific patterns of gene expression and gene function is now prompted.

Keywords: human papillomavirus; tropism; diversity; evolution; tissue stem cells; niche; carcinogenesis

---

1. Introduction

Papillomaviruses have been discovered in a wide array of vertebrates. More than 300 papillomaviruses have been identified and completely sequenced, including over 200 human papillomaviruses (PaVE: Papillomavirus Episteme [1]). One of the most distinctive characteristics of the papillomavirus group is their genotype-specific host-restriction, and the preference of particular papillomavirus types for distinct anatomical sites, where they cause lesions with distinctive clinical pathologies [2]. These include benign hyper-proliferative lesions such as warts, as well as unapparent or asymptomatic precursor lesions, that can in some instances progress to high-grade neoplasia and invasive malignant cancer. The association of "high-risk" human papillomavirus (HPV) types (see legend to Figure 1) with cervical cancer is now well established, and provides a rationale for the introduction of HPV DNA testing in cervical screening, as well as the development of prophylactic vaccines against HPV16 and 18 which are the major papillomavirus types responsible for cervical cancer. Such typing studies have also revealed a plethora of HPV types, both high and low-risk, in oral mouthwash samples despite the absence of apparent clinical disease [3], as well as in skin swabs and plucked hairs taken from immunocompetent individuals [4–9]. The predominant asymptomatic skin HPV types come primarily from the genera Betapapillomavirus and Gammapapillomavirus, and at a population level, members of these genera are very successful, infecting children at a young age to produce persistent subclinical infections [4]. Changes in the epithelial micro-environment, as can occur following immunosuppression or in individuals suffering from epidermodysplasia verruciformis (EV), can allow these HPV types to produce visible papillomas, and in some situations can facilitate the development of cancers [10]. Certain Beta HPV types are a significant cause of non-Melanoma skin cancer in susceptible individuals, although the molecular mechanism by which they facilitate cancer progression appears to be somewhat different from what has been worked out for the Alphapapillomavirus types [11]. When considered together, it appears that different papillomavirus types have evolved distinct life-cycle strategies, which allow them to thrive and produce viral progeny at different epithelial sites. At least part of this variation reflects the different ability of papillomaviruses to interact with the immune system, and to produce productive infections that are visible at the macroscopic level. The complex immune evasion strategies that underlie the ability to produce such lesions are a particular characteristic of the Genus Alphapapillomavirus, with low-risk Alphapapillomavirus types in particular (Figure 1), often being responsible for recalcitrant warts even in immunocompetent hosts [12]. By contrast, most members of the genera β- and Gammapapillomavirus only cause such visible lesions when the normal immune response of the host is compromised [13–16]. The clinical importance of papillomaviruses, and their relatively small genomic size, has led to many full genomic sequences becoming available in recent years. The availability of such extensive sequence information, combined with a developing clinical and biochemical understanding of disease-biology, means that papillomaviruses are an ideal model system to understand how evolution can influence viral tropisms, pathogenicity, and the underlying molecular processes that govern disease outcome [17–20]. As discussed below, this "natural experiment" in infection is also providing us with insight into epithelial cell biology and immunology.

2. Papillomavirus Diversity at the Level of Genotype, Epithelial Tropism and Pathogenicity

Papillomaviruses comprise a diverse group of viruses that infect both humans and animals. Their origin is linked to changes in the epithelium of their ancestral host that occurred at least 350 million years ago. Since then, they have co-evolved as their different host species have evolved, with little cross-transfer between species [17,18]. They are now found in birds, reptiles, marsupials and other mammals, pointing to an earlier evolutionary appearance than was initially suspected. Recent phylogenetic analysis suggests, however, that the "generalist" ancestral papillomavirus may not have followed an identical evolutionary path to that of their hosts, but paralleled the evolution of host resources or attributes, such as the presence or absence of fur or the evolution of sweat glands. These host-adaptations are thought to have created new ecological niches for papillomavirus to colonise, which in turn drove viral diversity followed by co-speciation with their hosts [17]. Through this route, papillomaviruses have developed their remarkable species specificity as well as a great diversity of epithelial tropisms. With over 240 distinct papillomavirus types classified into 37 genera, papillomavirus may perhaps be considered as one of the most successful families of vertebrate viruses [17,21,22].

The classification of papillomaviruses is based on nucleotide sequence comparison rather than on serology, with individual HPVs being referred to as genotypes [22]. Data from vaccine trials has shown that there is limited antibody cross-reactivity, except between closely related genotypes [23], with the major coat protein of the virus (L1) containing hypervariable loops that are exposed on the virion surface [24,25]. The L1 gene was chosen early on as the standard for PV classification, and for some papillomavirus types, there is little sequence information outside of this region. To be classified as distinct types, individual papillomaviruses must be at least 10% divergent from each other in their L1 nucleotide sequence. These papillomavirus "types" are grouped into larger phylogenetic groupings or genera, which are categorised with a Greek letter followed by a number that indicates the species (Figure 1) [22].

Thus the species Alphapapillomavirus 9 includes HPV types 16, 31, 35, 33, 52, 58 and 67. Ideally, papillomavirus (PV) classification should integrate phylogeny, genome organization, biology and pathogenicity as a single property, rather than being based simply on genomic sequence analysis, or the analysis of genomic fragments [21]. This phylogenetic species concept, although potentially useful, is complex to implement, however, and for many papillomavirus types, detailed information regarding their biology is only poorly defined.

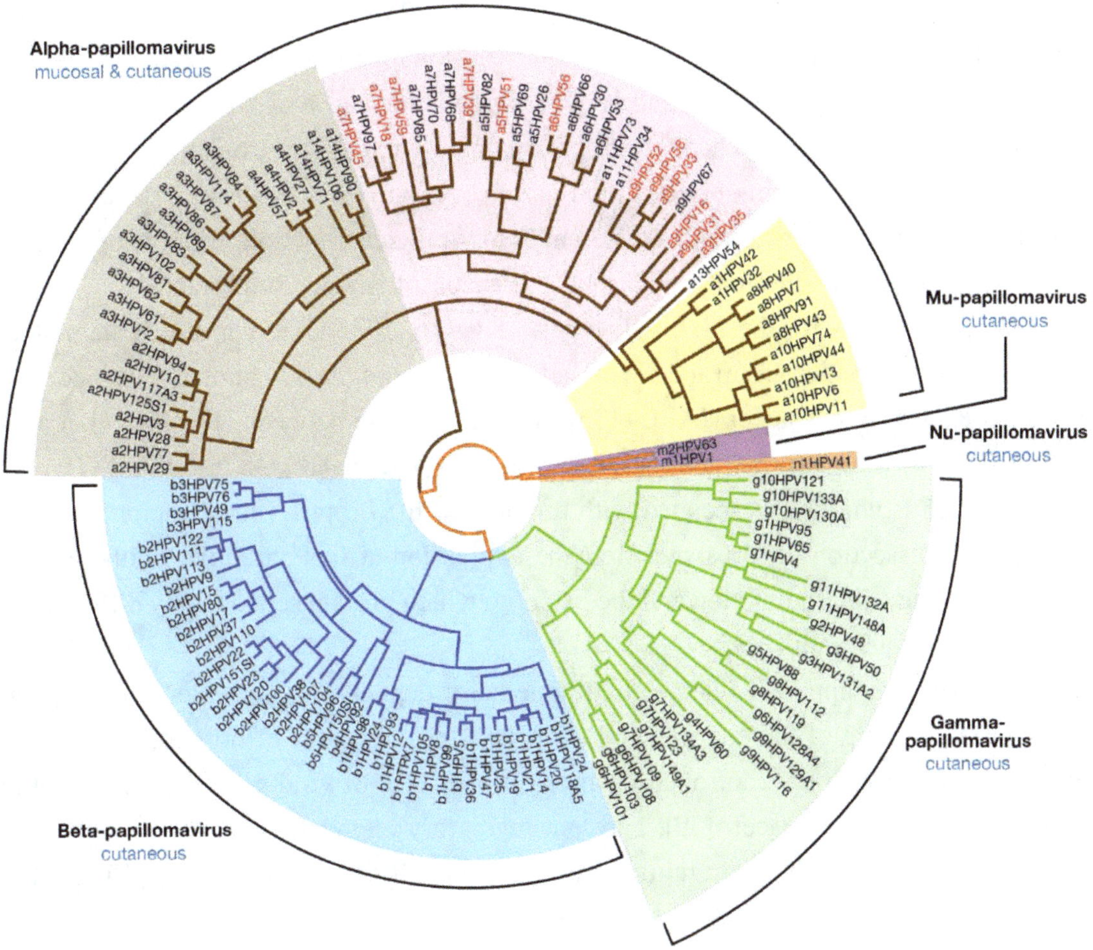

Figure 1. Evolutionary Relationship between Human Papillomaviruses. The human papillomaviruses types found in humans fall into five genera, with the Alpha-, Beta- (**blue**) and Gammapapillomavirus (**green**) representing the largest groups; Human papillomaviruses types from the Alphapapillomavirus genus are often classified as low-risk cutaneous (**light brown**); low-risk mucosal (**yellow**); or high-risk (**pink**) according to their association with the development of cancer. The high-risk types highlighted with red text are confirmed as "human carcinogens" on the basis of epidemiological data. The remaining high-risk types are "probable" or "possible" carcinogens. Although the predominant tissue associations of each genus are listed as either cutaneous or mucosal, these designations do not necessarily hold true for every member of the genus. The evolutionary tree is based on alignment of the *E1*, *E2*, *L1*, and *L2* genes [26]. HPV sequence data was be obtained from PaVE [1].

In general, sequence-based phylogeny does provide some useful insight into disease association, although closely related types can in some instances show distinct pathologies. HPV4, 65 and 95 are encompassed in the Gammapapillomavirus 1 species, for instance, but while HPV4 and 65 induce indistinguishable pigmented wart-like lesions mainly on the palmoplantar or lateral surface of hands and feet [27–29], HPV95 induces less obvious unpigmented papules primarily on plantar epithelial surfaces [30]. HPV6 and 11 are similarly contained within a common species-grouping (Alphapapillomavirus 10), and although both cause papillomas of similar appearance, HPV6 shows a marked predilection for genital sites, when compared to HPV11, which is the most prominent type at oral sites [31–34]. A third example comes from the Alphapapillomavirus 8 species which includes HPV40, which causes mucosal lesions, and HPV7, which is the cause of "butchers" warts that develop at cutaneous sites, particularly the hands [35]. Explaining such subtle tropism differences is beyond our current understanding of virus biology, and is not of obvious medical importance. It is however likely that such tropism differences reflect differences in viral gene function, patterns of gene expression and epithelial regulation at different body sites. Perhaps of greater importance are the differences in cancer risk associated with the high-risk types. HPV16, 31 and 35 are all contained within the Alphapapillomavirus 9 species group and are classified as "carcinogenic to humans" by The International Agency for the Research on Cancer (IARC) [36]. The association between HPV16 and cervical cancer is more than 10 times stronger than that between either HPV31 or HPV35 however [37], and of these three types, HPV16 is uniquely associated with tumours of the oropharyngeal region [38]. To explain this will require a dissection of virus-specific gene expression at this particular epithelial site, and an understanding of virus protein function and the extent to which proteins encoded by different HPV types affect common molecular pathways.

From the above, it is apparent that viral pathogenicity depends on multiple factors, including the virus genotype, the nature of the cell infected (tropism) and the status of host immunity. Our current thinking suggest that tropism is controlled primarily at the level of viral gene expression rather than at the level of viral entry into the cell [39], and that regulatory elements within the long control region (LCR) are of key importance in determining the tissue range of different HPV types [40,41]. Differences in infectivity may however be a contributing factor, and it has been suggested that this may correlate with differences in surface charge distribution between cutaneous and mucosal virions [42]. Although the diseases caused by specific HPV types sometimes occur at non-typical sites, this is uncommon, with such lesions often exhibiting non-typical morphology and pathology [43]. The idea that papillomaviruses have epithelial sites where they have evolved to complete their productive life-cycle, and epithelial sites where they do this less-well or not at all, makes good sense when we consider the small number of instances where cross-species infection has been documented. Bovine Papillomavirus type 1 infection of cattle leads to the development of benign cutaneous lesions that may regress, whereas infection of horses typically results in the development of locally aggressive, non-regressing equine sarcoids that are non-permissive for virus production [44–47]. In this case, it appears that the BPV E5 gene, which is important for the production of fibropapillomas in cattle, can stimulate aberrant cell proliferation in the dermal layers in the horse [47]. Although cottontail rabbit papillomavirus (CRPV) is not a fibropapillomavirus like BPV, a similar concept explains its ability to generate non-productive lesions in domestic rabbits, that have a tendency to develop over time into neoplasia and cancer [48,49]. In this case, it is the E6 and E7 proteins, along with the viral transcription factor E2, that are ultimately important for the development of the cancer phenotype [50,51]. Historically, these ideas are not new to the field of tumour virus biology, with a large body of experimental work using animal models to understand how members of the polyoma and adenoviruses families can cause tumours [52,53]. In the case of adenoviruses, it is the E1A and E1B proteins, and with polyomaviruses it is the T antigens, that when deregulated can cause tumours in experimental systems [54,55], and it is now well known that these proteins share functional similarity with the E6 and E7 proteins of the high-risk papillomaviruses [56,57]. In fact, our current knowledge suggests that it is the deregulated expression of the high-risk E6 and E7 proteins that leads to the development of neoplasia at specific epithelial sites, and that these infections should be regarded as "non-productive or abortive infections" rather than "ordered" productive infections, where the level and pattern of viral gene expression is properly controlled [58,59]. It has been reported that several factors such as the type of cell, hormone as well as inflammatory cytokines control viral gene expression [41,60–62]. With this in mind, it is clearly important to understand how epithelial environment, cell type and host immunity act together to drive neoplasia, and we suspect that this will be an important topic of future research. Although this line of thinking fits well with our understanding of how high-risk HPV types cause neoplasia and cancer at specific sites, including the cervix, anus and oropharynx, the same broad principles also explain the elevated risk of non-melanoma skin cancer posed by Betapapillomaviruses, even though the molecular detail of how these viruses cause cancer is different [11]. Betapapillomavirus types are prevalent as asymptomatic infections in normal skin and mucosa in the general population [3,63,64], with infection occurring soon after birth [9]. In immunocompromised individuals, including those suffering from epidermodysplasia verruciformis, it appears that normal patterns of viral gene expression can become deregulated, allowing a level of viral gene expression that would not be tolerated in immune competent individuals (Figure 2) [11].

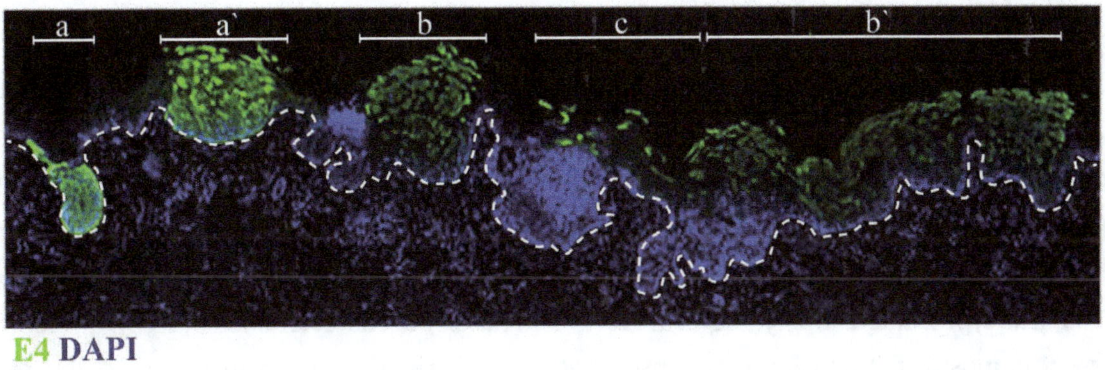

Figure 2. Viral gene-expression in adjacent Betapapillomavirus lesions. Immunostaining for the Betapapillomavirus E4 protein (**green**) reveals distinct patterns of expression in different lesions in an immunosuppressed individual. Lesion (**a**) and (**a´**) are atypical, and show marked basal and suprabasal staining; This pattern of E4 expression is distinct from typical E4 pattern of expression, which is usually restricted to the mid/upper epithelial layers as seen in region (**c**); Lesions (**b**) and (**b´**) show an intermediate pattern of E4 staining with expression close to the basal layer, as well as in the suprabasal cell layers (see also review [11]).

Interestingly, we have also seen that certain papillomaviruses, which are usually associated with symptomatic lesions following infection, can persist at the site of infection following immune regression, with reactivation occurring as the immune environment changes [65,66]. For both α- and Betapapillomavirus types, this work suggests that the immune system provides an important check on the extent of viral gene expression, and that overexpression of viral gene products can predispose to cancer progression following infection by certain β HPV types as well as for the high-risk Alphapapillomaviruses. The existence of latent papillomavirus infections remains to be conclusively validated in humans, but experiments in animal models suggest that this is likely [67,68].

3. Genome Structure and the Classification of Viral Gene Products

As outlined above, papillomaviruses can complete their life-cycle at many different anatomical sites, including the skin, anogenital tract and the oral cavity, but do not always produce clinically apparent lesions, sometimes persisting in the epithelium as non-productive latent infections. To progress beyond these basic observations requires an understanding of viral protein function and the expression patterns of the viral gene products in the epithelium. The viral genome is a circular double-stranded DNA episome, which ranges in length from 6953 bp for Cheloniamydas papillomavirus type 1 (CmPV1) to 8607 bp for Canine papillomavirus type 1 (CPV1). Viral genomes generally contain one regulatory region designated as the URR (upstream regulatory region) or LCR (long control region), which contains transcription factor-binding sites and the replication origin, and two groups of ORFs, which are designated early (E) or late (L) [69]. Some papillomavirus types, such as CPV, contain a second regulatory region between the end of the early region and the start of the late regions [70,71]. Despite variation in the size and number of ORFs, all PV members include a URR, along with a group of proteins with a high level of conservation that are found in all sequenced papillomavirus types (Figure 3A).

These "core" genes include the E1 and E2 proteins necessary for viral replication [72,73], and the viral late proteins L1 and L2 [24,74]. The remaining viral genes (E6, E7, E5) may be considered as "accessory" genes that have evolved to facilitate replication in stratified epithelium (Figure 3B) [56,57,75]. These early gene products are generally more divergent than E1 and E2, both functionally and at the primary amino acid sequence level, and are not universally present in all papillomavirus types. Interestingly, the viral E4 protein has some characteristics of a core protein, in that it is present in most if not all papillomaviruses, but is also variable at the primary amino acid sequence level, which at first site could suggest a divergent function [76]. It is thought however that E4 plays a key role in virus escape from the cornified epithelial layers, and that evolution has driven E4 divergence to allow it to carry out its common function at different anatomical sites where epithelial structure differs. In general, the viral core genes are thought to have existed early during papillomavirus evolution, and carry out essential functions during the virus life cycle in the epithelium. L1 encodes primary structural protein in the virus capsid [77], with the minor capsid protein L2 binding to the circular viral DNA to facilitate optimal genome encapsidation [78]. E1 encodes a virus-specific DNA helicase [72], while E2 functions in viral transcription, replication and genome partitioning [73]. The remaining genes (E6, E7 and E5) encode proteins that modify the cellular environment, and in many cases perform similar but not necessarily identical functions during the life cycle of different papillomaviruses to support the production of progeny virions and to affect virulence. As such, it is thought that a major determinant of virus tropism may lie in the function of these accessory genes as well as in their regulation.

A

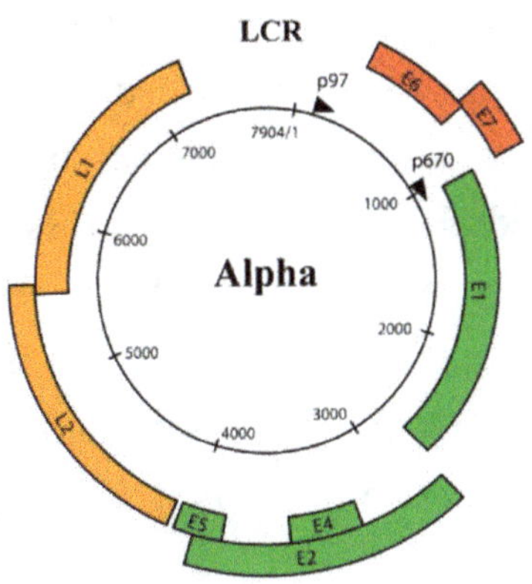

B

Core Proteins	
E1	ATP-dependent helicase. Role in papillomavirus genome replication.
E2	Coactivator of viral genome replication through the recruitment of E1 to the viral replication origin. Transcription factor of E6 and E7, also important for viral genome segregation.
L1	Major capsid protein. Assembles into pentomeric capsomeres, which are the primary components of the icosahedral virion shell.
L2	Minor capsid protein. Involved in encapsidation of viral DNA. Facilitate virus entry and trafficikng to the nucleus.
E4	E4 gene is embedded within the E2 gene, and is expressed abundantly as an E1^E4 fusion protein during the late stages of the viral life cycle. Binds to cytokeratin filaments and disrupts their structure. E4 is thought also to contribute to virus release and transmission.
Accessory Proteins	
E5	Small transmembrane protein. In Alpha-PVs, E5 interacts with the EGF receptor and activates mitogenic signaling pathways. Has a role in evading the immune response and apoptosis. Beta-, Gamma- and Mu-PVs lack E5 gene.
E6	Drives cell cycle entry to allow genome amplification in the upper epithelial layers. E6 of high-risk Alpha-PV types binds and degrades p53 and can also activate telomerase and contribute to transformation. Also involved in immune evasion. Some Gamma-PVs lack E6 gene.
E7	Drives cell cycle entry to allow genome amplification in the upper epithelial layers. E7 of high-risk Alpha-PV types binds and degrades pRb and can induces chromosomal instability. E7 is necessary for cell transformation.
	Both E6 and E7 have a large number of cellular substrates, with the identity of these substrates differing between HPV types [78].

Figure 3. Alphapapillomavirus genome organization and the function of HPV proteins. (**A**) Genome organization typical of the high-risk Alphapapillomavirus types is illustrated by the genome of HPV16. The early (p97) and late (p670) promoters are marked by arrows. The six early ORFs (E1, E2, E4 and E5 (**in green**) and E6 and E7 (**in red**)) are expressed from the different promoters at different stages during epithelial cell differentiation. The late ORFs (L1 and L2 (**in yellow**)) are expressed from the p670 promoter in the upper epithelial layers as result of changes in splicing. The LCR/URR also contains the replication origin as well as post-transcriptional control sequences that contribute to viral gene expression. (**B**) The function of viral proteins. All known papillomavirus encodes a group of "core" proteins that were present early on during papillomavirus evolution, and which are conserved in sequence and in function between PV types. These include E1, E2, L2 and L1. The E4 protein may also be a core protein that has evolved to meet papillomaviruses epithelial specialization. The accessory proteins have evolved in each papillomavirus type during adaptation to different epithelial niches. The sequence and function of these genes are divergent between types. In general, these proteins are involved in modifying the cellular environment to facilitate virus life cycle completion, contributing to the virulence and pathogenicity. Knowledge of accessory protein function comes primarily from the study of Alphapapillomavirus types.

4. Productive Papillomavirus Life Cycle and Non-Productive Infection

Because the study of papillomaviruses has been driven by the association of the high-risk Alphapapillomavirus types with anogenital and oropharyngeal cancers, our knowledge of these types is perhaps more complete. However, there are some general principles that extend across the different genera that are worth overviewing before commenting further on the specific characteristics of different papillomavirus groups [79]. It is widely accepted that papillomavirus infection occurs once virus particles gain access to the epithelial basal cells or stem cells, which in many cases involves some level of epithelial trauma. In all cases, it is thought that virions bind initially to the glycosaminoglycan (GAG) chains of heparan sulfate proteoglycan (HSPG) in a charge-based manner, and that this leads to conformational changes in the virion which expose a furin/proprotein convertase cleavage site at the amino terminus of L2. It is generally thought that virus entry requires interaction with a secondary receptor, which still remains to be properly characterised [39]. Importantly, these early HSPG-dependent events have been shown to occur on the extracellular basement membrane (BM) in the murine cervico-vaginal model of HPV16 infection [80], close to where the target basal cells reside.

After PV infection, an initial phase of genome amplification takes place prior to maintenance of the viral episome at low copy number in the infected basal cells (Figure 4A) [81,82].

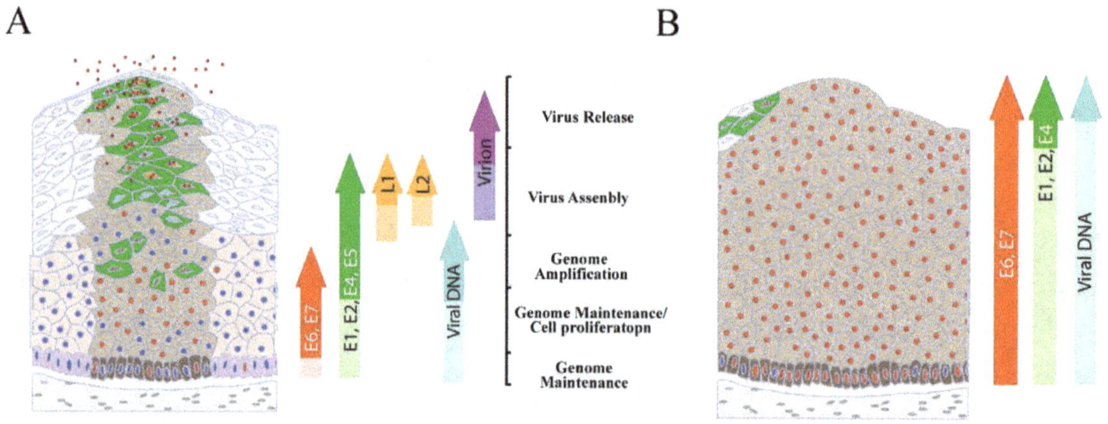

Figure 4. Regulation and deregulation of the high-risk Alphapapillomavirus life cycle. (**A**) The papillomavirus life cycle is regulated during epithelial cell differentiation and is shown diagrammatically. Cells that are driven through the cell cycle as a result of E6 and E7 expression are marked with red nuclei. The up-regulation of viral proteins necessary for genome amplification (*i.e.*, E1 and E2) requires activation of the viral late promoter in the upper epithelial layers (cells shown in green with red nuclei), with virus particles subsequently being released from the epithelial surface; (**B**) In HPV-associated neoplasia, late gene expression is retarded, and although the order of events remains the same, the production of infectious virions is restricted to smaller and smaller areas close to the epithelial surface. This situation is thought to be accompanied elevated E6/E7 expression, and represents a non-productive or poorly productive abortive infection. Integration of HPV DNA into the host cell genome is facilitated by deregulated E6/E7 expression. If integration disrupts the E1/E2 region this can allow the persistent high-level expression of E6 and E7 and the accumulation of genetic errors in the host genome. Eventually, the productive virus life cycle is no longer supported and viral episomes are lost (reviewed in [83]).

The viral replication proteins E1 and E2 are thought to be essential for this initial amplification, but E1 may be dispensable for maintenance-replication once copy number has stabilised at 50–100 [65]. E2 has an established role in genome partitioning, replication and viral gene expression. Experimental systems have shown at least a two-log increase in viral copy number during genome amplification [65], with E1, E2 and cellular DNA replication proteins being crucial for viral genome amplification *in vitro* [72,73,84]. The extent of genome amplification may be higher (four-log increase) during infection *in vivo*, as suggested from laser capture analysis of productive infections in rabbits [65]. The essential role of E6 and E7 in the viral lifecycle is primarily to modify the cellular environment to allow viral genome amplification, mainly by driving S-phase re-entry in the upper epithelial layers. Genome amplification occurs as the infected cell moves from an S to a G2-like phase before committing to full differentiation. In the case of high-risk types, E6 and E7 appear also to drive cell proliferation in the basal and parabasal layers [83]. By contrast, in the case of low-risk types (HPV6, HPV11 or other HPV types that have a tendency to cause benign lesions), the precise role of these proteins in the infected basal cells is unclear. In fact, functional differences in E6 and E7 represent a major determinant of HPV disease pathogenicity between HPV types [85]. During the virus life cycle, E5 also contributes to viral genome amplification as a result of its ability to stabilize epidermal growth factor (EGF) receptor and to enhance mitogen-activated protein (MAP) kinase activity. E5 also modulates both extracellular-signal-regulated kinase 1/2 (ERK 1/2) and p38 independently of EGF receptor [75]. Interestingly, the nuclear localisation and export signals in E1 are phosphorylated by these MAP kinases, which in turn enhances the nuclear localisation of E1 protein which is necessary for genome amplification [86,87]. In the upper layers of the epithelium, amplified viral genomes are packaged into virus particles produced from the major (L1) and minor (L2) virus coat proteins. The E4 protein, which accumulates at very high levels in cells supporting virus synthesis [76], appears to have a primary function in virus release and/or transmission, but acts also to optimise the success of virus genome amplification. In high-risk HPV types, the E4 protein assembles into amyloid fibrils that can disrupt keratin structure and compromise the normal assembly of the cornified envelope [88,89]. Although not yet precisely defined, E4 amyloid fibres may contribute to virion release from the upper epithelial layers, and therefore infectivity and transmission.

Although high-risk HPV infection is common, cervical cancer arises rarely as a result of infection, with most infections being cleared by the host without clinical symptoms. Regression of anogenital warts is accompanied by a CD4+ T cell-dominated Th1 response, which is also seen in animal models [90–95]. In general, HPV infections evade both the adaptive and innate immune response, with the life cycle being totally intra-epithelial, without viraemia, cell lysis or inflammation. During persistent infection, pro-inflammatory cytokines are not released, and the signals for Langerhans cell and dendritic cell activation and recruitment are largely absent [96]. In fact, cells supporting viral late gene expression, and which may contain high levels of viral proteins, are shed from the surface of the epithelium away from immune surveillance. In general, a failure to develop an effective host immune response correlates with persistent infection and an increased probability of progression toward invasive cancer.

In HPV-associated neoplasias, the ordered expression of viral gene products necessary for virus synthesis does not occur, leading to a non-productive or abortive infection rather than a productive infection (Figure 4B). In this situation, the deregulated expression of the high-risk E7 protein can stimulate host genome instability through deregulation of the centrosome cycle, with the deregulated expression of the high-risk E6 protein contributing to the accumulation of cellular mutations as a result of inhibition or loss of E6 function. This deregulation and the subsequent effects on the cell can eventually lead to the development of cancer (reviewed in [2]).

5. Epithelial Stem Cells and Their Postulated Role in Papillomavirus-Associated Disease

Current thinking suggests that the development of papillomavirus-associated disease requires the infection not just of an epithelial basal cell, but more specifically an epithelial tissue stem cell at a pluristratified cutaneous or mucosal site [97–99]. In general, papillomavirus-associated lesions often persist for many years. Epithelial tissue renewal is achieved by proliferation of stem or stem-like cells in the basal layer, to produce transit amplifying cells that have a limited proliferative capacity, and which subsequently go on to terminally differentiate [100]. Once committed to differentiate, these cells are pushed towards the cell surface by the production of new cells beneath them, and are eventually lost from the epithelial surface as terminally differentiated squames. This movement comprises the "epidermal flow", which occurs over a shorter time period than the life span of a papillomavirus infection [101]. Thus, we assume that papillomaviruses target basal cells with stem cell-like properties [97], or in the case of the high-risk papillomaviruses, they confer such properties on the cells that they infect. The idea that papillomaviruses generally reside in an epithelial stem cell following infection, is compatible with our understanding of latency and reactivation from latency [68], and the clonal origin of papillomas which was established several decades ago [102]. Indeed, studies on animal models have shown that CRPV primarily targets the bulge region of the hair follicle, where epithelial stem cells reside [103], and in cervical neoplasia, the epithelial reserve cells have long been considered the target cell from which cervical disease arises [99,104]. However, the cellular targets of infection have not yet been mapped more precisely, and this still remains a hypothesis, albeit a plausible one.

6. Local Epithelial Structure and Sites of Papillomavirus Infection

Epithelial tissue is composed of three components; epidermis, dermis and subepidermal tissue (subcutaneous tissue at skin sites). The epidermis is composed of multiple keratinocyte layers, and is the component that papillomaviruses target. In addition, the skin also consists of various functional appendages, including hair follicles, sebaceous glands, eccrine and apocrine sweat glands, finger and toe nails, as well as the inter-appendageal epidermis. Specialised epithelial sites contain additional appendages, such as the salivary glands of the oral cavity and the tonsillar crypts of the oropharynx. For papillomaviruses, these "specialist" structures represent particularly vulnerable sites, as they lack the highly structured barrier function usually associated with the epithelium. An additional level of complexity resides at transformation zone regions, where stratified epithelium abuts columnar epithelium, and it is generally accepted that high-risk HPV-associated neoplasias develop primarily at these sites [105]. High-risk HPV types are associated with the vast majority of cervical cancers (>99%), most of which arise at the cervical transformation zone, as well as the more than 90% of cancers that arise at the anal transformation zone. It is reasonable to suspect that transformation zones at other anatomical sites, such as at the boundary between the oesophagus and the stomach, may also be susceptible to HPV-associated neoplasia, but that these sites only rarely become infected because of their location. At the cervix, the transformation zone is maintained by a specialised type of cell known as the reserve cell [104], and possibly also by a cluster of cuboidal cells localised more precisely at the squamo-columnar junction [98]. Our current thinking suggests that these cell types represent the stem cells that maintain either the columnar epithelium of the endocervix, or the stratified epithelium of the transformation zone depending on their extracellular environment. These cells are thought to respond differently to signals from neighbouring epithelial cells and from the dermis, when compared to the more conventional epithelial stem cells that populate the stratified layers of the ectocervix. Indeed, our current model suggests that cervical neoplasia develops primarily at the squamo-columnar junction because these cells fail to properly regulate viral gene expression, leading to a non-productive or abortive infection rather than a productive infection (Figure 5) [59,106].

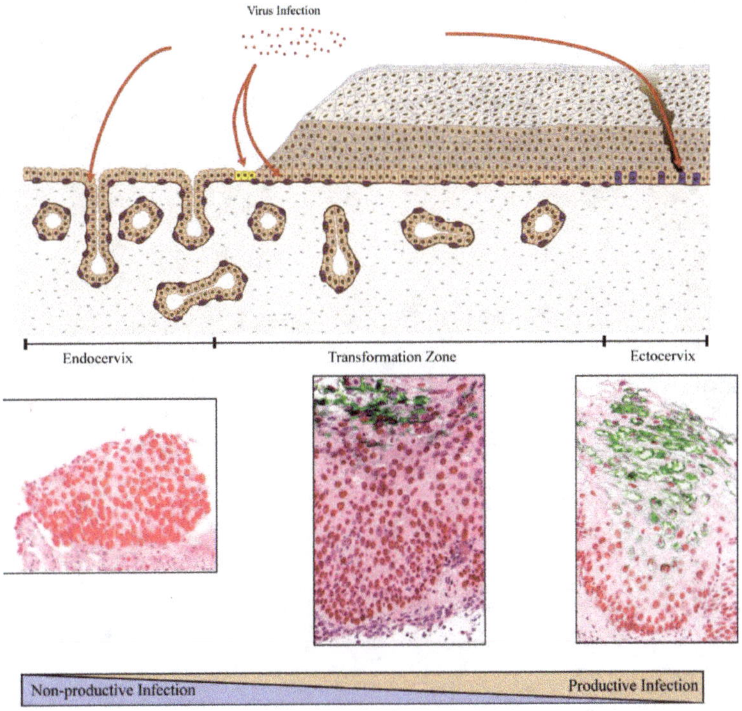

Figure 5. The difference of host cells (the site of infection) affects viral pathogenicity. Most cervical cancers arise at the cervical transformation zone. The transformation zone is maintained by a specialized type of tissue stem cell known as the reserve cell (shown in purple in the transformation zone), and possibly also by a cluster of cuboidal cells (**yellow**) localized more precisely at the squamo-columnar junction. These cells can maintain either the columnar epithelium of the endocervix or the stratified epithelium of transformation zone depending on their extracellular environment. In the ectocervix, the epithelium is populated by conventional epithelial tissue stem cells (purple in the ectocervix). The different characteristics of the various tissue stem cells that HPV infects are thought to influence the pattern of viral gene expression differently [41]. Current thinking suggests that productive infection is favoured at the ectocervix, while a non-productive or abortive infection is more likely at the endocervix. In the immunostains, MCM expression (**red**) indicates the expression of viral E7 protein. E4 expression (**green**) indicates the productive infection [59].

In this situation, deregulated viral gene expression facilitates the accumulation of genetic errors in the infected cell that no longer supports a productive infection (as described previously), leading eventually to the development of cancer.

By comparison with the cervical reserve cells, the stem cells that populate cutaneous epithelial sites are better characterised, and are known to reside in the bulge region of the hair follicle (Figure 6A) [107,108].

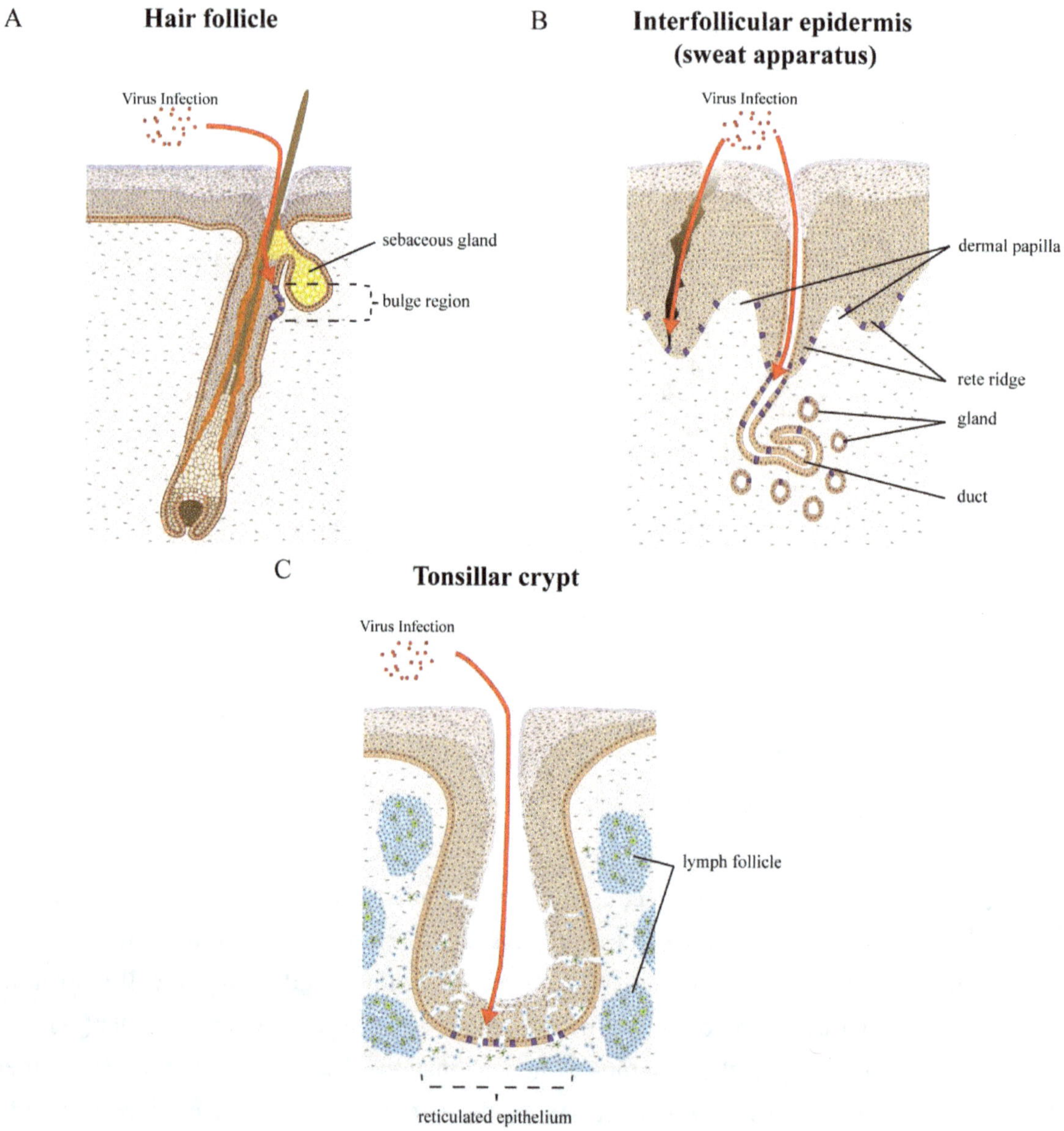

Figure 6. Epithelial tissue sites and tissue stem cells as targets for HPV infection. HPVs infect a variety of epithelial tissue sites, and can cause lesions in the vicinity of hair follicles, eccrine and apocrine sweat apparatus), nails, and also the inter-appendageal epidermis. Specialized epithelial sites contain other appendages, such as the salivary glands of the oral cavity and the tonsillar crypts of the oropharynx, where oropharyngeal cancers arise. The transformation zone regions, where stratified epithelium abuts columnar epithelium such as the cervical (Figure 5) or anal transformation zones, are other target sites where infection is

thought to be facilitated. (**A**) The bulge region of the hair follicle is a well characterized region where the stem cells that populate cutaneous epithelial sites reside. HPV virions are thought to gain access to the epithelial stem cells (coloured purple), either through a wound or possibly through the hair follicle; (**B**) Between the hair follicles, the tissue stem cells are thought to reside in both rete ridge and over the dermal papilla, and are not thought to be clustered at any specific location in the basal component [109]. With the sweat apparatus, at least two distinct stem cell populations have been identified that may be accessible for infection, either in the gland or the duct. These are able to repair damaged epidermis. HPV virions are thought to gain access to these stem cells (coloured purple), either through a wound or maybe through the eccrine duct; (**C**) The tonsillar crypts are a highly specialized lymphoepithelial tissue. A dense lymphocyte infiltrate generally obscures the junction between the lymphoid and epithelial components and splinters the epithelial sheath into irregular nests and cords. This reticulated epithelium may facilitate viral access to tissue stem cells at an immune-privileged site, which can inhibit virus-specific T cell activity and thereby facilitate immune evasion during initial HPV infection and subsequent virus-induced malignant transformation.

Because these cells can mediate the repair of damaged interfollicular epidermis, the interfollicular stem cells were for some time, thought to be supplied by follicular stem cells routinely [110]. However, recent work has shown that stem cells in the hair follicle do not contribute to epidermal homeostasis, but points instead to the presence of a distinct population of interfollicular epidermal stem cells [111]. This idea is supported by several observations [112], including the visualisation of discrete slow-cycling cells that are interspersed throughout the basal layer in mouse interfollicular epidermis [113] and in monkey palm epidermis [114], as well as the visualisation of clonal regenerating units of interfollicular epidermis (Figure 6B) [115]. In human skin, however, our inability to mark slow-cycling cells using *in situ* approaches, coupled with a lack of specific stem cell markers, has meant that the identification and location of interfollicular epidermal stem cells remains uncertain. Although it is generally accepted that eccrine sweat duct-derived cells can repair damaged epidermis [116], little attention has been paid to the sweat gland as an additional location of epidermal stem cells. Recently, stem cell populations in sweat glands and ducts have however been identified by lineage-tracing (Figure 6B) [117].

7. Examples of Papillomavirus Niche-Adaptation and Tropisms

Given the genotype-specific tropisms of papillomaviruses and the varied pathologies associated with infection, it is not unreasonable to think that different papillomaviruses have become well adapted to their respective epithelial niches. Although this has already been overviewed to some extent in the preceding paragraphs, the diversity of niche-adaptation can perhaps be appreciated by reference to particular examples that are outlined below.

Schmitt *et al.* [103] have shown that the primary target cells of CRPV co-localize with the hair follicle stem cells. In this study, E6 and E7 transcripts were detected at 11 days post-infection, despite the absence of apparent disease, with expression of these genes representing an early marker of infection. The subsequent finding that viable keratinocyte clones isolated from these infected follicles were CRPV mRNA-positive, suggests infection of a replication competent cell, which given the location, is suspected to be a bulge stem cell. A similar cellular target and epithelial tropism has also been suggested for the HPV types associated with epidermodysplasia verruciformis (EV). These HPV types usually come from the Genus Betapapillomavirus, and can be detected in plucked hair from different body sites. EV is a rare autosomal recessive genodermatosis associated with a high risk of skin carcinoma [11,118,119]. In many cases, the disease is linked to mutations in two genes (EVER1 and EVER2) that are expressed in the endoplasmic reticulum, and which form a complex with zinc-transporter-1 (ZnT-1), thereby controlling zinc balance [120]. Lesions generally start on the dorsa of the hands and the forehead, and spread progressively to the limb, neck and trunk. However, the mucous epithelium is not involved. EV skin lesions are hardly seen on the palmoplantar skin, even though they are frequently productive in nearby epithelium. At a clinical level, it is very clear that the Betapapillomavirus types associated with EV precisely "select" their preferential anatomical sites. The frequent detection of EV-PV in plucked hairs points to the hair follicle as an important site of infection for EV-PV [121,122].

HPV1 and 63 are members of the Genus Mupapillomavirus, and appear to target eccrine ducts in the palmoplantar skin. HPV1 causes typical myrmecia warts on the palms and soles [27,123], and it is quite rare for this HPV type to infect and cause lesions at extra-palmoplantar sites. The most characteristic histological feature is eosinophilic granular intracytoplasmic inclusion bodies (Gr-ICBs), which are larger and more numerous in the upper layer of the epidermis, and which are pathognomonic of infection by this virus. HPV1 infection provided a good example of how the site of infection influences clinical features and can affect viral gene expression [43]. Lesion development occurs on the skin surface ridges on the palms or soles. Histopathological studies and *in situ* hybridization analysis of early lesions have revealed that both HPV1-associated disease-pathology and *in situ* DNA-positivity are closely associated with eccrine ducts (Figure 7A, and our unpublished data).

HPV63, which is the second Mupapillomavirus type, induces tiny punctate warts (0.5 to 2 mm) characterised by the presence of heavily-stained tonofibril-like structures referred to as filamentous inclusion bodies [27,29]. To date, HPV63-induced warts have only been reported on the sole, with HPV63 DNA being detected both in keratinocytes around acrosyringiums (Figure 7B) and also in the uppermost portion of the eccrine dermal duct, which was hypertrophied with the HPV infection [124].

The final example focuses on HPV6 and 11, which share 85% sequence identity and belong to same HPV species (Alphapapillomavirus 2). Interestingly, in contrast to EV-HPVs from the Genus Betapapillomavirus, and which are both detectable in plucked pubic and eyebrow hairs, HPV6 and 11 could be detected only in hair plucked from pubic and perianal regions of patients with genital warts, but not in eyebrow hairs of the same patients. It has been suggested that HPV6 and 11 have a more limited epithelial distribution [125]. In contrast to this, Kocjan *et al.* [126], showed the presence of four genital HPVs (HPV6, 11 31 and 58) in plucked eyebrow hairs from immunocompetent individuals, suggesting that these viruses may sometimes be more widely distributed, but that they develop lesions preferentially at anogenital or oral sites. Since HPV6 and 11 are well-known causative agents for condyloma acuminatum, and can be detected in pubic and perianal hairs, a follicular distribution for this virus may exist. In fact, hair follicle-associated papules are sometimes observed in conjunction with the larger more prominent lesions at anogenital sites, with hair follicles being present widely at many epithelial sites. Interestingly, histological studies show that HPV6/11 DNA can also be detected in association with hair follicles as well as the vicinity of sweat apparatus or inter-appendageal epidermis, along with associated histological changes (Figure 7C, and our unpublished data). HPV6 and 11 are also causative agents of laryngeal papillomatosis, although in this instance the target cells remain unclear. The vocal cord, where HPV6 and 11 can also produce papillomatosis consists of squamous epithelium, pseudostratified epithelium and a transitional zone, which may facilitate access to stem-like cells at this site.

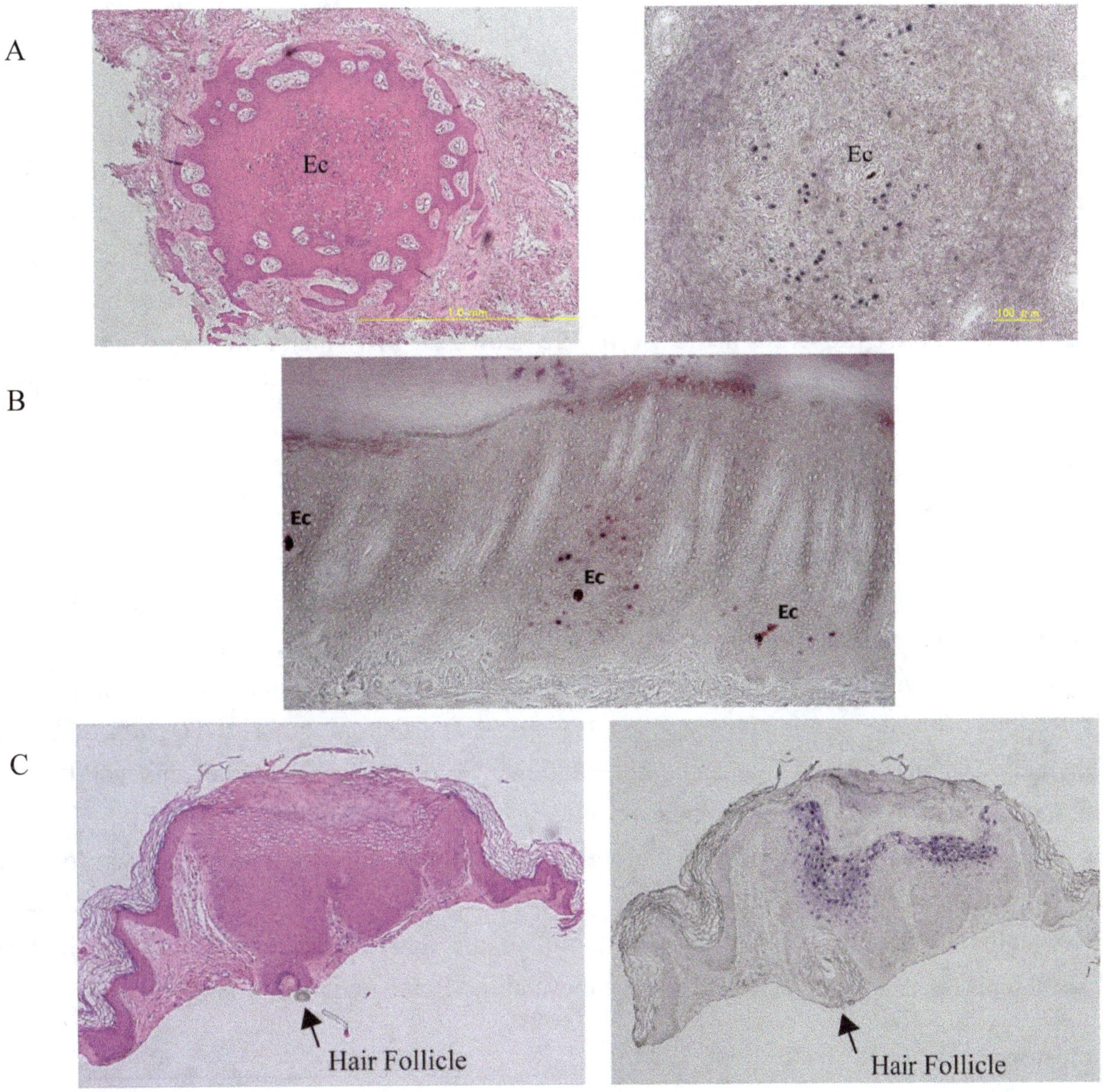

Figure 7. Examples for HPV targeting cutaneous appendages. (**A**) Haemotoxylin & eosin stain (**left**) of a horizontal section of a tiny wart. An eccrine (Ec)-centered distribution of histological changes is observed. HPV1 DNAs are identified within the pathology changes following DNA *in situ* hybridization (**right**); (**B**) HPV63 DNA is identified in resident keratinocytes in the vicinity of eccrine ducts (Ec) in a ridge of the plantar skin following DNA *in situ* hybridization; (**C**) HPV6/11 histopathological changes are identified in the resident keratinocytes in and around the hair follicle (arrow) by haemotoxylin & eosin staining (**left**) and DNA *in situ* hybridization (**right**).

8. High-Risk Mucosal HPV Types

The high-risk mucosal HPVs, such as HPV16, 18, 31 and 33 appear to have evolved a number of additional characteristics that are not shared by low-risk papillomaviruses. These relate primarily to the function of the E5, E6 and E7 gene products, and the regulatory mechanisms that govern their expression (reviewed in [2]). Many functional studies have however focused on the contribution of these viral proteins to cancer development rather than life-cycle completion, and a detailed comparison of the role of these proteins in the life cycles of high and low-risk papillomaviruses remains to be done. A prominent characteristic of high-risk E6 proteins is the presence of a C-terminal PDZ-binding motif [127–131], along with an ability to bind and degrade the cellular p53 protein [132–134]. In addition, the high-risk HPV types have been shown to express their E6 and E7 proteins from a single promoter, with the levels of these two proteins being regulated by differential splicing [1,135]. This contrasts with the presence of separate promoters that regulate E6 and E7 expression in low-risk HPV types, such as those from the Alphpapillomavirus genus. Although there are additional key differences between these broad groups of papillomaviruses, these properties in themselves are known to have a major impact on high-risk virus pathogenesis. Although the precise advantage that the high-risk HPV types gain from these additional functions remains unclear, it is very likely to be related to particular sites of infection and their different strategies for productive infection at these sites. Clearly, the high-risk viruses have an ability to drive cell cycle entry as well as cell proliferation, which may be an important part of their normal life cycle at mucosal sites [83]. High-risk HPV-associated cancers occur predominantly within the cervical and anal transformation zone, as well as in the crypts of the oropharynx (Figure 6C) [136], which are thought to be sites where viral gene expression is poorly controlled. Given the preferential tissue distributions of different papillomaviruses, it is not surprising that particular HPV types may sometimes infect sites where full productive infection is either not supported or supported only poorly. The different cancer risk at the penis, vagina and vulva, when compared to the cervix or anus, illustrates this well [137]. In addition, the different risk of cancer progression associated with different HPV types (e.g., HPV16, 18 and 45) must reflect the different basic tropisms or tissue-specificities of the species Alphapapillomavirus 7 and Alphapapillomaviru 9 [138], and the different ways in which their genes are expressed and achieve their effects at these different epithelial sites. In addition to infection at these genital sites, some high-risk types can be found at other cutaneous sites where they cause "Bowenoid papulosis" [139,140].

9. Conclusions

Papillomaviruses have evolved over many millions of years to propagate themselves in a range of different species including humans. The evolution of skin glands, hair follicles and other ecological niches has provided papillomaviruses with new opportunities for infection. These have been followed by niche-adaptation, and it is thought that through this route, the great diversity of papillomaviruses has arisen. In general, β- and Gammapapillomavirus types have evolved a strategy of causing chronic asymptomatic infections accompanied by long-term virion-production and shedding from infected epidermis. This strategy minimises the risk of immune clearance, and depends on a balance between immune suppression and virus synthesis without any marked effect on host-fitness. By contrast, other papillomaviruses, such as those from the Genus Alphapapillomavirus, have evolved an array of sophisticated immune evasion strategies that allow them to cause prominent and persistent papillomas, even in immune competent individuals. Immune clearance of such lesions can however lead to asymptomatic or latent infections, with the possibility of an increase in viral copy number upon immunosuppression. Thus, both the cellular environment and the site of infection are important determinants of viral gene expression and virus activity. HPV pathogenicity, however, also reflects differences in viral gene function, which is evidenced most significantly when high and low-risk HPV types are compared. The genotype-specific association with disease, and more specifically with neoplasia, provides the basis for the recent introduction of DNA testing in cervical screening, and underlies the introduction of HPV 16/18 vaccines to protect against cervical cancer. High-risk mucosal HPVs do however have different cancer associations at different sites, prompting a detailed analysis of site-specific patterns of gene expression and gene function at different epithelial sites, such as the endocervix, the cervical transformation zone and the ectocervix, as well as the tonsillar crypts and other oropharyngeal sites where HPV-associated neoplasia can develop. An understanding of the site-specific aspects of HPV infection should facilitate the development of better strategies for disease treatment (e.g., target antivirals, immunotherapeutics) and disease management (e.g., risk assessment), and is very likely to provide new insight into epithelial biology and immunology.

Acknowledgments

Thanks to Ignacio Bravo (Catalan Institute of Oncology, Barcelona, Spain) for the evolutionary tree, which is modified from [26]. Our understanding of HPV immunology has been significantly enhanced through discussion with Margaret Stanley (University of Cambridge, UK) and Merilyn Hibma (University of Otago, New Zealand). The support and encouragement of Geoffrey Smith, Head of Department (Department of Pathology, University of Cambridge, UK) are greatly acknowledged. Thanks to Isao Murakami and Christian Kranjec (University of Cambridge, UK) for helpful discussion. The Human Papillomavirus Research Group at the University of Cambridge is funded by the UK Medical Research Council.

Author Contributions

Nagayasu Egawa and John Doorbar wrote the manuscript. Kiyofumi Egawa wrote the section of “Examples of Papillomavirus Niche-Adaptation and Tropisms” and provided the figures. Heather Griffin wrote the section relating to β-papillomavirus infection and deregulation and provided the figure.

References

1. PaVE: Papillomavirus Episteme. Available online: http://pave.niaid.nih.gov/ (accessed on 11 July 2015).
2. Doorbar, J.; Egawa, N.; Griffin, H.; Kranjec, C.; Murakami, I. Human papillomavirus molecular biology and disease association. *Rev. Med. Virol.* **2015**, *25* (Suppl. 1), 2–23. [CrossRef] [PubMed]

3. Bottalico, D.; Chen, Z.; Dunne, A.; Ostoloza, J.; McKinney, S.; Sun, C.; Schlecht, N.F.; Herrero, R.; Fatahzadeh, M.; Schiffman, M.; *et al.* The oral cavity contains abundant known and novel human papillomaviruses from the betapapillomavirus and gammapapillomavirus genera. *J. Infect. Dis.* **2011**, *204*, 787–792. [CrossRef] [PubMed]
4. De Koning, M.N.; Quint, K.D.; Bruggink, S.C.; Gussekloo, J.; Bouwes Bavinck, J.N.; Quint, W.G.; Feltkamp, M.C.; Eekhof, J.A. High prevalence of cutaneous warts in elementary school children and the ubiquitous presence of wart-associated human papillomavirus on clinically normal skin. *Br. J. Dermatol.* **2015**, *172*, 196–201. [CrossRef] [PubMed]
5. Poljak, M.; Kocjan, B.J.; Potocnik, M.; Seme, K. Anogenital hairs are an important reservoir of α-papillomaviruses in patients with genital warts. *J. Infect. Dis.* **2009**, *199*, 1270–1274. [CrossRef] [PubMed]
6. Potocnik, M.; Kocjan, B.J.; Seme, K.; Luzar, B.; Babic, D.Z.; Poljak, M. β-papillomaviruses in anogenital hairs plucked from healthy individuals. *J. Med. Virol.* **2006**, *78*, 1673–1678. [CrossRef] [PubMed]
7. De Koning, M.N.; Struijk, L.; Bavinck, J.N.; Kleter, B.; ter Schegget, J.; Quint, W.G.; Feltkamp, M.C. Betapapillomaviruses frequently persist in the skin of healthy individuals. *J. Gen. Virol.* **2007**, *88*, 1489–1495. [CrossRef] [PubMed]
8. Antonsson, A.; Erfurt, C.; Hazard, K.; Holmgren, V.; Simon, M.; Kataoka, A.; Hossain, S.; Hakangard, C.; Hansson, B.G. Prevalence and type spectrum of human papillomaviruses in healthy skin samples collected in three continents. *J. Gen. Virol.* **2003**, *84*, 1881–1886. [CrossRef] [PubMed]
9. Antonsson, A.; Karanfilovska, S.; Lindqvist, P.G.; Hansson, B.G. General acquisition of human papillomavirus infections of skin occurs in early infancy. *J. Clin. Microbiol.* **2003**, *41*, 2509–2514. [CrossRef] [PubMed]
10. Jablonska, S.; Orth, G. Epidermodysplasia verruciformis. *Clin. Dermatol.* **1985**, *3*, 83–96. [CrossRef]
11. Quint, K.D.; Genders, R.E.; de Koning, M.N.; Borgogna, C.; Gariglio, M.; Bouwes Bavinck, J.N.; Doorbar, J.; Feltkamp, M.C. Human β-papillomavirus infection and keratinocyte carcinomas. *J. Pathol.* **2015**, *235*, 342–354. [CrossRef] [PubMed]
12. Goon, P.; Sonnex, C.; Jani, P.; Stanley, M.; Sudhoff, H. Recurrent respiratory papillomatosis: An overview of current thinking and treatment. *Eur. Arch. Oto-Rhino-Laryngol.* **2008**, *265*, 147–151. [CrossRef] [PubMed]
13. Cubie, H.A. Diseases associated with human papillomavirus infection. *Virology* **2013**, *445*, 21–34. [CrossRef] [PubMed]
14. Harwood, C.A.; Spink, P.J.; Surentheran, T.; Leigh, I.M.; de Villiers, E.M.; McGregor, J.M.; Proby, C.M.; Breuer, J. Degenerate and nested PCR: A highly sensitive and specific method for detection of human papillomavirus infection in cutaneous warts. *J. Clin. Microbiol.* **1999**, *37*, 3545–3555. [PubMed]
15. Rogers, H.D.; Macgregor, J.L.; Nord, K.M.; Tyring, S.; Rady, P.; Engler, D.E.; Grossman, M.E. Acquired epidermodysplasia verruciformis. *J. Am. Acad. Dermatol.* **2009**, *60*, 315–320. [CrossRef] [PubMed]

16. Bouwes Bavinck, J.N.; Feltkamp, M.; Struijk, L.; ter Schegget, J. Human papillomavirus infection and skin cancer risk in organ transplant recipients. *J. Investig. Dermatol. Symp. Proc. Soc.* **2001**, *6*, 207–211. [CrossRef] [PubMed]
17. Van Doorslaer, K. Evolution of the papillomaviridae. *Virology* **2013**, *445*, 11–20. [CrossRef] [PubMed]
18. Bravo, I.G.; Felez-Sanchez, M. Papillomaviruses: Viral evolution, cancer and evolutionary medicine. *Evol. Med. Public Health* **2015**, *2015*, 32–51. [CrossRef] [PubMed]
19. Van Doorslaer, K.; Burk, R.D. Evolution of human papillomavirus carcinogenicity. *Adv. Virus Res.* **2010**, *77*, 41–62. [PubMed]
20. Burk, R.D.; Chen, Z.; van Doorslaer, K. Human papillomaviruses: Genetic basis of carcinogenicity. *Public Health Genomics* **2009**, *12*, 281–290. [CrossRef] [PubMed]
21. Bernard, H.U.; Burk, R.D.; Chen, Z.; van Doorslaer, K.; zur Hausen, H.; de Villiers, E.M. Classification of papillomaviruses (PVS) based on 189 PV types and proposal of taxonomic amendments. *Virology* **2010**, *401*, 70–79. [CrossRef] [PubMed]
22. De Villiers, E.M.; Fauquet, C.; Broker, T.R.; Bernard, H.U.; zur Hausen, H. Classification of papillomaviruses. *Virology* **2004**, *324*, 17–27. [CrossRef] [PubMed]
23. Drolet, M.; Benard, E.; Boily, M.C.; Ali, H.; Baandrup, L.; Bauer, H.; Beddows, S.; Brisson, J.; Brotherton, J.M.; Cummings, T.; *et al.* Population-level impact and herd effects following human papillomavirus vaccination programmes: A systematic review and meta-analysis. *Lancet. Infect. Dis.* **2015**, *15*, 565–580. [CrossRef]
24. Buck, C.B.; Day, P.M.; Trus, B.L. The papillomavirus major capsid protein L1. *Virology* **2013**, *445*, 169–174. [CrossRef] [PubMed]
25. Dasgupta, J.; Bienkowska-Haba, M.; Ortega, M.E.; Patel, H.D.; Bodevin, S.; Spillmann, D.; Bishop, B.; Sapp, M.; Chen, X.S. Structural basis of oligosaccharide receptor recognition by human papillomavirus. *J. Biol. Chem.* **2011**, *286*, 2617–2624. [CrossRef] [PubMed]
26. Doorbar, J.; Quint, W.; Banks, L.; Bravo, I.G.; Stoler, M.; Broker, T.R.; Stanley, M.A. The biology and life-cycle of human papillomaviruses. *Vaccine* **2012**, *30*, F55–F70. [CrossRef] [PubMed]
27. Egawa, K. New types of human papillomaviruses and intracytoplasmic inclusion bodies: A classification of inclusion warts according to clinical features, histology and associated HPV types. *Br. J. Dermatol.* **1994**, *130*, 158–166. [CrossRef] [PubMed]
28. Egawa, K.; Honda, Y.; Inaba, Y.; Ono, T. Pigmented viral warts: A clinical and histopathological study including human papillomavirus typing. *Br. J. Dermatol.* **1998**, *138*, 381–389. [CrossRef] [PubMed]
29. Egawa, K.; Delius, H.; Matsukura, T.; Kawashima, M.; de Villiers, E.M. Two novel types of human papillomavirus, HPV 63 and HPV 65: Comparisons of their clinical and histological features and DNA sequences to other HPV types. *Virology* **1993**, *194*, 789–799. [CrossRef] [PubMed]
30. Egawa, K.; Kimmel, R.; de Villiers, E.M. A novel type of human papillomavirus (HPV 95): Comparison with infections of closely related human papillomavirus types. *Br. J. Dermatol.* **2005**, *153*, 688–689. [CrossRef] [PubMed]

31. Ball, S.L.; Winder, D.M.; Vaughan, K.; Hanna, N.; Levy, J.; Sterling, J.C.; Stanley, M.A.; Goon, P.K. Analyses of human papillomavirus genotypes and viral loads in anogenital warts. *J. Med. Virol.* **2011**, *83*, 1345–1350. [CrossRef] [PubMed]
32. Dickens, P.; Srivastava, G.; Loke, S.L.; Larkin, S. Human papillomavirus 6, 11, and 16 in laryngeal papillomas. *J. Pathol.* **1991**, *165*, 243–246. [CrossRef] [PubMed]
33. Syrjanen, S. Human papillomavirus infections and oral tumors. *Med. Microbiol. Immunol. Berl* **2003**, *192*, 123–128. [CrossRef] [PubMed]
34. De Villiers, E.M. Human pathogenic papillomavirus types: An update. *Curr. Top. Microbiol. Immunol.* **1994**, *186*, 1–12. [PubMed]
35. Orth, G.; Jablonska, S.; Favre, M.; Croissant, O.; Obalek, S.; Jarzabek-Chorzelska, M.; Jibard, N. Identification of papillomaviruses in butchers' warts. *J. Investig. Dermatol.* **1981**, *76*, 97–102. [CrossRef] [PubMed]
36. International Agency for the Research on Cancer. Avilable online: http://monographs.iarc.fr/ENG/ Monographs/vol90/ (acessed on 11 July 2015).
37. Munoz, N.; Bosch, F.X.; de Sanjose, S.; Herrero, R.; Castellsague, X.; Shah, K.V.; Snijders, P.J.; Meijer, C.J.; International Agency for Research on Cancer Multicenter Cervical Cancer Study Group. Epidemiologic classification of human papillomavirus types associated with cervical cancer. *N. Engl. J. Med.* **2003**, *348*, 518–527. [CrossRef] [PubMed]
38. Herrero, R.; Castellsague, X.; Pawlita, M.; Lissowska, J.; Kee, F.; Balaram, P.; Rajkumar, T.; Sridhar, H.; Rose, B.; Pintos, J.; *et al.* Human papillomavirus and oral cancer: The international agency for research on cancer multicenter study. *J. Natl. Cancer Inst.* **2003**, *95*, 1772–1783. [CrossRef] [PubMed]
39. Day, P.M.; Schelhaas, M. Concepts of papillomavirus entry into host cells. *Curr. Opin. Virol.* **2014**, *4*, 24–31. [CrossRef] [PubMed]
40. Steinberg, B.M.; Auborn, K.J.; Brandsma, J.L.; Taichman, L.B. Tissue site-specific enhancer function of the upstream regulatory region of human papillomavirus type 11 in cultured keratinocytes. *J. Virol.* **1989**, *63*, 957–960. [PubMed]
41. Ottinger, M.; Smith, J.A.; Schweiger, M.R.; Robbins, D.; Powell, M.L.; You, J.; Howley, P.M. Cell-type specific transcriptional activities among different papillomavirus long control regions and their regulation by E2. *Virology* **2009**, *395*, 161–171. [CrossRef] [PubMed]
42. Mistry, N.; Wibom, C.; Evander, M. Cutaneous and mucosal human papillomaviruses differ in net surface charge, potential impact on tropism. *Virol. J.* **2008**, *5* [CrossRef] [PubMed]
43. Egawa, K.; Inaba, Y.; Yoshimura, K.; Ono, T. Varied clinical morphology of HPV-1-induced warts, depending on anatomical factors. *Br. J. Dermatol.* **1993**, *128*, 271–276. [CrossRef] [PubMed]
44. Trenfield, K.; Spradbrow, P.B.; Vanselow, B. Sequences of papillomavirus DNA in equine sarcoids. *Equine Vet. J.* **1985**, *17*, 449–452. [CrossRef] [PubMed]
45. Otten, N.; von Tscharner, C.; Lazary, S.; Antczak, D.F.; Gerber, H. DNA of bovine papillomavirus type 1 and 2 in equine sarcoids: Pcr detection and direct sequencing. *Arch. Virol.* **1993**, *132*, 121–131. [CrossRef] [PubMed]
46. Angelos, J.A.; Marti, E.; Lazary, S.; Carmichael, L.E. Characterization of BPV-like DNA in equine sarcoids. *Arch. Virol.* **1991**, *119*, 95–109. [CrossRef] [PubMed]

47. Chambers, G.; Ellsmore, V.A.; O'Brien, P.M.; Reid, S.W.; Love, S.; Campo, M.S.; Nasir, L. Association of bovine papillomavirus with the equine sarcoid. *J. Gen. Virol.* **2003**, *84*, 1055–1062. [CrossRef] [PubMed]
48. Rous, P.; Beard, J.W. The progression to carcinoma of virus-induced rabbit papillomas (shope). *J. Exp. Med.* **1935**, *62*, 523–548. [CrossRef] [PubMed]
49. Syverton, J.T. The pathogenesis of the rabbit papilloma-to-carcinoma sequence. *Ann. N. Y. Acad. Sci.* **1952**, *54*, 1126–1140. [CrossRef] [PubMed]
50. Jeckel, S.; Huber, E.; Stubenrauch, F.; Iftner, T. A transactivator function of cottontail rabbit papillomavirus E2 is essential for tumor induction in rabbits. *J. Virol.* **2002**, *76*, 11209–11215. [CrossRef] [PubMed]
51. Meyers, C.; Harry, J.; Lin, Y.L.; Wettstein, F.O. Identification of three transforming proteins encoded by cottontail rabbit papillomavirus. *J. Virol.* **1992**, *66*, 1655–1664. [PubMed]
52. Gjoerup, O.; Chang, Y. Update on human polyomaviruses and cancer. *Adv. Cancer Res.* **2010**, *106*, 1–51. [PubMed]
53. Schlesinger, R.W. Adenoviruses: The nature of the virion and of controlling factors in productive or abortive infection and tumorigenesis. *Adv. Virus Res.* **1969**, *14*, 1–61. [PubMed]
54. Pipas, J.M. SV40: Cell transformation and tumorigenesis. *Virology* **2009**, *384*, 294–303. [CrossRef] [PubMed]
55. Endter, C.; Dobner, T. Cell transformation by human adenoviruses. *Curr. Top. Microbiol. Immunol.* **2004**, *273*, 163–214. [PubMed]
56. Vande Pol, S.B.; Klingelhutz, A.J. Papillomavirus E6 oncoproteins. *Virology* **2013**, *445*, 115–137. [CrossRef] [PubMed]
57. Roman, A.; Munger, K. The papillomavirus E7 proteins. *Virology* **2013**, *445*, 138–168. [CrossRef] [PubMed]
58. Middleton, K.; Peh, W.; Southern, S.; Griffin, H.; Sotlar, K.; Nakahara, T.; El-Sherif, A.; Morris, L.; Seth, R.; Hibma, M.; *et al.* Organization of human papillomavirus productive cycle during neoplastic progression provides a basis for selection of diagnostic markers. *J. Virol.* **2003**, *77*, 10186–10201. [CrossRef] [PubMed]
59. Griffin, H.; Soneji, Y.; van Baars, R.; Arora, R.; Jenkins, D.; van de Sandt, M.; Wu, Z.; Quint, W.; Jach, R.; Okon, K.; *et al.* Stratification of HPV-induced cervical pathology using the virally encoded molecular marker E4 in conbination with p16 or mcm. *Mod. Pathol.* **2015**. in press [CrossRef] [PubMed]
60. Khare, S.; Pater, M.M.; Tang, S.C.; Pater, A. Effect of glucocorticoid hormones on viral gene expression, growth, and dysplastic differentiation in HPV16-immortalized ectocervical cells. *Exp. Cell Res.* **1997**, *232*, 353–360. [CrossRef] [PubMed]
61. Mittal, R.; Tsutsumi, K.; Pater, A.; Pater, M.M. Human papillomavirus type 16 expression in cervical keratinocytes: Role of progesterone and glucocorticoid hormones. *Obstet. Gynecol.* **1993**, *81*, 5–12. [PubMed]
62. Kyo, S.; Inoue, M.; Hayasaka, N.; Inoue, T.; Yutsudo, M.; Tanizawa, O.; Hakura, A. Regulation of early gene expression of human papillomavirus type 16 by inflammatory cytokines. *Virology* **1994**, *200*, 130–139. [CrossRef] [PubMed]

63. Antonsson, A.; Forslund, O.; Ekberg, H.; Sterner, G.; Hansson, B.G. The ubiquity and impressive genomic diversity of human skin papillomaviruses suggest a commensalic nature of these viruses. *J. Virol.* **2000**, *74*, 11636–11641. [CrossRef] [PubMed]
64. Antonsson, A.; Hansson, B.G. Healthy skin of many animal species harbors papillomaviruses which are closely related to their human counterparts. *J. Virol.* **2002**, *76*, 12537–12542. [CrossRef] [PubMed]
65. Maglennon, G.A.; McIntosh, P.; Doorbar, J. Persistence of viral DNA in the epithelial basal layer suggests a model for papillomavirus latency following immune regression. *Virology* **2011**, *414*, 153–163. [CrossRef] [PubMed]
66. Maglennon, G.A.; McIntosh, P.B.; Doorbar, J. Immunosuppression facilitates the reactivation of latent papillomavirus infections. *J. Virol.* **2014**, *88*, 710–716. [CrossRef] [PubMed]
67. Doorbar, J. Latent papillomavirus infections and their regulation. *Curr. Opin. Virol.* **2013**, *3*, 416–421. [CrossRef] [PubMed]
68. Gravitt, P.E. Evidence and impact of human papillomavirus latency. *Open Virol. J.* **2012**, *6*, 198–203. [CrossRef] [PubMed]
69. De Villiers, E.M. Cross-roads in the classification of papillomaviruses. *Virology* **2013**, *445*, 2–10. [CrossRef] [PubMed]
70. Delius, H.; van Ranst, M.A.; Jenson, A.B.; zur Hausen, H.; Sundberg, J.P. Canine oral papillomavirus genomic sequence: A unique 1.5-kb intervening sequence between the E2 and L2 open reading frames. *Virology* **1994**, *204*, 447–452. [CrossRef] [PubMed]
71. Terai, M.; Burk, R.D. Felis domesticus papillomavirus, isolated from a skin lesion, is related to canine oral papillomavirus and contains a 1.3 kb non-coding region between the E2 and L2 open reading frames. *J. Gen. Virol.* **2002**, *83*, 2303–2307. [PubMed]
72. Bergvall, M.; Melendy, T.; Archambault, J. The E1 proteins. *Virology* **2013**, *445*, 35–56. [CrossRef] [PubMed]
73. McBride, A.A. The papillomavirus E2 proteins. *Virology* **2013**, *445*, 57–79. [CrossRef] [PubMed]
74. Wang, J.W.; Roden, R.B. L2, the minor capsid protein of papillomavirus. *Virology* **2013**, *445*, 175–186. [CrossRef] [PubMed]
75. DiMaio, D.; Petti, L.M. The E5 proteins. *Virology* **2013**, *445*, 99–114. [CrossRef] [PubMed]
76. Doorbar, J. The E4 protein; structure, function and patterns of expression. *Virology* **2013**, *445*, 80–98. [CrossRef] [PubMed]
77. Chen, X.S.; Garcea, R.L.; Goldberg, I.; Casini, G.; Harrison, S.C. Structure of small virus-like particles assembled from the L1 protein of human papillomavirus 16. *Mol. Cell* **2000**, *5*, 557–567. [CrossRef]
78. Holmgren, S.C.; Patterson, N.A.; Ozbun, M.A.; Lambert, P.F. The minor capsid protein L2 contributes to two steps in the human papillomavirus type 31 life cycle. *J. Virol.* **2005**, *79*, 3938–3948. [CrossRef] [PubMed]
79. Doorbar, J. The papillomavirus life cycle. *J. Clin. Virol.* **2005**, *32*, S7–S15. [CrossRef] [PubMed]
80. Kines, R.C.; Thompson, C.D.; Lowy, D.R.; Schiller, J.T.; Day, P.M. The initial steps leading to papillomavirus infection occur on the basement membrane prior to cell surface binding. *Proc. Natl. Acad. Sci. USA* **2009** *106*, 20458–20463. [CrossRef] [PubMed]

81. Pyeon, D.; Pearce, S.M.; Lank, S.M.; Ahlquist, P.; Lambert, P.F. Establishment of human papillomavirus infection requires cell cycle progression. *PLoS Pathog.* **2009**, *5*, e1000318. [CrossRef] [PubMed]
82. Parish, J.L.; Bean, A.M.; Park, R.B.; Androphy, E.J. Chlr1 is required for loading papillomavirus E2 onto mitotic chromosomes and viral genome maintenance. *Mol. Cell* **2006**, *24*, 867–876. [CrossRef] [PubMed]
83. Doorbar, J. Molecular biology of human papillomavirus infection and cervical cancer. *Clin. Sci. Lond.* **2006**, *110*, 525–541. [CrossRef] [PubMed]
84. Melendy, T.; Sedman, J.; Stenlund, A. Cellular factors required for papillomavirus DNA replication. *J. Virol.* **1995**, *69*, 7857–7867. [PubMed]
85. White, E.A.; Howley, P.M. Proteomic approaches to the study of papillomavirus-host interactions. *Virology* **2013**, *435*, 57–69. [CrossRef] [PubMed]
86. Yu, J.H.; Lin, B.Y.; Deng, W.; Broker, T.R.; Chow, L.T. Mitogen-activated protein kinases activate the nuclear localization sequence of human papillomavirus type 11 E1 DNA helicase to promote efficient nuclear import. *J. Virol.* **2007**, *81*, 5066–5078. [CrossRef] [PubMed]
87. Fradet-Turcotte, A.; Moody, C.; Laimins, L.A.; Archambault, J. Nuclear export of human papillomavirus type 31 E1 is regulated by CDK2 phosphorylation and required for viral genome maintenance. *J. Virol.* **2010**, *84*, 11747–11760. [CrossRef] [PubMed]
88. McIntosh, P.B.; Laskey, P.; Sullivan, K.; Davy, C.; Wang, Q.; Jackson, D.J.; Griffin, H.M.; Doorbar, J. E1–E4-mediated keratin phosphorylation and ubiquitylation: A mechanism for keratin depletion in HPV16-infected epithelium. *J. Cell Sci.* **2010**, *123*, 2810–2822. [CrossRef] [PubMed]
89. McIntosh, P.B.; Martin, S.R.; Jackson, D.J.; Khan, J.; Isaacson, E.R.; Calder, L.; Raj, K.; Griffin, H.M.; Wang, Q.; Laskey, P.; *et al.* Structural analysis reveals an amyloid form of the human papillomavirus type 16 E1–E4 protein and provides a molecular basis for its accumulation. *J. Virol.* **2008**, *82*, 8196–8203. [CrossRef] [PubMed]
90. Nicholls, P.; Klaunberg, B.; Moore, R.A.; Santos, E.B.; Parry, N.R.; Gough, G.W.; Stanley, M.A. Naturally occurring, nonregressing canine oral papillomavirus infection: Host immunity, virus characterization, and experimental infection. *Virology* **1999**, *265*, 365–374. [CrossRef] [PubMed]
91. Wilgenburg, B.J.; Budgeon, L.R.; Lang, C.M.; Griffith, J.W.; Christensen, N.D. Characterization of immune responses during regression of rabbit oral papillomavirus infections. *Comp. Med.* **2005**, *55*, 431–439. [PubMed]
92. Nicholls, P.K.; Moore, P.F.; Anderson, D.M.; Moore, R.A.; Parry, N.R.; Gough, G.W.; Stanley, M.A. Regression of canine oral papillomas is associated with infiltration of CD4+ and CD8+ lymphocytes. *Virology* **2001**, *283*, 31–39. [CrossRef] [PubMed]
93. Coleman, N.; Birley, H.D.; Renton, A.M.; Hanna, N.F.; Ryait, B.K.; Byrne, M.; Taylor-Robinson, D.; Stanley, M.A. Immunological events in regressing genital warts. *Am. J. Clin. Pathol.* **1994**, *102*, 768–774. [PubMed]
94. Monnier-Benoit, S.; Mauny, F.; Riethmuller, D.; Guerrini, J.S.; Capilna, M.; Felix, S.; Seilles, E.; Mougin, C.; Pretet, J.L. Immunohistochemical analysis of CD4+ and CD8+ T-cell subsets in high risk human papillomavirus-associated pre-malignant and malignant lesions of the uterine cervix.

Gynecol. Oncol. **2006**, *102*, 22–31. [CrossRef] [PubMed]

95. Stanley, M.A. Epithelial cell responses to infection with human papillomavirus. *Clin. Microbiol. Rev.* **2012**, *25*, 215–222. [CrossRef] [PubMed]
96. Kanodia, S.; Fahey, L.M.; Kast, W.M. Mechanisms used by human papillomaviruses to escape the host immune response. *Curr. Cancer Drug Targets* **2007**, *7*, 79–89. [CrossRef] [PubMed]
97. Egawa, K. Do human papillomaviruses target epidermal stem cells? *Dermatology* **2003**, *207*, 251–254. [CrossRef] [PubMed]
98. Herfs, M.; Vargas, S.O.; Yamamoto, Y.; Howitt, B.E.; Nucci, M.R.; Hornick, J.L.; McKeon, F.D.; Xian, W.; Crum, C.P. A novel blueprint for "top down" differentiation defines the cervical squamocolumnar junction during development, reproductive life, and neoplasia. *J. Pathol.* **2013**, *229*, 460–468. [CrossRef] [PubMed]
99. Herfs, M.; Yamamoto, Y.; Laury, A.; Wang, X.; Nucci, M.R.; McLaughlin-Drubin, M.E.; Munger, K.; Feldman, S.; McKeon, F.D.; Xian, W.; *et al.* A discrete population of squamocolumnar junction cells implicated in the pathogenesis of cervical cancer. *Proc. Natl. Acad. Sci. USA* **2012**, *109*, 10516–10521. [CrossRef] [PubMed]
100. Watt, F.M. Epidermal stem cells: Markers, patterning and the control of stem cell fate. *Philos. Trans. R. Soc. Lond. Ser. B Biol. Sci.* **1998**, *353*, 831–837. [CrossRef] [PubMed]
101. Potten, C.S. Cell replacement in epidermis (keratopoiesis) via discrete units of proliferation. *Int. Rev. Cytol.* **1981**, *69*, 271–318. [PubMed]
102. Feuerman, E. Verruca vulgaris—Benign tumor of viral etiology and clonal development. *Harefuah* **1972**, *83*, 211–212. [PubMed]
103. Schmitt, A.; Rochat, A.; Zeltner, R.; Borenstein, L.; Barrandon, Y.; Wettstein, F.O.; Iftner, T. The primary target cells of the high-risk cottontail rabbit papillomavirus colocalize with hair follicle stem cells. *J. Virol.* **1996**, *70*, 1912–1922. [PubMed]
104. Martens, J.E.; Smedts, F.M.; Ploeger, D.; Helmerhorst, T.J.; Ramaekers, F.C.; Arends, J.W.; Hopman, A.H. Distribution pattern and marker profile show two subpopulations of reserve cells in the endocervical canal. *Int. J. Gynecol. Pathol.* **2009**, *28*, 381–388. [CrossRef] [PubMed]
105. Mirkovic, J.; Howitt, B.E.; Roncarati, P.; Demoulin, S.; Suarez-Carmona, M.; Hubert, P.; McKeon, F.D.; Xian, W.; Li, A.; Delvenne, P.; *et al.* Carcinogenic HPV infection in the cervical squamo-columnar junction. *J. Pathol.* **2015**, *236*, 265–271. [CrossRef] [PubMed]
106. Isaacson Wechsler, E.; Wang, Q.; Roberts, I.; Pagliarulo, E.; Jackson, D.; Untersperger, C.; Coleman, N.; Griffin, H.; Doorbar, J. Reconstruction of human papillomavirus type 16-mediated early-stage neoplasia implicates E6/E7 deregulation and the loss of contact inhibition in neoplastic progression. *J. Virol.* **2012**, *86*, 6358–6364. [CrossRef] [PubMed]
107. Cotsarelis, G.; Sun, T.T.; Lavker, R.M. Label-retaining cells reside in the bulge area of pilosebaceous unit: Implications for follicular stem cells, hair cycle, and skin carcinogenesis. *Cell* **1990**, *61*, 1329–1337. [CrossRef]
108. Cotsarelis, G. Epithelial stem cells: A folliculocentric view. *J. Investig. Dermatol.* **2006**, *126*, 1459–1468. [CrossRef] [PubMed]
109. Ghazizadeh, S.; Taichman, L.B. Organization of stem cells and their progeny in human epidermis. *J. Investig. Dermatol.* **2005**, *124*, 367–372. [CrossRef] [PubMed]

110. Taylor, G.; Lehrer, M.S.; Jensen, P.J.; Sun, T.T.; Lavker, R.M. Involvement of follicular stem cells in forming not only the follicle but also the epidermis. *Cell* **2000**, *102*, 451–461. [CrossRef]
111. Ito, M.; Liu, Y.; Yang, Z.; Nguyen, J.; Liang, F.; Morris, R.J.; Cotsarelis, G. Stem cells in the hair follicle bulge contribute to wound repair but not to homeostasis of the epidermis. *Nat. Med.* **2005**, *11*, 1351–1354. [CrossRef] [PubMed]
112. Kaur, P. Interfollicular epidermal stem cells: Identification, challenges, potential. *J. Investig. Dermatol.* **2006**, *126*, 1450–1458. [CrossRef] [PubMed]
113. Braun, K.M.; Niemann, C.; Jensen, U.B.; Sundberg, J.P.; Silva-Vargas, V.; Watt, F.M. Manipulation of stem cell proliferation and lineage commitment: Visualisation of label-retaining cells in wholemounts of mouse epidermis. *Development* **2003**, *130*, 5241–5255. [CrossRef] [PubMed]
114. Lavker, R.M.; Sun, T.T. Epidermal stem cells. *J. Investig. Dermatol.* **1983**, *81*, 121s–127s. [CrossRef] [PubMed]
115. Ghazizadeh, S.; Taichman, L.B. Multiple classes of stem cells in cutaneous epithelium: A lineage analysis of adult mouse skin. *EMBO J.* **2001**, *20*, 1215–1222. [CrossRef] [PubMed]
116. Miller, S.J.; Burke, E.M.; Rader, M.D.; Coulombe, P.A.; Lavker, R.M. Re-epithelialization of porcine skin by the sweat apparatus. *J. Investig. Dermatol.* **1998**, *110*, 13–19. [CrossRef] [PubMed]
117. Lu, C.P.; Polak, L.; Rocha, A.S.; Pasolli, H.A.; Chen, S.C.; Sharma, N.; Blanpain, C.; Fuchs, E. Identification of stem cell populations in sweat glands and ducts reveals roles in homeostasis and wound repair. *Cell* **2012**, *150*, 136–150. [CrossRef] [PubMed]
118. Jablonska, S.; Dabrowski, J.; Jakubowicz, K. Epidermodysplasia verruciformis as a model in studies on the role of papovaviruses in oncogenesis. *Cancer Res.* **1972**, *32*, 583–589. [PubMed]
119. Orth, G. Genetics of epidermodysplasia verruciformis: Insights into host defense against papillomaviruses. *Semin. Immunol.* **2006**, *18*, 362–374. [CrossRef] [PubMed]
120. Lazarczyk, M.; Dalard, C.; Hayder, M.; Dupre, L.; Pignolet, B.; Majewski, S.; Vuillier, F.; Favre, M.; Liblau, R.S. Ever proteins, key elements of the natural anti-human papillomavirus barrier, are regulated upon t-cell activation. *PLoS ONE* **2012**, *7*, e39995. [CrossRef] [PubMed]
121. Boxman, I.L.; Berkhout, R.J.; Mulder, L.H.; Wolkers, M.C.; Bouwes Bavinck, J.N.; Vermeer, B.J.; ter Schegget, J. Detection of human papillomavirus DNA in plucked hairs from renal transplant recipients and healthy volunteers. *J. Investig. Dermatol.* **1997**, *108*, 712–715. [CrossRef] [PubMed]
122. Boxman, I.L.; Mulder, L.H.; Russell, A.; Bouwes Bavinck, J.N.; Green, A.; Ter Schegget, J. Human papillomavirus type 5 is commonly present in immunosuppressed and immunocompetent individuals. *Br. J. Dermatol.* **1999**, *141*, 246–249. [CrossRef] [PubMed]
123. Jablonska, S.; Orth, G.; Obalek, S.; Croissant, O. Cutaneous warts. Clinical, histologic, and virologic correlations. *Clin. Dermatol.* **1985**, *3*, 71–82. [CrossRef]
124. Egawa, K. Eccrine-centred distribution of human papillomavirus 63 infection in the epidermis of the plantar skin. *Br. J. Dermatol.* **2005**, *152*, 993–996. [CrossRef] [PubMed]
125. Boxman, I.L.; Hogewoning, A.; Mulder, L.H.; Bouwes Bavinck, J.N.; ter Schegget, J. Detection of human papillomavirus types 6 and 11 in pubic and perianal hair from patients with genital warts. *J. Clin. Microbiol.* **1999**, *37*, 2270–2273. [PubMed]

126. Kocjan, B.J.; Poljak, M.; Seme, K.; Potocnik, M.; Fujs, K.; Babic, D.Z. Distribution of human papillomavirus genotypes in plucked eyebrow hairs from slovenian males with genital warts. *Infect. Genet. Evol. J. Mol. Epidemiol. Evol. Genet. Infect. Dis.* **2005**, *5*, 255–259. [CrossRef] [PubMed]
127. Javier, R.T. Cell polarity proteins: Common targets for tumorigenic human viruses. *Oncogene* **2008**, *27*, 7031–7046. [CrossRef] [PubMed]
128. Kranjec, C.; Banks, L. A systematic analysis of human papillomavirus (HPV) E6 pdz substrates identifies magi-1 as a major target of HPV type 16 (HPV-16) and HPV-18 whose loss accompanies disruption of tight junctions. *J. Virol.* **2011**, *85*, 1757–1764. [CrossRef] [PubMed]
129. Massimi, P.; Narayan, N.; Thomas, M.; Gammoh, N.; Strand, S.; Strand, D.; Banks, L. Regulation of the hdlg/hscrib/hugl-1 tumour suppressor complex. *Exp. Cell Res.* **2008**, *314*, 3306–3317. [CrossRef] [PubMed]
130. Pim, D.; Bergant, M.; Boon, S.S.; Ganti, K.; Kranjec, C.; Massimi, P.; Subbaiah, V.K.; Thomas, M.; Tomaic, V.; Banks, L. Human papillomaviruses and the specificity of pdz domain targeting. *FEBS J.* **2012**, *279*, 3530–3537. [CrossRef] [PubMed]
131. Thomas, M.; Dasgupta, J.; Zhang, Y.; Chen, X.; Banks, L. Analysis of specificity determinants in the interactions of different HPV E6 proteins with their pdz domain-containing substrates. *Virology* **2008**, *376*, 371–378. [CrossRef] [PubMed]
132. Fu, L.; van Doorslaer, K.; Chen, Z.; Ristriani, T.; Masson, M.; Trave, G.; Burk, R.D. Degradation of p53 by human alphapapillomavirus E6 proteins shows a stronger correlation with phylogeny than oncogenicity. *PLoS ONE* **2010**, *5*, e12816. [CrossRef] [PubMed]
133. Zanier, K.; ould M'hamed ould Sidi, A.; Boulade-Ladame, C.; Rybin, V.; Chappelle, A.; Atkinson, A.; Kieffer, B.; Trave, G. Solution structure analysis of the HPV16 E6 oncoprotein reveals a self-association mechanism required for E6-mediated degradation of p53. *Structure* **2012**, *20*, 604–617. [CrossRef] [PubMed]
134. Pim, D.; Banks, L. Interaction of viral oncoproteins with cellular target molecules: Infection with high-risk *vs.* low-risk human papillomaviruses. *Apmis* **2010**, *118*, 471–493. [CrossRef] [PubMed]
135. Zheng, Z.M.; Baker, C.C. Papillomavirus genome structure, expression, and post-transcriptional regulation. *Front. Biosci.* **2006**, *11*, 2286–2302. [CrossRef] [PubMed]
136. Westra, W.H. The morphologic profile of HPV-related head and neck squamous carcinoma: Implications for diagnosis, prognosis, and clinical management. *Head Neck Pathol.* **2012**, *6*, S48–S54. [CrossRef] [PubMed]
137. Parkin, D.M. The global health burden of infection-associated cancers in the year 2002. *Int. J. Cancer J. Int. Cancer* **2006**, *118*, 3030–3044. [CrossRef] [PubMed]
138. Munoz, N.; Bosch, F.X.; Castellsague, X.; Diaz, M.; de Sanjose, S.; Hammouda, D.; Shah, K.V.; Meijer, C.J. Against which human papillomavirus types shall we vaccinate and screen? The international perspective. *Int. J. Cancer J. Int. Cancer* **2004**, *111*, 278–285. [CrossRef] [PubMed]
139. Gross, G.; Hagedorn, M.; Ikenberg, H.; Rufli, T.; Dahlet, C.; Grosshans, E.; Gissmann, L. Bowenoid papulosis. Presence of human papillomavirus (HPV) structural antigens and of HPV 16-related DNA sequences. *Arch. Dermatol.* **1985**, *121*, 858–863. [CrossRef] [PubMed]
140. Tschandl, P.; Rosendahl, C.; Kittler, H. Cutaneous human papillomavirus infection: Manifestations and diagnosis. *Curr. Probl. Dermatol.* **2014**, *45*, 92–97. [PubMed]

4

Activation of DNA Damage Response Pathways during Lytic Replication of KSHV

Robert Hollingworth [1], George L. Skalka [1], Grant S. Stewart [1], Andrew D. Hislop [1], David J. Blackbourn [2] and Roger J. Grand [1,*]

[1] School of Cancer Sciences, the College of Medicine and Dentistry, University of Birmingham, Birmingham B15 2TT, UK; E-Mails: rxh291@student.bham.ac.uk (R.H.); gls210@student.bham.ac.uk (G.L.S.); g.s.stewart@bham.ac.uk (G.S.S.); a.d.hislop@bham.ac.uk (A.D.H.)

[2] School of Biosciences and Medicine, University of Surrey, Surrey GU2 7XH, UK; E-Mail: d.blackbourn@surrey.ac.uk

* Author to whom correspondence should be addressed; E-Mail: r.j.a.grand@bham.ac.uk;

Academic Editor: Eric O. Freed

Abstract: Kaposi's sarcoma-associated herpesvirus (KSHV) is the causative agent of several human malignancies. Human tumour viruses such as KSHV are known to interact with the DNA damage response (DDR), the molecular pathways that recognise and repair lesions in cellular DNA. Here it is demonstrated that lytic reactivation of KSHV leads to activation of the ATM and DNA-PK DDR kinases resulting in phosphorylation of multiple downstream substrates. Inhibition of ATM results in the reduction of overall levels of viral replication while inhibition of DNA-PK increases activation of ATM and leads to earlier viral release. There is no activation of the ATR-CHK1 pathway following lytic replication and CHK1 phosphorylation is inhibited at later times during the lytic cycle. Despite evidence of double-strand breaks and phosphorylation of H2AX, 53BP1 foci are not consistently observed in cells containing lytic virus although RPA32 and MRE11 localise to sites of viral DNA synthesis. Activation of the DDR following KSHV lytic reactivation does not result in a G1 cell cycle block and cells are able to proceed to S-phase during the lytic cycle. KSHV appears then to selectively activate DDR pathways, modulate cell cycle progression and recruit DDR proteins to sites of viral replication during the lytic cycle.

Keywords: Kaposi's sarcoma-associated herpesvirus; KSHV; DNA damage response; DDR; lytic replication; ATM; ATR; DNA-PK

1. Introduction

Kaposi's sarcoma-associated herpesvirus (KSHV) is a γ-2 herpesvirus identified as the etiological agent of several human malignancies. Transformation of endothelial cells by KSHV is associated with the development of Kaposi's sarcoma (KS) [1], while infection of B cells can lead to the lymphoproliferative diseases primary effusion lymphoma (PEL) and multicentric Castleman's disease (MCD) [2,3].

Like all herpesviruses, KSHV has a double-stranded DNA genome and a biphasic lifecycle that consists of latent and lytic stages. During latent infection, the virus persists as an extrachromosomal episome that is replicated by host replication machinery. Latency is characterised by expression of a limited subset of viral genes required for episomal maintenance and immune evasion that include the latency-associated nuclear antigen (LANA). In order to propagate, the virus must switch to the lytic phase, during which the majority of viral genes are expressed, viral DNA is amplified and infectious virus is released following lysis of the host cell. The viral replication and transcription activator (RTA), encoded by open reading frame 50 (ORF50), is a lytic switch protein as expression is necessary and sufficient for initiation of the full lytic replication programme [4]. Lytic viral genes are expressed in an ordered cascade and the lytic cycle can be divided into several stages that include immediate-early gene expression, delayed-early gene expression, viral DNA amplification, late gene expression and finally, assembly and release of infectious virions [5]. Significantly, lytic replication has been shown to play a major role in the progression of KSHV-related malignancies [6,7].

The DNA damage response (DDR) has evolved to respond to the multitude of lesions inflicted on cellular DNA by both endogenous biological processes and exogenous agents. Three phosphoinositide-3-kinase-related kinases (PIKKs), ataxia telangiectasia mutated (ATM), ATM- and Rad3-related (ATR) and DNA-dependent protein kinase (DNA-PK), can orchestrate activation of the DDR via phosphorylation of multiple target proteins involved in cell cycle regulation, apoptosis and DNA repair. ATM and DNA-PK are primarily activated following formation of double-strand breaks (DSBs) in DNA. DSBs are recognised and bound by the MRE11-RAD50-NBS1 (MRN) complex that facilitates ATM recruitment and activation. ATM subsequently activates effector molecules that include H2AX, CHK2, KAP1, SMC1 and NBS1 that mediate cell cycle arrest and DNA repair. DNA-PK is a core component of the non-homologous end-joining (NHEJ) pathway that acts throughout the cell cycle to repair DSBs [8]. DNA-PK is activated after the Ku70/Ku80 heterodimer binds DNA ends and recruits the DNA-PK catalytic subunit (DNA-PKcs) to form the DNA-PK holoenzyme that is critical for completion of NHEJ [9]. In conjunction with ATR, DNA-PK also plays a role in maintaining genome stability following replication stress [10]. ATR is activated by a number of different lesions that result in persistent single-stranded DNA (ssDNA) that is first coated by replication protein A (RPA) before recruitment of ATR via its binding partner, ATR-interacting protein (ATRIP) [11]. The recruitment of DNA topoisomerase 2-binding protein 1 (TOPBP1) contributes to activation of ATR which subsequently orchestrates activation of cell cycle checkpoints via phosphorylation of CHK1 [12,13].

Several species of herpesvirus are known to interact with the DDR during their lifecycles. These interactions can involve the selective activation and deactivation of DDR pathways and the use of specific DDR proteins in the replication of viral genomes. Since the DDR has evolved to protect the genome from the accumulation of harmful mutations, the modulation of these pathways by human tumour viruses may contribute to the malignant transformation of host cells. KSHV has previously been shown to activate the DDR during *de novo* infection of primary endothelial cells and this plays a role in establishing latency [14]. More recently, it has been demonstrated that lytic replication of KSHV in B cells results in increased phosphorylation of H2AX, a sensitive marker for the presence of DNA damage [15,16].

It has also been demonstrated that expression of immediate-early lytic protein ORF57 alone can cause DNA damage through sequestration of the hTREX complex leading to R-loop formation and ultimately DSBs [16]. Here a more detailed assessment of DDR pathways activated during lytic replication of KSHV is presented and the effect of inhibition of the major DDR kinases on replication of viral DNA is examined. In addition, changes in the localisation of several DDR proteins in cells containing lytic virus is assessed.

2. Materials and Methods

2.1. Cell Culture

TRE-BCBL-1-RTA cells (generously provided by Jae Jung, USC, Los Angeles, CA, USA) and BCBL-1 cells were cultured in RPMI (Sigma, St. Louis, MO, USA) supplemented with 10% fetal bovine serum (FBS) (Sigma) and 1% penicillin-streptomycin (Gibco, Grand Island, NY, USA). TRE-BCBL-1-RTA cells were also cultured in the presence of 100 μg/mL of Hygromycin B (Roche, Burgess Hill, UK). The endothelial cell line, EA.hy926 (purchased from ATCC, Manassas, VA, USA), was grown in DMEM (Sigma) supplemented with 10% FBS and 1% penicillin-streptomycin. EA.hy926-RTA cells, transduced with an Inducer 20 lentivirus [17] which expresses RTA under the control of the tetracycline promoter, were cultured in the presence of 250 μg/mL of G418 (Sigma). rKSHV-EA.hy926-RTA cells, which contain the RTA expression construct and are also infected with recombinant rKSHV.219 virus [18], were cultured in the presence of 250 μg/mL of G418 and 1 μg/mL Puromycin (Sigma).

2.2. Induction of Lytic Reactivation in KSHV-Infected Cell Lines

To assess DDR activation in response to KSHV lytic reactivation, TRE-BCBL-1-RTA cells and rKSHV-EA.hy926-RTA cells, as well as corresponding controls, were treated with 0.5 μg/mL doxycycline (Sigma) and subsequently harvested at the indicated times for western blot analysis. To generate positive controls for DDR activation, TRE-BCBL-1-RTA cells were either exposed to 6 Gy ionising radiation (IR) and harvested after 1 h or exposed to 20 Jm^{-2} ultraviolet light (UV) and harvested after 6 h. To inhibit viral DNA synthesis, TRE-BCBL-1-RTA cells were first treated with 100 μM ganciclovir (Cayman Chemical, Ann Arbor, MI, USA) for 2 h prior to the addition of 0.5 μg/mL doxycycline.

2.3. *Inhibition of DDR Kinases during Lytic Replication*

The ATR inhibitor VE-821, ATM inhibitor KU55933 and DNA-PK inhibitor NU7441 were purchased from Tocris Bioscience (Bristol, UK). TRE-BCBL-1-RTA cells were treated with specified concentrations of kinase inhibitors, or equivalent DMSO control, 1 h prior to the addition of 0.5 μg/mL doxycycline. Cells were harvested after 24 and 48 h for western blot or immunofluorescence microscopy analysis while supernatants were collected and stored at 4 °C for assessment of infectious virus production.

2.4. *Infection of EA.hy926 Cells with TRE-BCBL-1-RTA-Derived KSHV Virus*

Supernatants collected from TRE-BCBL-1-RTA cells were added to EA.hy926 cells cultured in 6-well plates or on coverslips in 24-well plates. Cells were centrifuged (330× *g*, 20 min, ambient temperature) and following 4 h incubation at 37 °C, medium containing virus was removed and replaced with supplemented DMEM medium. After 48 h, cells were harvested for western blot analysis or fixed for immunofluorescence microscopy analysis of LANA expression.

2.5. *Cell Cycle Analysis*

Propidium iodide (PI) staining was used to determine cell cycle distribution in TRE-BCBL-1-RTA cells. Cells were treated with 100 μM ganciclovir for 1 h followed by DDR kinase inhibitors or DMSO for 1 h prior to addition of 0.5 μg/mL doxycycline. TRE-BCBL-1-RTA cells treated with ganciclovir and DMSO but not doxycycline were used as un-reactivated controls. At each time point specified, cells were washed in phosphate buffered saline (PBS) and fixed in cold 70% ethanol before storage at −20 °C. Following two PBS washes, cells were treated with PBS containing RNase A (20 μg/mL) (Sigma) and PI (10 μg/mL) (Sigma) before being analysed using an Accuri C6 flow cytometer (BD, Oxford, UK).

2.6. *Immunofluorescence Microscopy (IF)*

Following treatment with 0.5 μg/mL doxycycline for 24 h, TRE-BCBL-1-RTA cells were washed in PBS and allowed to adhere on poly-L-lysine coated glass slides (Sigma). EA.hy926-RTA cells, cultured on coverslips, were infected with KSHV derived from TRE-BCBL-1-RTA cells as described above. After 48 h, EA.hy926-RTA cells were treated with 0.5 μg/mL doxycycline for 24 h. Both cell lines were fixed with 4% paraformaldehyde and permeabilised with 0.5% Triton X-100. Cells were then blocked in 10% heat-inactivated goat serum (HINGS) before addition of primary antibodies diluted in 10% HINGS for 1 h. Cells were washed 3 times in PBS before addition of appropriate secondary antibodies diluted in 10% HINGS for 1 h. Following three PBS washes, cells were stained with DAPI nucleic acid stain (Life Technologies, Grand Island, NY, USA) and cover slides were applied using ProLong Gold antifade reagent (Life Technologies). Images were taken on a Leica DM6000B epifluorescence microscope with Leica Application Suite Advanced Fluorescence software (LAS AF) (Leica, Milton Keynes, UK).

For BrdU staining, TRE-BCBL-1-RTA cells were treated with 10 μl BrdU (Sigma) for 1 h prior to adherence on poly-L-lysine coated glass slides. Cells were then fixed in 70% ethanol for 30 min followed by treatment with 0.07 M NaOH for 2 min prior to addition of FITC-conjugated BrdU antibody for 30 min. Visualisation of viral proteins was then carried out as above.

The following primary antibodies were used for immunofluorescence microscopy: anti-γH2AX (S139) (05-636, Merck Millipore, Billerica, MA, USA), anti-RPA32 (NA19L, Calbiochem, Billerica, MA, USA), anti-MRE11 (GTX70212, Genetex, Irvine, USA), anti-53BP1 (ab36823, Abcam, Cambridge, UK), anti-K8α (SAB5300152, Sigma), anti-ORF6 (Provided by Gary Hayward) anti-ORF59 (in house), anti-LANA (NCL-HHV8-LNA, Novacastra, Newcastle, UK), anti-BrdU (347583, BD).

2.7. Western Blot Analysis

Lysates were prepared by re-suspending cell pellets in 8 M urea, 50 mM Tris HCl (pH 7.4) buffer containing 1% β-mercaptoethanol. Samples were then sonicated, centrifuged (16,300× *g*, 20 min, 4 °C) and stored at −80 °C. Protein determination was carried using Bradford reagent (Bio-Rad, Hercules, CA, USA) and protein standards of known concentration. Lysates were then subjected to Sodium Dodecyl Sulphate-Polyacrylamide Gel Electrophoresis (SDS-PAGE).

The following primary antibodies were used for Western blotting: anti-DNA-PKcs (04-1024, Merck Millipore), anti-phospho-DNA-PKcs (S2056) (ab124918, Abcam), anti-ATM (2873, Cell Signaling, Danvers, MA, USA), anti-phospho-ATM (S1981) (AF1655, R&D Systems, Minneapolis, MN, USA), anti-SMC1 (A300-055A, Bethyl, Montgomery, AL, USA) anti-phospho-SMC1 (S966) (A300-050A, Bethyl), anti-KAP1 (A300-274A, Bethyl), anti-phospho-KAP1 (S824) (A300-767A, Bethyl), anti-NBS1 (ab23996, Abcam), anti-phospho-NBS1 (S343) (ab47272, Abcam), anti-CHK1 (sc-8408, Santa Cruz, Dallas, TX, USA), anti-phospho-CHK1 (S345) (2341, Cell Signaling), anti-phospho-CHK1 (S317) (2344, Cell signaling), anti-CHK2 (2662, Cell Signaling), anti-phospho-CHK2 (T68) (2661, Cell Signaling), anti-RPA32 (NA19L, Calbiochem), anti-phospho-RPA32 (S4/S8) (A300-245A, Bethyl), anti-phospho-RPA32 (S33) (ab87278, Abcam), anti-H2AX (7631, Cell Signaling), anti-γH2AX (S139) (05-636, Merck Millipore), anti-β-Actin (A2228, Sigma), anti-LANA (NCL-HHV8-LNA, Novacastra), anti-RTA (in house), anti-ORF57 (AP15004a, Abgent, San Diego, CA, USA), anti-K8.1A (in house).

The following HRP conjugated secondary antibodies were also used: Polyclonal Goat Anti-Mouse (Dako Laboratories, Glostrup, Denmark), polyclonal Swine Anti-Rabbit (Dako Laboratories) and polyclonal Rabbit Anti-Goat (Dako Laboratories). Proteins were visualised using a Fusion SL chemiluminescence imaging system (Vilber Lourmat, Marne-la-Vallée, France).

3. Results

3.1. Lytic Reactivation of KSHV in B Cells Activates DDR Pathways

Analysis of DDR pathway activation during KSHV lytic replication was initially performed on a derivative of the BCBL-1 PEL line that is latently infected with KSHV. These cells, called TRE-BCBL-1-RTA, have been modified to include the ORF50/RTA gene under the control of a tetracycline promoter [19]. Addition of doxycycline to TRE-BCBL-1-RTA cells reactivates KSHV into the lytic cycle resulting in expression of immediate-early lytic proteins such as ORF57 followed by late proteins such as envelope glycoprotein K8.1A and eventually release of infectious virions (Figure 1A). Using this cell line and control BCBL-1 cells lacking the RTA-expression construct, levels of phosphorylated DDR proteins were assessed by western blotting at 5 time points following addition of doxycycline. TRE-BCBL1-RTA cells exposed to either IR or UV were used as positive controls for

DDR activation. Addition of doxycycline to control BCBL-1 cells did not result in phosphorylation of any of the DDR proteins examined. While addition of doxycycline to TRE-BCBL-1-RTA cells resulted in minimal phosphorylation of SMC1 and CHK1 compared with IR and UV treated controls, after 12 h there was a notable increase in levels of phosphorylated ATM, DNA-PKcs, CHK2, KAP1, NBS1, RPA32 and H2AX indicating widespread activation of the DDR during the KSHV lytic cycle (Figure 1B).

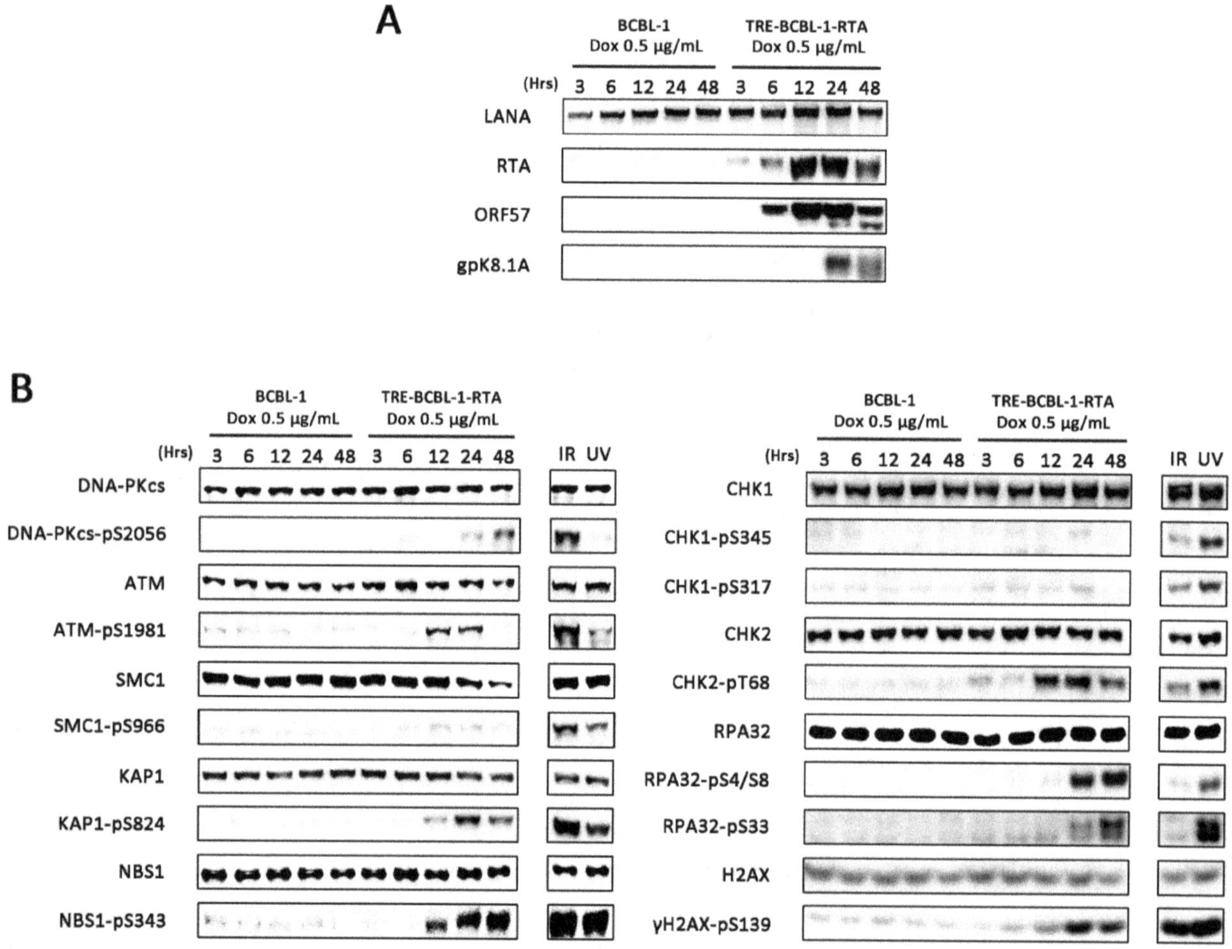

Figure 1. Activation of the DDR during lytic replication of KSHV in TRE-BCBL-1-RTA cells. (**A**) Expression of immediate-early lytic proteins RTA and ORF57 and late lytic glycoprotein K8.1A in TRE-BCBL-1-RTA cells following addition of 0.5 µg/mL doxycycline; (**B**) Phosphorylation of DDR proteins in TRE-BCBL-1-RTA cells following addition of 0.5 µg/mL doxycycline. TRE-BCBL-1-RTA cells treated with ionising radiation (IR) and ultraviolet light (UV) represent positive controls for DDR activation.

3.2. Amplification of Viral DNA and Late Viral Gene Expression Is Not Required for DDR Activation

To determine whether amplification of viral DNA or late viral gene expression is required for DDR activation in TRE-BCBL-1-RTA cells, the antiviral compound ganciclovir was employed. Ganciclovir inhibits viral DNA synthesis without affecting the expression of early lytic proteins or replication of host DNA [20]. TRE-BCBL-1-RTA cells were treated with and without 100 µM ganciclovir prior to the addition of doxycycline. Cells were also treated with ganciclovir alone to ensure that this compound in isolation did not activate the DDR. To ensure that ganciclovir was efficiently inhibiting production of infectious virus, TRE-BCBL-1-RTA supernatants from each condition were collected after 48 h and used to infect EA.hy926 cells. Expression of LANA was assessed by immunofluorescence microscopy as a marker of KSHV infection. Minimal LANA expression was observed in EA.hy926 cells infected with supernatants from TRE-BCBL-1-RTA cells treated with doxycycline and ganciclovir or ganciclovir alone (Figure 2A). Western blots confirmed that the cells treated with ganciclovir and doxycycline expressed the immediate-early lytic proteins RTA and ORF57 but not the late envelope glycoprotein K8.1A (Figure 2B). Levels of phosphorylated H2AX and RPA32 were unchanged in the doxycycline-treated cells despite the presence of ganciclovir suggesting that DDR activation is mediated by early viral gene expression and does not require amplification of viral DNA or expression of late lytic proteins.

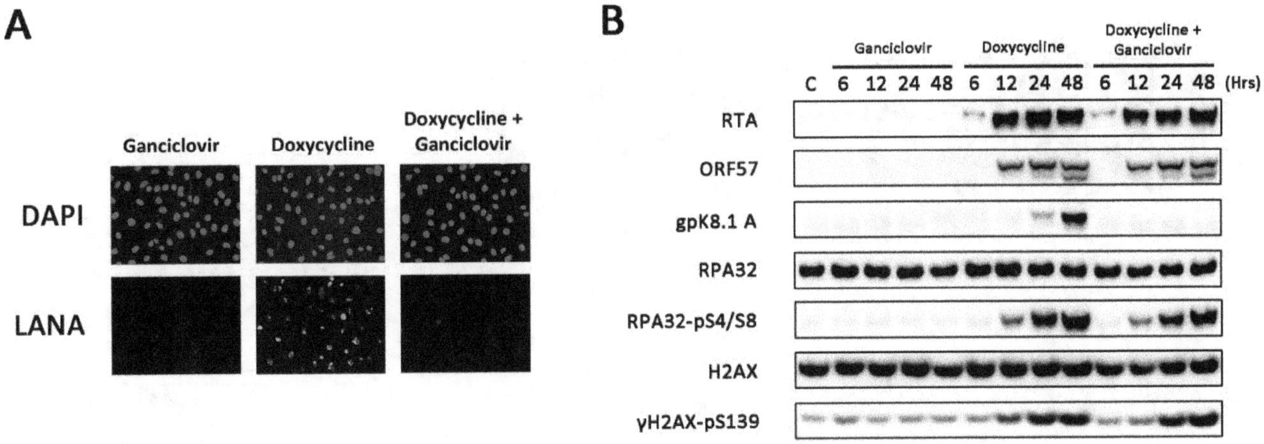

Figure 2. DDR activation following inhibition of viral DNA synthesis and late viral gene expression. (**A**) Immunofluorescence microscopy analysis of LANA expression in EA.hy926 cells following infection with supernatants obtained from TRE-BCBL-1-RTA cells collected 48 h after treatment with 100 μM ganciclovir alone, 0.5 μg/mL doxycycline alone or both compounds in combination; (**B**) Phosphorylation of RPA32 and H2AX in TRE-BCBL-1-RTA cells treated with 100 μM ganciclovir alone, 0.5 μg/mL doxycycline alone or both compounds in combination.

3.3. Inhibition of DDR Kinases Results in Alterations in Production of Infectious Virus

To determine what effect inhibition of DDR kinases has on production of infectious virus, TRE-BCBL-1-RTA cells were treated with two concentrations of ATR, ATM and DNA-PK inhibitors or an equivalent concentration of DMSO 1 h prior to the addition of 0.5 μg/mL doxycycline. After 24 and 48 h, expression of late lytic glycoprotein K8.1A was initially assessed as an indicator of completed viral replication (Figure 3A). At 24 h, expression of K8.1A was relatively low compared to 48 h but was clearly elevated following inhibition of DNA-PK. After 48 h, expression was similar between the DMSO-treated and DNA-PK inhibitor-treated cells but clearly reduced in the cells treated with the higher concentrations of ATR and ATM inhibitors.

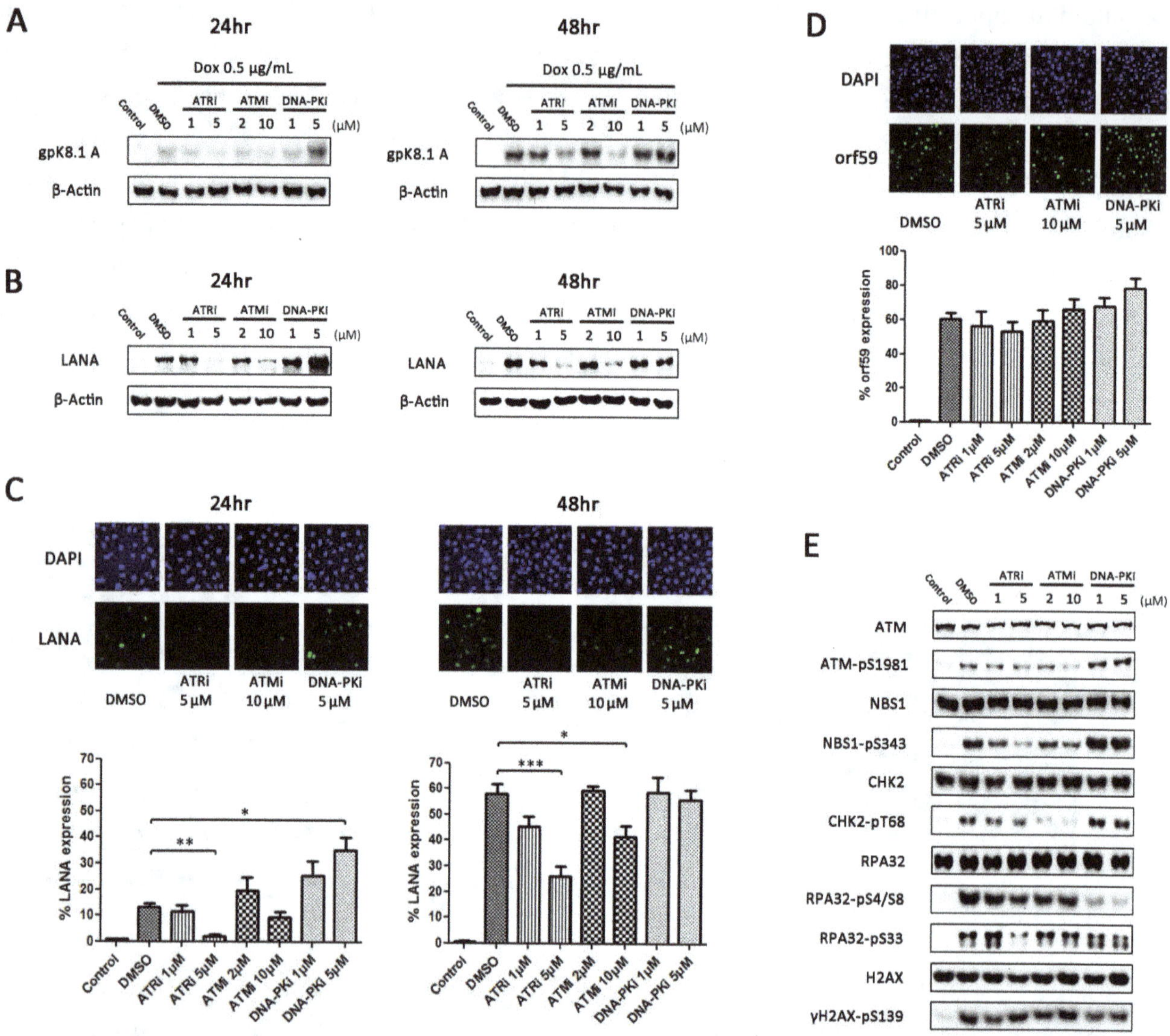

Figure 3. Effect of DDR inhibition on production of infectious virus. (**A**) Expression of late lytic glycoprotein K8.1A in TRE-BCBL-1-RTA cells 24 and 48 h following treatment with DDR kinase inhibitors and doxycycline; (**B**) Expression of LANA in EA.hy926 cells following infection with supernatants collected from TRE-BCBL-1-RTA cells 24 and 48 h after treatment with DDR kinase inhibitors and doxycycline; (**C**) Immunofluorescence microscopy analysis of the percentage of EA.hy926 cells expressing LANA following infection with supernatants collected from TRE-BCBL-1-RTA cells 24 and 48 h after treatment with DDR kinase inhibitors and doxycycline. Each column represents the mean of three independent experiments while the error bars represent the standard error of the mean (SEM). A minimum of 500 cells were analysed for each repetition. * $p < 0.05$; ** $p < 0.01$; *** $p < 0.001$ (statistical analyses were performed using a two-tailed and unpaired Student's *t*-test); (**D**) Percentage of TRE-BCBL-1-RTA cells expressing early lytic protein ORF59 24 h following treatment with DDR kinase inhibitors and doxycycline. Each column represents the mean of three independent experiments while the error bars represent the standard error of the mean (SEM). A minimum of 500 cells were analysed for each repetition; (**E**) Levels of phosphorylated DDR proteins in TRE-BCBL-1-RTA cells 24 h following treatment with DDR kinase inhibitors and doxycycline.

To ensure that levels of K8.1A expression were representative of the amount of infectious virus produced from TRE-BCBL1-RTA cells, the medium supernatants were collected from the cells after 24 and 48 h and used to infect the EA.hy926 endothelial cell line. After 48 h, western blotting was used to assess expression of LANA as a marker of KSHV infection (Figure 3B). The expression levels of LANA in the EA.hy926 cells correlated well with the levels of K8.1A expression in TRE-BCBL-1-RTA cells at both 24 and 48 h. To quantify further the level of virus contained in the supernatants, the proportion of EA.hy926 cells expressing LANA was calculated using immunofluorescence microscopy (Figure 3C). In the EA.hy926 cells treated with the 24 h supernatants there was a significant increase in the proportion of cells expressing LANA following infection with the 5 μM DNA-PKi supernatants and a significant decrease following infection with the 5 μM ATRi supernatants. In the EA.hy926 cells treated with the 48 h supernatants there was a significant decrease in the proportion of cells expressing LANA following infection with the 5 μM ATRi and 10 μM ATMi supernatants.

Since not all TRE-BCBL-1-RTA cells contain lytically replicating virus following treatment with doxycycline, it is possible that the differences observed in infectious virus production are due to changes in the percentages of cells containing lytic virus rather than changes in the amount of virus produced from individual cells. To quantify the percentage of cells containing lytic virus following treatment with DDR inhibitors and doxycycline, expression of delayed-early lytic protein ORF59 was assessed using immunofluorescence microscopy (Figure 3D). Although the percentage of cells expressing ORF59 appears elevated following the addition of DNA-PK inhibitor there were no significant differences between any of the conditions. This suggests that the changes in production of infectious virus are not because of differing numbers of cells containing lytic virus but because of changes in the efficiency of viral replication.

Several proteins involved in DDR signalling can be phosphorylated by more than one of the three key DDR kinases. To examine which kinase was responsible for the phosphorylation events observed during lytic replication of KSHV, changes in phosphorylation level of several DDR proteins in TRE-BCBL-1-RTA cells was assessed 24 h following addition of DDR inhibitors and doxycycline (Figure 3E). Inhibition of DNA-PK markedly reduced phosphorylation of RPA32 at S4/S8 and moderately reduced phosphorylation of H2AX at S139 and RPA32 at S33. DNA-PK inhibition also led to an increase in ATM, NBS1 and CHK2 phosphorylation. Inhibition of ATM strongly reduced CHK2 phosphorylation as expected but only partially reduced phosphorylation of NBS1. Inhibition of ATR reduced phosphorylation of RPA32 at S33 and reduced NBS1 phosphorylation to a greater extent than the ATM inhibitor. This indicates that DNA-PK and ATM are activating downstream targets during lytic replication but also suggests active ATR despite the lack of CHK1 phosphorylation.

3.4. CHK1 Activation is Inhibited at Later Times during Lytic Replication

While there is evidence of ATR activation during lytic replication, substantial CHK1 phosphorylation is not observed (Figure 1B). To determine whether ATR-CHK1 signalling is functional during lytic replication, TRE-BCBL-1-RTA cells were exposed to 20 Jm^{-2} UV at several time points following initiation of lytic replication (Figure 4). Expression of RTA and ORF57 were used to confirm lytic reactivation of KSHV. Exposure to UV at 3 and 6 h post-doxycycline treatment led to phosphorylation of CHK1 at S345 and S317 which was comparable to the un-reactivated control. However, when TRE-BCBL-1-RTA cells were treated with UV at 12, 24 and 48 h following addition of doxycycline, levels of phosphorylated CHK1 were noticeably lower than in the un-reactivated control. This suggests that at later times in the lytic cycle, when phosphorylation of other DDR substrates occurs, activation of CHK1 is specifically inhibited by the virus.

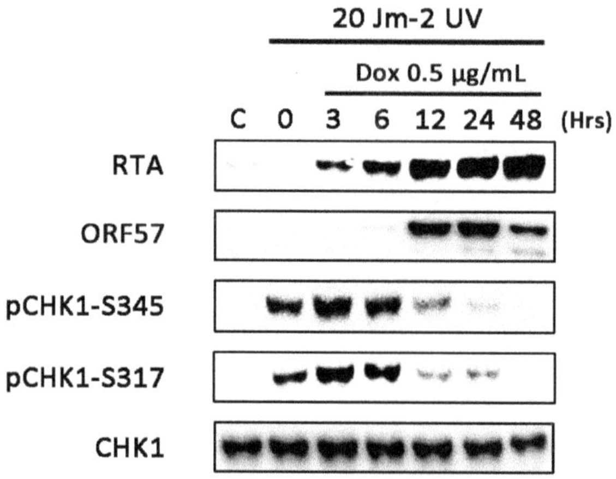

Figure 4. Inhibition of CHK1 signalling at late times during KSHV lytic replication. Levels of phosphorylated CHK1 (S317 and S345) following UV treatment of TRE-BCBL-1-RTA cells treated with doxycycline for varying lengths of time. At each time point following the addition of doxycycline, cells were treated with 20 Jm^{-2} UV and levels of phosphorylated CHK1 were assessed by western blot.

3.5. DDR Activation Does Not Result in a G1 Block Following Lytic Reactivation

Since viruses are known to modulate the cell cycle to facilitate viral replication and DDR activation can vary throughout the cell cycle, an assessment of cell cycle changes during lytic replication and in the presence of DDR kinase inhibitors was undertaken (Figure 5). TRE-BCBL-1-RTA cells were treated with DMSO or the higher concentrations of DDR kinase inhibitors 1 h prior to the addition of doxycycline. Cells were harvested after 6, 12, 18 and 24 h and subjected to PI staining. Because production of viral DNA by herpesviruses has been shown to interfere with PI staining [21], all TRE-BCBL-1-RTA cells were also treated with ganciclovir 1 h prior to the addition of DDR inhibitors or DMSO. At the 6 and 12 h time points the experiment was also conducted without ganciclovir to confirm that this compound alone has no significant effects on the cell cycle distribution following addition of doxycycline (data not shown). Cell counts also confirmed that ganciclovir alone had no significant effect on the growth rate of TRE-BCBL-1-RTA cells over 24 h (data not shown).

A

B

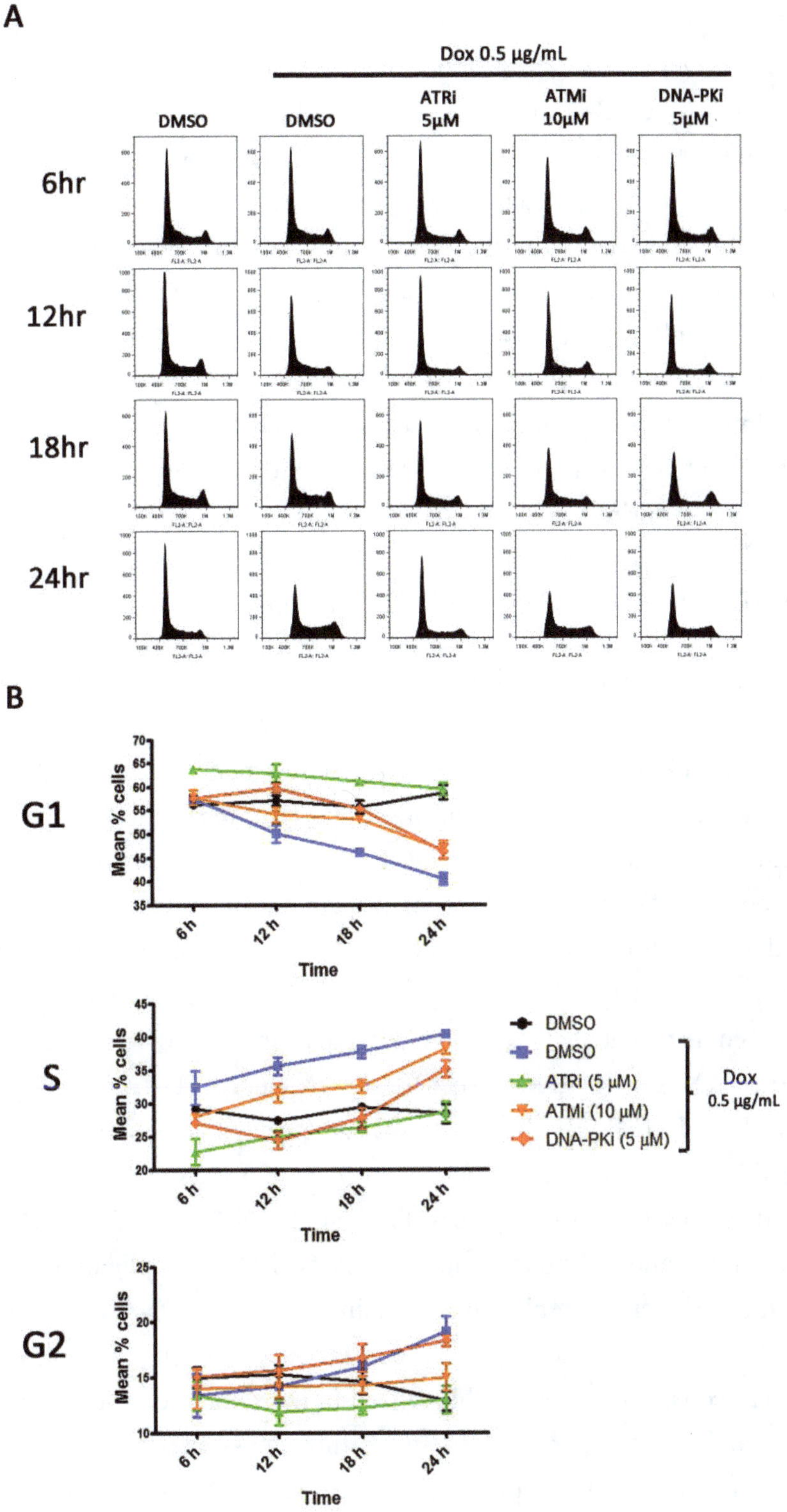

Figure 5. Cell cycle changes during lytic replication of KSHV. (**A**) Representative cell cycle profiles following PI staining of TRE-BCBL-1-RTA cells after addition of doxycycline in the presence and absence of DDR kinase inhibitors; (**B**) Percentage of TRE-BCBL-1-RTA cells in different phases of the cell cycle at 4 different time points following addition of doxycycline in the presence and absence of DDR kinase inhibitors. Each data point represents the mean of three independent experiments while the error bars represent the standard error of the mean (SEM).

The addition of doxycycline to cells treated with DMSO resulted in a decrease in the proportion of cells in G1 and an increase in the proportion in S-phase during the time course compared with the un-reactivated control. By 24 h there was also a notable increase in the proportion of cells in G2 following doxycycline treatment. Addition of the ATR inhibitor prior to doxycycline increased the proportion of cells in G1 and decreased the proportion in S and G2 compared with the cells treated with doxycycline and DMSO. By 24 h, the cell cycle profile in the presence of the ATR inhibitor and doxycycline was almost identical to the un-reactivated control. While treatment with the ATM and DNA-PK inhibitors also initially increased the proportion of cells in G1, by 24 h the difference between these conditions and the cells treated with doxycycline and DMSO was minimal. It appears then that DDR activation following lytic activation does not cause a G1 cell cycle block and instead cells are able to proceed to S and G2 phases. Addition of the ATR inhibitor, however, appears to inhibit the cell cycle changes normally induced during the lytic cycle.

3.6. RPA32 and MRE11 Localise to Sites of Viral Replication

Several DDR proteins are known to form discrete foci at sites of DNA damage [22]. In addition, several herpesviruses are known to recruit DDR proteins to sites of viral replication where they may be involved in viral DNA synthesis [23–25]. An assessment of the localisation of several DDR proteins was undertaken 24 h after induction of KSHV lytic replication (Figure 6). As well as using TRE-BCBL-1-RTA cells (Figure 6A), EA.hy926-RTA cells were examined as their larger size and flat morphology allowed for clearer visualisation of protein localization (Figure 6B). Expression of lytic proteins ORF6 and K8α were used as markers of KSHV lytic replication. The delayed-early lytic protein ORF6 has been shown previously to localise to sites of viral DNA replication in BCBL-1 cells [26]. BrdU staining was used to confirm that ORF6-positive domains were sites of viral DNA synthesis (Figure 6A).

Phosphorylated H2AX is a sensitive marker for the presence of DNA damage and γH2AX foci were consistently observed in TRE-BCBL-1-RTA and EA.hy926 cells positive for ORF6 expression. When ORF6 was localised to discrete replication bodies in EA.hy926-RTA cells, γH2AX foci typically formed outside of these bodies in cellular DNA while in TRE-BCBL-1-RTA cells γH2AX foci appear to form on the margins of these replication compartments. In cells with larger replication bodies, γH2AX staining could be seen on the periphery of replication domains as cellular DNA is marginalised to the edge of the nucleus. RPA32, which binds to single-stranded DNA, also forms foci following DNA damage. In this case, RPA32 was consistently observed localised in the same areas of the nucleus as ORF6 in both TRE-BCBL-1-RTA and EA.hy926-RTA cells, suggesting an association with viral replication domains. In addition, MRE11, part of the MRN complex that localises to DSBs, was also found to localise to viral replication compartments in both cell lines.

The localisation of 53BP1 was also examined as this protein is known to form foci at sites of DSBs [27]. Despite the activation of ATM and DNA-PK in TRE-BCBL-1-RTA cells, consistent formation of 53BP1 foci was not observed in cells positive for K8α after 24 h. In EA.hy926-RTA cells, where it is possible to accurately quantify the number of foci present, less than 30% of cells positive for K8α contained more than ten 53BP1 foci. As K8α did not appear to localise to replication domains in EA.hy926-RTA cells, and since RPA32 was consistently observed in association with ORF6, RPA32 was used as surrogate marker for KSHV replication domains when staining for 53BP1. When 53BP1 did form foci there was no evidence of localisation to KSHV replication domains.

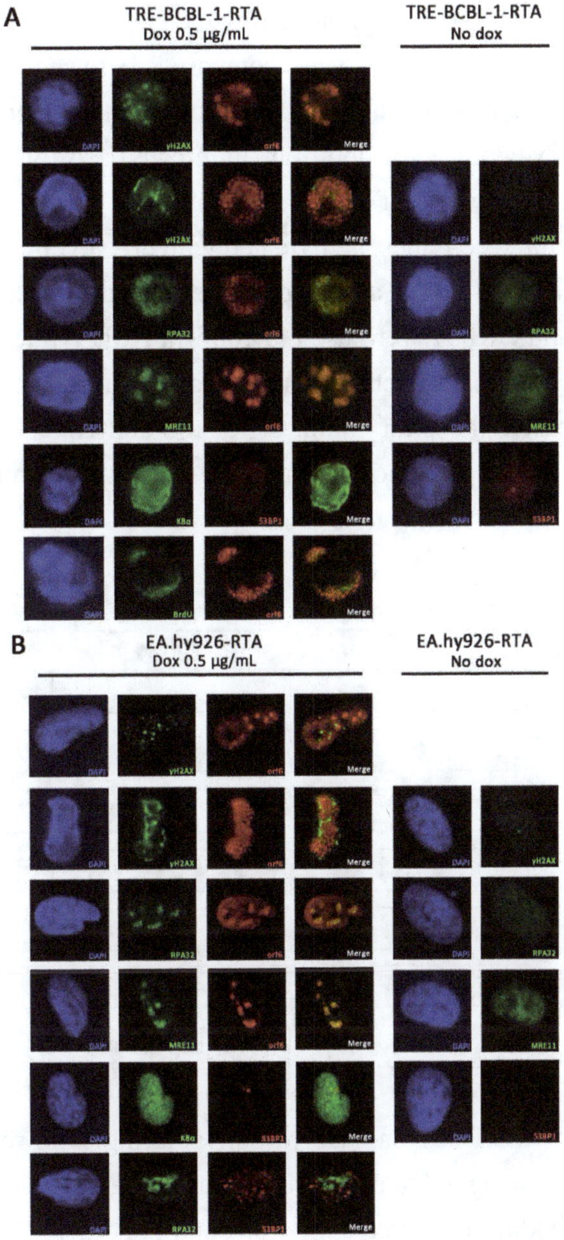

Figure 6. Localisation of DDR proteins during lytic replication of KSHV. (**A**) Localisation of γH2AX, RPA32, MRE11 and 53BP1 in TRE-BCBL-1-RTA cells 24 h following addition of doxycycline and in cells without doxycycline treatment. KSHV lytic proteins K8α and ORF6 were used as markers of lytic reactivation. In the bottom panels, BrdU was used to confirm that ORF6 localises to sites of viral replication; (**B**) Localisation of γH2AX, RPA32, MRE11 and 53BP1 in KSHV-infected EA.hy926-RTA cells 24 h following addition of doxycycline and in cells without doxycycline treatment. KSHV lytic proteins K8α and ORF6 were used as markers of lytic reactivation. In the bottom panels, RPA32 was used as a surrogate marker for sites of viral replication. DAPI staining is only shown in the left hand set of panels in each case for clarity.

3.7. Lytic Reactivation of KSHV in an Endothelial Cell Line Activates the DDR

Since KSHV targets both B cells and endothelial cells *in vivo*, activation of the DDR during KSHV lytic replication was also assessed in the EA.hy926 endothelial cell line (Figure 7). As withthe TRE-BCBL-1-RTA cells, DDR activation was compared between uninfected EA.hy926 cells and KSHV-infected EA.hy926 cells containing an RTA expression construct (termed rKSHV-EA.hy926-RTA) following treatment with doxycycline. In addition, uninfected EA.hy926 cells containing the RTA expression construct (termed EA.hy926-RTA) were also used to assess the effect of RTA expression alone on DDR activation. All three cell lines were treated with doxycycline and levels of phosphorylated H2AX and RPA32 were used to assess DDR activation at the same times examined in TRE-BCBL-1-RTA cells. Expression of LANA and ORF57 were used to confirm KSHV infection and lytic reactivation in the rKSHV-EA.hy926-RTA cell line. Induction of lytic replication in rKSHV-EA.hy926-RTA cells led to DDR activation with increased phosphorylation of RPA32 and H2AX. Expression of RTA alone in EA.hy926-RTA cells also increased phosphorylation of H2AX but to a limited extent compared to cells containing KSHV.

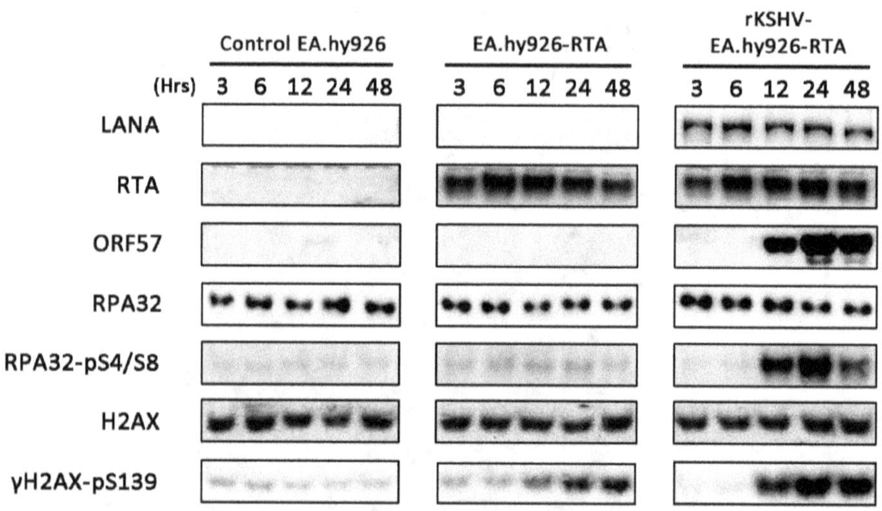

Figure 7. Activation of the DNA damage response during lytic replication of KSHV in EA.hy926 cells and following RTA expression alone. Levels of phosphorylated H2AX and RPA32 following addition of doxycyline to control EA.hy926 cells, EA.hy926 cells containing an ORF50 expression construct (EA.hy926-RTA) and KSHV-infected EA.hy926 cells containing an ORF50 expression construct (rKSHV-EA.hy926-RTA). Expression of LANA and ORF57 confirm presence of KSHV and lytic reactivation of the virus respectively.

4. Discussion

It has been demonstrated here that during lytic replication of KSHV, the ATM and DNA-PK kinases are activated and phosphorylate several downstream targets. The timing of some of these phosphorylation events suggests that immediate-early or delayed-early lytic gene expression is responsible for DDR activation. The use of ganciclovir to inhibit viral DNA synthesis and late viral gene expression confirms that these stages of the lytic cycle are not required for the observed activation of the

DDR. In accordance with this, it was recently reported that expression of KSHV immediate early lytic protein ORF57 can cause DNA damage and phosphorylation of H2AX when expressed in isolation [16].

It has also been shown here that inhibition of ATR and ATM results in reduced production of infectious virus following induction of lytic replication in B cells. Inhibition of ATM signalling has also been shown to reduce replication of the related gamma herpesvirus Epstein-Barr virus (EBV) in several studies [28–30]. Although the reduction in viral replication following ATM inhibition was moderate, DNA-PK inhibition led to increased phosphorylation of ATM and downstream substrates and increased production of infectious virus after 24 h. This observation also suggests that activation of the ATM-CHK2 arm of the DDR can promote efficient KSHV replication in B cells. The abrogation of ATM signalling was not completely efficient even at the higher concentration of ATM inhibitor. While increased concentrations of inhibitor were avoided due to concerns about toxicity and off-target effects, it would be interesting to see if a more complete knockdown of ATM could result in a more dramatic inhibitory effect on viral replication. This could potentially be achieved using Crispr/Cas in further investigations.

The inhibition of ATR resulted in the largest reduction in virus production although the lack of CHK1 phosphorylation prompts the question of whether this kinase is activated during the lytic cycle. While ATR inhibition reduced phosphorylation of NBS1 and RPA32, both of which are known ATR substrates [31,32], it is possible that cell cycle changes induced by the ATR inhibitor could contribute to a reduction in phosphorylation of these proteins by ATM and DNA-PK as well as the observed decline in virus production, assuming that progression into S-phase is advantageous (Figure 5). Whereas phosphorylation of CHK1 at serines 317 and 345 are typical markers for ATR activation in response to replication stress [33], the ATR-CHK1 pathway can also be activated when repair of DSBs during S and G2 phases generates RPA-coated ssDNA [34,35]. It was interesting therefore to observe that there was minimal CHK1 phosphorylation even at late times during lytic replication. In herpes simplex virus 1 (HSV-1), ATR signalling is disabled during viral replication and proteins involved in the ATR-CHK1 pathway are recruited to viral replication centres [25]. It appears that ATR-CHK1 signalling is disrupted at later times during KSHV lytic replication following treatment with UV. It is not clear at this stage whether inhibition of CHK1 is a deliberate viral strategy or merely a consequence of wider DDR deregulation during lytic replication.

It was notable that a G1 block was not observed during the first 24 h following lytic replication considering that this has been reported in several studies of herpesviruses including KSHV [21,36–39]. KSHV lytic proteins RTA and K8α have both been shown to induce a G1 block when expressed in isolation [37–39]. However, KSHV also encodes a D-cyclin homolog, known as v-cyclin, that has been reported to induce cell cycle progression via inactivation of $p27^{KIP1}$ [40]. v-cyclin is expressed throughout the viral lifecycle but expression is increased following lytic reactivation [41]. It has also been shown to activate the DDR in endothelial cells by promoting deregulated S-phase entry [42]. Considering the apparent opposing effects of these viral proteins on cell cycle progression, and the large number of genes expressed during the lytic cycle, it is clear that single gene expression studies could lead to contradictory finding in this area. While it has been postulated that replication in G1 is ideal during the lytic cycle as the virus avoids competition for DNA replication resources [37], there is also evidence that S-phase can provide KSHV with a favourable environment for viral replication [43]. The data presented here suggest that, despite the presence of DNA damage, cells containing lytic virus can still progress into S-phase and that when a G1 block is induced by inhibition of ATR it has a negative effect on the efficient production of viral DNA.

The activation of ATM and DNA-PK suggests the formation of DSBs during KSHV replication. Increased phosphorylation of H2AX and the presence of γH2AX foci have previously been used to confirm the presence of DSBs in B cells following induction of the lytic cycle [15,16]. The formation of γH2AX foci was also observed during this study but since γH2AX foci can also form at single-stranded DNA breaks and stalled replication forks [44], the presence of 53BP1 foci which form rapidly at sites of DSBs was also examined. Curiously, we did not observe consistent formation of 53BP1 foci in cells positive for lytic virus. Although 53BP1 localisation has been implicated in ATM activation it is not strictly required following high levels of DNA damage [45]. In EBV, 53BP1 has been shown to be important for viral replication [46] while in human cytomegalovirus (HCMV), overall 53BP1 levels decrease during infection [24]. In HSV-1, degradation of the E3 ubiquitin ligases RNF8 and RNF168 inhibits localisation of 53BP1 to incoming viral genomes [47]. It will be interesting to assess further whether expression and localisation of this protein is deregulated during the KSHV lifecycle.

RPA32 and MRE11 can also form foci following DNA damage and both proteins were consistently observed localised to areas of viral replication; this was particularly evident in EA.hy926 cells where ORF6 staining can be seen as discrete bodies that occupy a smaller proportion of the nucleus than in B cells. Both RPA32 and MRE11 have been shown to localise to EBV replication compartments where they are loaded onto newly synthesised viral DNA along with HR factors Rad51 and Rad52 [23]. Further work will be required to determine if any other DDR factors are recruited to KSHV replication compartments and what role they play in viral replication.

Overall, it appears that lytic reactivation of KSHV leads to selective activation of the DDR and this plays a positive role in the viral lifecycle. In addition, the localisation of DDR proteins to areas of viral replication suggests that individual DDR proteins may contribute to viral DNA synthesis, as is the case with other herpesviruses. Although the data presented here do not contradict the demonstration that expression of ORF57 can elicit a DDR, our observations using an endothelial cell line suggest that RTA alone can also modestly increase phosphorylation of H2AX. It is therefore possible that expression of several early lytic proteins could be responsible for DDR activation which then contributes to efficient production of viral progeny.

Acknowledgments

We are most grateful to Cancer Research UK (CRUK) for funding this study. We would also like to thank Jae Jung for kindly providing the TRE-BCBL-1-RTA cells and Gary Hayward for generously supplying the ORF6 antibody.

Author Contributions

Roger J. Grand and Robert Hollingworth conceived and designed the experiments. Robert Hollingworth conducted all experiments in B cells and wrote the manuscript. George L. Skalka conducted all experiments in endothelial cells. David J. Blackbourn, Andrew D. Hislop and Grant S. Stewart provided materials and reagents as well as critical evaluation of experimental procedures. All authors reviewed and approved the final manuscript.

References

1. Chang, Y.; Cesarman, E.; Pessin, M.S.; Lee, F.; Culpepper, J.; Knowles, D.M.; Moore, P.S. Identification of herpesvirus-like DNA sequences in aids-associated kaposi's sarcoma. *Science* **1994**, *266*, 1865–1869. [CrossRef] [PubMed]
2. Cesarman, E.; Chang, Y.; Moore, P.S.; Said, J.W.; Knowles, D.M. Kaposi's sarcoma-associated herpesvirus-like DNA sequences in aids-related body-cavity-based lymphomas. *N. Engl. J. Med.* **1995**, *332*, 1186–1191. [CrossRef] [PubMed]
3. Soulier, J.; Grollet, L.; Oksenhendler, E.; Cacoub, P.; Cazals-Hatem, D.; Babinet, P.; D'Agay, M.F.; Clauvel, J.P.; Raphael, M.; Degos, L.; *et al.* Kaposi's sarcoma-associated herpesvirus-like DNA sequences in multicentric castleman's disease. *Blood* **1995**, *86*, 1276–1280. [PubMed]
4. Sun, R.; Lin, S.F.; Gradoville, L.; Yuan, Y.; Zhu, F.; Miller, G. A viral gene that activates lytic cycle expression of kaposi's sarcoma-associated herpesvirus. *Proc. Natl. Acad. Sci. USA* **1998**, *95*, 10866–10871. [CrossRef] [PubMed]
5. Guito, J.; Lukac, D.M. Kshv reactivation and novel implications of protein isomerization on lytic switch control. *Viruses* **2015**, *7*, 72–109. [CrossRef] [PubMed]
6. Martin, D.F.; Kuppermann, B.D.; Wolitz, R.A.; Palestine, A.G.; Li, H.; Robinson, C.A. Oral ganciclovir for patients with cytomegalovirus retinitis treated with a ganciclovir implant. Roche ganciclovir study group. *N. Engl. J. Med.* **1999**, *340*, 1063–1070. [CrossRef] [PubMed]
7. Grundhoff, A.; Ganem, D. Inefficient establishment of kshv latency suggests an additional role for continued lytic replication in kaposi sarcoma pathogenesis. *J. Clin. Investig.* **2004**, *113*, 124–136. [CrossRef] [PubMed]
8. Rothkamm, K.; Kruger, I.; Thompson, L.H.; Lobrich, M. Pathways of DNA double-strand break repair during the mammalian cell cycle. *Mol. Cell. Biol.* **2003**, *23*, 5706–5715. [CrossRef] [PubMed]
9. Lieber, M.R. The mechanism of double-strand DNA break repair by the nonhomologous DNA end-joining pathway. *Annu. Rev. Biochem.* **2010**, *79*, 181–211. [CrossRef] [PubMed]
10. Ashley, A.K.; Shrivastav, M.; Nie, J.; Amerin, C.; Troksa, K.; Glanzer, J.G.; Liu, S.; Opiyo, S.O.; Dimitrova, D.D.; Le, P.; *et al.* DNA-pk phosphorylation of rpa32 ser4/ser8 regulates replication stress checkpoint activation, fork restart, homologous recombination and mitotic catastrophe. *DNA Repair Amst.* **2014**, *21*, 131–139. [CrossRef] [PubMed]
11. Zou, L.; Elledge, S.J. Sensing DNA damage through atrip recognition of rpa-ssdna complexes. *Science* **2003**, *300*, 1542–1548. [CrossRef] [PubMed]
12. Chini, C.C.; Chen, J. Human claspin is required for replication checkpoint control. *J. Biol. Chem.* **2003**, *278*, 30057–30062. [CrossRef] [PubMed]
13. Kumagai, A.; Lee, J.; Yoo, H.Y.; Dunphy, W.G. Topbp1 activates the atr-atrip complex. *Cell* **2006**, *124*, 943–955. [CrossRef] [PubMed]
14. Singh, V.V.; Dutta, D.; Ansari, M.A.; Dutta, S.; Chandran, B. Kaposi's sarcoma-associated herpesvirus induces the ATM and H2AX DNA damage response early during de novo infection of primary endothelial cells, which play roles in latency establishment. *J. Virol.* **2014**, *88*, 2821–2834. [CrossRef] [PubMed]
15. Xiao, Y.; Chen, J.; Liao, Q.; Wu, Y.; Peng, C.; Chen, X. Lytic infection of kaposi's

sarcoma-associated herpesvirus induces DNA double-strand breaks and impairs non-homologous end joining. *J. Gen. Virol.* **2013**, *94*, 1870–1875. [CrossRef] [PubMed]

16. Jackson, B.R.; Noerenberg, M.; Whitehouse, A. A novel mechanism inducing genome instability in kaposi's sarcoma-associated herpesvirus infected cells. *PLoS Pathog.* **2014**, *10*, e1004098. [CrossRef] [PubMed]
17. Meerbrey, K.L.; Hu, G.; Kessler, J.D.; Roarty, K.; Li, M.Z.; Herschkowitz, J.I.; Burrows, A.E.; Fang, J.E.; Ciccia, A.; Sun, T.; *et al.* The pinducer lentiviral toolkit for inducible rna interference *in vitro* and *in vivo*. *Proc. Natl. Acad. Sci. USA* **2011**, *108*, 3665–3670. [CrossRef] [PubMed]
18. Vieira, J.; O'Hearn, P.M. Use of the red fluorescent protein as a marker of kaposi's sarcoma-associated herpesvirus lytic gene expression. *Virology* **2004**, *325*, 225–240. [CrossRef] [PubMed]
19. Nakamura, H.; Lu, M.; Gwack, Y.; Souvlis, J.; Zeichner, S.L.; Jung, J.U. Global changes in kaposi's sarcoma-associated virus gene expression patterns following expression of a tetracycline-inducible rta transactivator. *J. Virol.* **2003**, *77*, 4205–4220. [CrossRef] [PubMed]
20. Matthews, T.; Boehme, R. Antiviral activity and mechanism of action of ganciclovir. *Rev. Infect. Dis.* **1988**, *10*, S490–S494. [CrossRef] [PubMed]
21. Bresnahan, W.A.; Boldogh, I.; Thompson, E.A.; Albrecht, T. Human cytomegalovirus inhibits cellular DNA synthesis and arrests productively infected cells in late g1. *Virology* **1996**, *224*, 150–160. [CrossRef] [PubMed]
22. Polo, S.E.; Jackson, S.P. Dynamics of DNA damage response proteins at DNA breaks: A focus on protein modifications. *Genes Dev.* **2011**, *25*, 409–433. [CrossRef] [PubMed]
23. Kudoh, A.; Iwahori, S.; Sato, Y.; Nakayama, S.; Isomura, H.; Murata, T.; Tsurumi, T. Homologous recombinational repair factors are recruited and loaded onto the viral DNA genome in epstein-barr virus replication compartments. *J. Virol.* **2009**, *83*, 6641–6651. [CrossRef] [PubMed]
24. Luo, M.H.; Rosenke, K.; Czornak, K.; Fortunato, E.A. Human cytomegalovirus disrupts both ataxia telangiectasia mutated protein (ATM)- and ATM-rad3-related kinase-mediated DNA damage responses during lytic infection. *J. Virol.* **2007**, *81*, 1934–1950. [CrossRef] [PubMed]
25. Mohni, K.N.; Dee, A.R.; Smith, S.; Schumacher, A.J.; Weller, S.K. Efficient herpes simplex virus 1 replication requires cellular atr pathway proteins. *J. Virol.* **2013**, *87*, 531–542. [CrossRef] [PubMed]
26. Wang, Y.; Li, H.; Tang, Q.; Maul, G.G.; Yuan, Y. Kaposi's sarcoma-associated herpesvirus ori-lyt-dependent DNA replication: Involvement of host cellular factors. *J. Virol.* **2008**, *82*, 2867–2882. [CrossRef] [PubMed]
27. Anderson, L.; Henderson, C.; Adachi, Y. Phosphorylation and rapid relocalization of 53bp1 to nuclear foci upon DNA damage. *Mol. Cell. Biol.* **2001**, *21*, 1719–1729. [CrossRef] [PubMed]
28. Li, R.; Zhu, J.; Xie, Z.; Liao, G.; Liu, J.; Chen, M.R.; Hu, S.; Woodard, C.; Lin, J.; Taverna, S.D.; *et al.* Conserved herpesvirus kinases target the DNA damage response pathway and tip60 histone acetyltransferase to promote virus replication. *Cell Host Microbe* **2011**, *10*, 390–400. [CrossRef] [PubMed]
29. Hagemeier, S.R.; Barlow, E.A.; Meng, Q.; Kenney, S.C. The cellular ataxia telangiectasia-mutated kinase promotes epstein-barr virus lytic reactivation in response to multiple different types of lytic

reactivation-inducing stimuli. *J. Virol.* **2012**, *86*, 13360–13370. [CrossRef] [PubMed]

30. Hau, P.M.; Deng, W.; Jia, L.; Yang, J.; Tsurumi, T.; Chiang, A.K.; Huen, M.S.; Tsao, S.W. Role of atm in the formation of the replication compartment during lytic replication of epstein-barr virus in nasopharyngeal epithelial cells. *J. Virol.* **2015**, *89*, 652–668. [CrossRef] [PubMed]
31. Liu, S.; Bekker-Jensen, S.; Mailand, N.; Lukas, C.; Bartek, J.; Lukas, J. Claspin operates downstream of TOPBP1 to direct atr signaling towards chk1 activation. *Mol. Cell. Biol.* **2006**, *26*, 6056–6064. [CrossRef] [PubMed]
32. Liu, S.; Opiyo, S.O.; Manthey, K.; Glanzer, J.G.; Ashley, A.K.; Amerin, C.; Troksa, K.; Shrivastav, M.; Nickoloff, J.A.; Oakley, G.G. Distinct roles for DNA-pk, atm and atr in rpa phosphorylation and checkpoint activation in response to replication stress. *Nucleic Acids Res.* **2012**, *40*, 10780–10794. [CrossRef] [PubMed]
33. Cimprich, K.A.; Cortez, D. ATR: An essential regulator of genome integrity. *Nat. Rev. Mol. Cell. Biol.* **2008**, *9*, 616–627. [CrossRef] [PubMed]
34. Jazayeri, A.; Falck, J.; Lukas, C.; Bartek, J.; Smith, G.C.; Lukas, J.; Jackson, S.P. ATM- and cell cycle-dependent regulation of atr in response to DNA double-strand breaks. *Nat. Cell Biol.* **2006**, *8*, 37–45. [CrossRef] [PubMed]
35. Shibata, A.; Barton, O.; Noon, A.T.; Dahm, K.; Deckbar, D.; Goodarzi, A.A.; Lobrich, M.; Jeggo, P.A. Role of ATM and the damage response mediator proteins 53bp1 and mdc1 in the maintenance of G_2/M checkpoint arrest. *Mol. Cell. Biol.* **2010**, *30*, 3371–3383. [CrossRef] [PubMed]
36. Rodriguez, A.; Jung, E.J.; Flemington, E.K. Cell cycle analysis of epstein-barr virus-infected cells following treatment with lytic cycle-inducing agents. *J. Virol.* **2001**, *75*, 4482–4489. [CrossRef] [PubMed]
37. Wu, F.Y.; Tang, Q.Q.; Chen, H.; ApRhys, C.; Farrell, C.; Chen, J.; Fujimuro, M.; Lane, M.D.; Hayward, G.S. Lytic replication-associated protein (RAP) encoded by kaposi sarcoma-associated herpesvirus causes p21CIP-1-mediated G1 cell cycle arrest through ccaat/enhancer-binding protein-alpha. *Proc. Natl. Acad. Sci. USA* **2002**, *99*, 10683–10688. [CrossRef] [PubMed]
38. Izumiya, Y.; Lin, S.F.; Ellison, T.J.; Levy, A.M.; Mayeur, G.L.; Izumiya, C.; Kung, H.J. Cell cycle regulation by kaposi's sarcoma-associated herpesvirus k-bzip: Direct interaction with cyclin-CDK2 and induction of G1 growth arrest. *J. Virol.* **2003**, *77*, 9652–9661. [CrossRef] [PubMed]
39. Kumar, P.; Wood, C. Kaposi's sarcoma-associated herpesvirus transactivator rta induces cell cycle arrest in G0/G1 phase by stabilizing and promoting nuclear localization of p27kip. *J. Virol.* **2013**, *87*, 13226–13238. [CrossRef] [PubMed]
40. Jarviluoma, A.; Koopal, S.; Rasanen, S.; Makela, T.P.; Ojala, P.M. Kshv viral cyclin binds to p27kip1 in primary effusion lymphomas. *Blood* **2004**, *104*, 3349–3354. [CrossRef] [PubMed]
41. Arias, C.; Weisburd, B.; Stern-Ginossar, N.; Mercier, A.; Madrid, A.S.; Bellare, P.; Holdorf, M.; Weissman, J.S.; Ganem, D. Kshv 2.0: A comprehensive annotation of the kaposi's sarcoma-associated herpesvirus genome using next-generation sequencing reveals novel genomic and functional features. *PLoS Pathog.* **2014**, *10*, e1003847. [CrossRef] [PubMed]
42. Koopal, S.; Furuhjelm, J.H.; Jarviluoma, A.; Jaamaa, S.; Pyakurel, P.; Pussinen, C.; Wirzenius, M.; Biberfeld, P.; Alitalo, K.; Laiho, M.; *et al.* Viral oncogene-induced DNA damage response is

activated in kaposi sarcoma tumorigenesis. *PLoS Pathog.* **2007**, *3*, 1348–1360. [CrossRef] [PubMed]

43. Bryan, B.A.; Dyson, O.F.; Akula, S.M. Identifying cellular genes crucial for the reactivation of kaposi's sarcoma-associated herpesvirus latency. *J. Gen. Virol.* **2006**, *87*, 519–529. [CrossRef] [PubMed]
44. Ward, I.M.; Chen, J. Histone H2AX is phosphorylated in an atr-dependent manner in response to replicational stress. *J. Biol. Chem.* **2001**, *276*, 47759–47762. [PubMed]
45. Fernandez-Capetillo, O.; Chen, H.T.; Celeste, A.; Ward, I.; Romanienko, P.J.; Morales, J.C.; Naka, K.; Xia, Z.; Camerini-Otero, R.D.; Motoyama, N.; *et al.* DNA damage-induced g2-m checkpoint activation by histone h2ax and 53bp1. *Nat. Cell Biol.* **2002**, *4*, 993–997. [CrossRef] [PubMed]
46. Bailey, S.G.; Verrall, E.; Schelcher, C.; Rhie, A.; Doherty, A.J.; Sinclair, A.J. Functional interaction between epstein-barr virus replication protein zta and host DNA damage response protein 53bp1. *J. Virol.* **2009**, *83*, 11116–11122. [CrossRef] [PubMed]
47. Lilley, C.E.; Chaurushiya, M.S.; Boutell, C.; Everett, R.D.; Weitzman, M.D. The intrinsic antiviral defense to incoming HSV-1 genomes includes specific DNA repair proteins and is counteracted by the viral protein ICP0. *PLoS Pathog.* **2011**, *7*, e1002084. [CrossRef] [PubMed]

5

The Subcellular Localisation of the Human Papillomavirus (HPV) 16 E7 Protein in Cervical Cancer Cells and its Perturbation by RNA Aptamers

Özlem Cesur, Clare Nicol, Helen Groves, Jamel Mankouri, George Eric Blair and Nicola J. Stonehouse *

School of Molecular and Cellular Biology, Faculty of Biological Sciences and Astbury Centre for Structural Molecular Biology, University of Leeds, Leeds LS2 9JT, UK;
E-Mails: bs09oc@leeds.ac.uk (Ö.C.); c.nicol@leeds.ac.uk (C.N.); h.groves14@imperial.ac.uk (H.G.); j.mankouri@leeds.ac.uk (J.M.); g.e.blair@leeds.ac.uk (G.E.B.)

* Author to whom correspondence should be addressed; E-Mail: n.j.stonehouse@leeds.ac.uk;

Academic Editor: Joanna Parish

Abstract: Human papillomavirus (HPV) is the most common viral infection of the reproductive tract, affecting both men and women. High-risk oncogenic types are responsible for almost 90% of anogenital and oropharyngeal cancers including cervical cancer. Some of the HPV "early" genes, particularly E6 and E7, are known to act as oncogenes that promote tumour growth and malignant transformation. Most notably, HPV-16 E7 interacts with the tumour suppressor protein pRb, promoting its degradation, leading to cell cycle dysregulation in infected cells. We have previously shown that an RNA aptamer (termed A2) selectively binds to HPV16 E7 and is able to induce apoptosis in HPV16-transformed cervical carcinoma cell lines (SiHa) through reduction of E7 levels. In this study, we investigated the effects of the A2 aptamer on E7 localisation in order to define its effects on E7 activity. We demonstrate for the first time that E7 localised to the plasma membrane. In addition, we show that A2 enhanced E7 localisation in the ER and that the A2-mediated reduction of E7 was not associated with proteasomal degradation. These data suggest that A2 perturbs normal E7 trafficking through promoting E7 ER retention.

Keywords: HPV16 E7; SELEX; RNA aptamers; cell surface localisation; ER retention

1. Introduction

Papillomaviruses have been discovered in many vertebrates including humans, cattle, dogs, birds and reptiles. Within the papillomavirus family, around 170 human and 130 animal genotypes have been sequenced, identified and subsequently classified into 37 genera to date (see Papillomavirus Episteme (PaVE) [1]. Human papillomaviruses (HPVs) are classified into five genera (Alpha, Beta, Gamma, Mu and Nu) [2]. The Alpha genus contains high-risk mucosal HPVs that are the main cause of cervical cancer [3]. Amongst high-risk genotypes, HPV16 and 18 are most frequently found in cervical biopsies [4]. The majority (70%–90%) of HPV infections with both high- and low-risk genotypes are asymptomatic and can be cleared spontaneously within one to two years. Only a small percentage of persistent infections (around ∼5%–10%) with high-risk types result in precancerous lesions. If untreated, these lesions may lead to squamous cell carcinoma (SCC) [5].

HPV-related anogenital and oropharyngeal cancers are a global health burden. Cancer Research UK reported around ∼3000 new cases of cervical cancer in 2011 alone in the UK; the twelfth most common female cancer and third most common gynaecological cancer after uterine and ovarian cancers. In a worldwide perspective, cervical cancer is the second most prevalent cancer in women with an estimated 530,000 new cases in 2012 and around 270,000 deaths mostly in the developing world, according to the World Health Organisation (WHO) [6]. There is no HPV-specific cervical cancer treatment. However, protection can be achieved by the use of barrier methods and vaccination. Currently, there are two prophylactic vaccines in use based on virus-like particles (VLPs): the bivalent Cervarix (HPV16 and 18 VLPs) and the quadrivalent Gardasil (HPV6, 11, 16 and 18 VLPs). A nine-valent vaccine covering five additional high-risk HPVs is undergoing a Phase 3 clinical trial (trial number NCT00943722).

HPV encodes oncoproteins termed E5, E6 and E7. E7 is a highly phosphorylated, acidic polypeptide of approximately 100 amino acid residues. The E7 phosphoprotein has two conserved regions: CR1, CR2 and a carboxy-terminal region containing two zinc finger domains. CR2 contains a conserved LXCXE (L, leucine; C, cysteine; E, glutamate; X, any amino acid) motif, which is required for the interaction with pRb. E7 shares sequence similarities with the adenovirus (Ad) E1A protein and the simian vacuolating virus 40 (SV40) large tumour (large T) antigen [7]. Structural characterisation of HPV45 E7 [8,9] indicates that the N-terminus is intrinsically disordered while the C-terminus is highly structured with the zinc-binding region possibly involved in dimerisation. E7 has been shown to be present in dimeric form when expressed in *Escherichia coli* by gel filtration and non-denaturing acrylamide gel electrophoresis [10]. It has also been reported to form tetramers [11] and higher order oligomers [12] by analytical ultracentrifugation sedimentation equilibrium experiments.

The intracellular localisation of E7 has been investigated in detail. Subcellular fractionation experiments in CaSki cells demonstrated the presence of E7 in soluble cytoplasmic fractions [13]. Nuclear [14] and nucleolar [15] distribution in HPV16+ CaSki cells has also been proposed. Using antibodies with high discrimination capacity against monomeric, dimeric or oligomeric forms of E7, E7 dimers were shown to distribute to the nucleus, whilst oligomeric E7 displayed cytoplasmic distribution [16]. The presence of nuclear localisation and export sequences led to the hypothesis that E7 shuttles between the cytoplasm and nucleus [17]. Consistent with this, leptomycin B treatment has been shown to lead to E7 accumulation in the nucleus [17,18]. Cell confluency has also been proposed to dictate E7 localisation, being predominantly cytoplasmic in confluent cells but locating to both the nucleus and cytoplasm in sub-confluent cells [18], suggesting that location may be cell cycle-dependent.

Aptamers are short (15–100 nucleotides), single-stranded RNA or DNA molecules generated by SELEX (Systematic Evolution of Ligands by Exponential Enrichment), reviewed in [19–21]. Aptamers fold into specific complex structures that bind target proteins in a conformation-dependent manner and can interfere with function. Aptamers have been identified which recognise a number of viral proteins including HPV16 E6 and E7 [22–24], the RNA-dependent RNA polymerase of foot-and-mouth disease virus [25,26] and hepatitis C virus non-structural protein 5B [27,28]. An aptamer, targeted to VEGF termed pegaptanib (Macugen) was approved by the Food and Drug Administration (FDA) for the treatment of age-related macular degeneration in 2004 and examples of aptamers with anti-proliferative effects in cancer cells are currently undergoing clinical trials, including a guanosine-rich DNA oligonucleotide, AS1411 [29] and a L-RNA aptamer (Spiegelmer), NOX-12 [30].

We previously described an HPV16 E7 aptamer (termed A2) that resulted in a loss of E7 expression after transfection into HPV16+ cells [24]. We postulated that E7 was being targeted for degradation. Here, we show that aptamers can endocytose into early/late endosomes and that A2 redistributes E7 to the ER from the plasma membrane. We therefore propose that A2 interferes with normal E7 trafficking and cellular localisation.

2. Materials and Methods

2.1. Cell Culture

The SiHa cell line (ATCC No. HTB-35) was derived from a human squamous cell carcinoma of the cervix and contained 1–2 copies of the integrated HPV16 genome. CaSki cells (ATCC No. CRL-1550) were derived from a human epidermoid carcinoma of the cervix, and contain approximately 600 integrated copies. The HeLa cell line (ATCC No. CCL-2) was derived from a human adenocarcinoma of the cervix and contains approximately 10–50 copies of HPV18 genome. HaCaT cells are spontaneously-immortalised human keratinocytes (HPV negative). SaOS-2 (ATCC No. HTB-85) is an osteosarcoma cell line and negative for HPV DNA. SaOS-2, CaSki, SiHa, HeLa and HaCaT cells were maintained in DMEM containing 1% L-glutamine (GE Healthcare, Little Chalfont, Buckinghamshire, UK) supplemented with 10% foetal bovine serum (FBS) (PAA, Pasching, Austria), 100 units/mL penicillin (Lonza, Slough, UK), 0.1 mg/mL streptomycin (Lonza) in T-25 flasks. Flasks were maintained in a horizontal position in a humidified incubator (37 °C; 5% CO_2). Cells were plated in 6-well (for protein extraction) or 12-well (for immunostaining) dishes for the experiments. In order to analyse the pathway of E7 degradation, CaSki cells were treated with a proteasome inhibitor, MG132 (Cayman Chemicals, Ann Arbor, MI, USA) at 100 μM for up to 6 h in the presence or absence of 100 nM aptamer.

2.2. Generation of 2′-Fluoro-Modified RNA Molecules

We have previously generated a library for templates of RNA aptamers selected against E7 [23]. A2 and SF1 aptamer templates were amplified by PCR and *in vitro* transcription was performed as previously described, incorporating 2′F U and C [22–24]. Aptamer 21-2 (5′-Cy5 and 3′-Cy3-labelled) and aptamer

47tr (5′-Cy3-labelled) both contained 2′F C and aptamer 21-2 also included 2′F U. 21-2 was purchased from Abgene (UK) and 47tr was synthesised by phosphoramidite chemistry in house [26,31].

2.3. Transfection of Cells with Aptamers Using Oligofectamine

Cells were transfected with aptamers at a final RNA concentrations of up to 100 nM using Oligofectamine (Invitrogen, Life Technologies, Waltham, MA, USA) according to the manufacturer's instructions.

2.4. Collection of Cells and Protein Extraction

Cells were lysed in radio-immunoprecipitation (RIPA) buffer [50 mM Tris-HCl (pH 8.0), 150 mM NaCl, 1% (*v/v*) Nonidet P-40, 0.5% (*w/v*) sodium deoxycholate, 0.1% (*w/v*) SDS] containing EDTA-free protease inhibitors (Roche, Penzberg, Germany) (1 tablet per 10 mL buffer), DNase I (5 μg/ mL) and 10 mM $MgCl_2$ on ice for 30 min. Protein samples were mixed with 2 × Laemmli buffer and boiled to denature at 95 °C for 5 min.

2.5. SDS-PAGE and Western Blotting

This was performed as previously described [23]. Membranes were probed with rabbit anti-GAPDH (Sigma-Aldrich, St. Louis, MO, USA, used at 1:6000), mouse monoclonal HPV16 anti-E7; clone NM2 (Santa Cruz Biotechnology, Inc., Dallas, TX, USA, used at 1:200) overnight at 4 °C. Membranes were labelled with goat anti-mouse IgG peroxidase conjugate (Sigma, USA used at 1:2000) and goat anti-rabbit IgG peroxidase (Sigma, St. Louis, MO, USA, used at 1:1000) in 5% (*w/v*) milk for 1 h at room temperature.

2.6. Immunostaining of Cells and Fluorescence Microscopy

SiHa, SaOS-2, HeLa and HaCaT cells were grown on coverslips, washed with PBS and fixed with 4% (*v/v*) formaldehyde in PBS for 10 min at room temperature. Permeabilisation of cells was performed by incubation in 0.1% (*v/v*) TritonX-100/PBS for 10 min. Cells were incubated in blocking solution [1% BSA/Triton X-100 in 1 x PBS (*w/v*)] for 1 h at room temperature. Mouse monoclonal HPV16 anti-E7; clone 289–17013 (Abcam, UK used at 1:2000), mouse monoclonal HPV16 anti-E7; cloneNM2 (Santa Cruz Biotechnology, Inc., Dallas, TX, USA, used at 1:200), mouse monoclonal HPV18 anti-E7; clone 8E2 (Abcam, Cambridge, UK, used at 1:200), rabbit polyclonal anti-EEA1 (Millipore, Billerica, MA, USA, used at 1:500), rabbit polyclonal anti-LAMP-1 (CD107a) (Millipore, Billerica, MA USA used at 1:500) or rabbit polyclonal anti-LC3 (Abcam, Cambridge, UK used at 1:2000) were added to cells and incubated overnight at 4 °C on a rotating platform. To analyse cell-surface staining, cells were incubated with anti-E7 at 4 °C prior to fixation for 1 h.

Cells were washed with PBS and incubated with fluorochrome-conjugated secondary antibodies AlexaFluor 568 F goat anti-mouse IgG (H+L), AlexaFluor 488 chicken anti-mouse IgG (H+L), AlexaFluor 488 goat anti-rabbit IgG (H+L). Secondary antibodies (all from Life Technologies, Waltham, MA, USA) were used at 1:500 in 1% BSA/Triton X-100 for 2 h at room temperature and kept in the dark. Glass coverslips were mounted on microscope slides in Vectashield-DAPI stain (Vector laboratories, Burlingame, CA, USA) and viewed on Zeiss LSM 510 upright or LSM 700 inverted confocal microscopes.

2.7. *Quantitation of Co-Localisation by Imeris Software*

Confocal images were analysed by Bitplane:Imeris image analysis software in order to calculate the Pearson's co-localisation coefficient values. Results are presented as % of co-localisation between two different channels and n refers to the number of cells analysed.

3. Results

3.1. *A2-Mediated Degradation of E7 Is Not Mediated via Proteasomal Pathways*

We have previously described a loss of E7 in A2-transfected HPV16+ CaSki cells. The effect was not observed with a control aptamer SF1, selected to an unrelated protein [24]. Here, the peptide-aldehyde proteasome inhibitor, MG132 (carbobenzoxyl-L-leucyl-L-leucyl-L-leucinal) was used to study E7 degradation in the presence or absence of A2. CaSki cells transfected with A2 or a control aptamer (SF1) for 14–16 h were treated with 100 μM MG132 for up to 6 h. Figure 1 demonstrates that transfection of the A2 aptamer appeared to result in a lower level of E7, as evidenced by the level at t = 0 (corresponding to 14–16 h post-transfection), in agreement with previous data [24]. Furthermore, in A2-transfected cells, E7 levels remained low. MG132 treatment clearly had little effect, indicating that newly-synthesised E7 was still being degraded. In contrast, the level of MG132-mediated inhibition appeared to be highly variable in the mock- or SF1-treated cells and E7 did appear to accumulate, suggesting that the protein normally undergoes proteasomal degradation. The clear differences between the E7 levels in the mock- or SF1-treated cells compared to A2-treated cells led to the suggestion that A2 acts to enhance E7 degradation by a non-proteasomal mechanism.

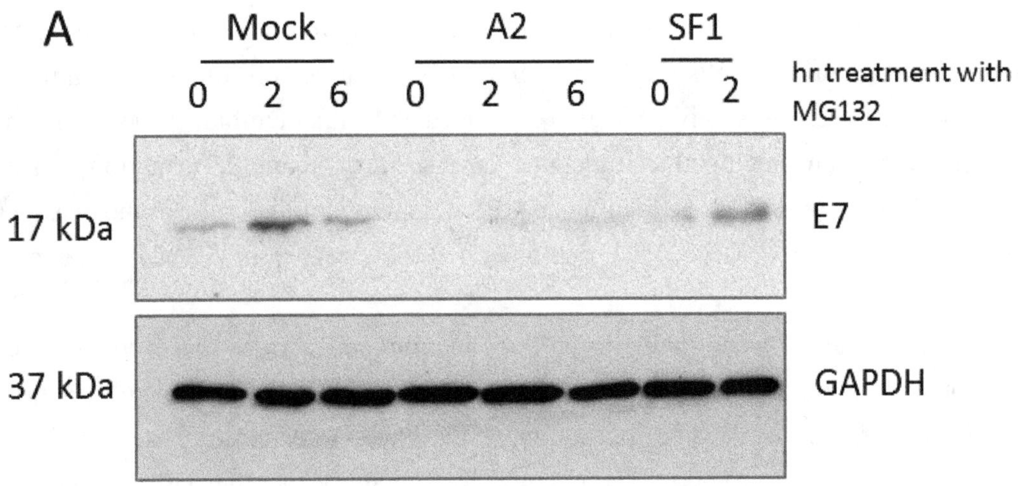

Figure 1. *Cont.*

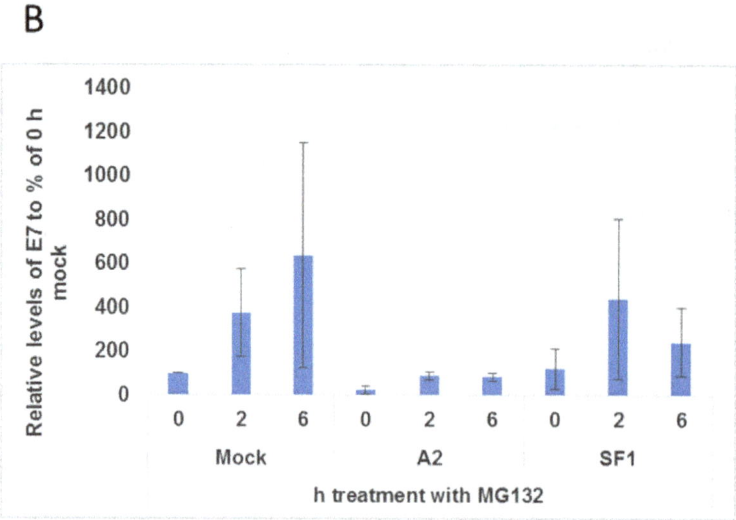

Figure 1. Proteasomal degradation of E7 was not affected by A2 treatment. CaSki cells were mock-transfected or transfected with 100 nM A2 or SF1 for 16 h. Cells were treated with MG132 (100 μM) for the indicated time points and immunoblot analysis of cell lysates was performed to detect E7 and GAPDH (as a housekeeping control) (**A**); Mean data from three independent experiments is shown, together with standard errors (**B**).

3.2. E7 Localises to the Plasma Membrane

We next sought to investigate the intracellular distribution of E7. Using HPV16 E7-specific antibodies in HPV16+ SiHa cells, we observed that E7 displayed diffuse cytoplasmic staining, as expected, however this appeared to extend to the cell periphery, characteristic of localisation to the plasma membrane or plasma membrane-associated sub-membrane cisternae (Figure 2A). It is interesting to note that HeLa cells (HPV18+) show a similar distribution of E7, Figure 2B. We aimed to confirm this observation by detecting E7 staining in unpermeabilised SiHa cells. These experiments (with two different anti-HPV16 antibodies) demonstrated E7 localisation at the cell surface (Figure 2A, i and ii). No such pattern of staining was evident in SaOS-2 cells or HaCaT cells (HPV-negative cell lines), confirming the staining to be E7 specific (Figure 2A, iii and iv). We also employed a plasma membrane-specific stain (CellMask Orange). This stain is an amphipathic molecule, consisting of a lipophilic region and a negatively charged hydrophilic dye for membrane loading and the attachment of the probe in the plasma membrane, respectively [32,33]. Use of CellMask also demonstrated the presence of E7 at the plasma membrane, Figure 3A.

It should be noted that we were unable to produce membrane fractions that were completely free of cytoplasmic contamination, therefore were unable to confirm E7 localisation by cell fractionation (data not shown). However, we investigated the ability of E7 to undergo internalisation and removal from the plasma membrane, using protocols documented for the study of other cell-surface proteins [34]. Cells were maintained at 4 °C to allow antibody attachment followed by incubation at 37 °C for 30 min to follow the internalisation of cell-surface E7. Redistribution of E7, from a peripheral cell surface localisation (observed at $t = 0$) to the peri-nuclear region of the cells (at $t = 30$ min) was observed. This strongly suggested that E7 is endocytosed from the plasma membrane to an intracellular compartment, indicative of rapid internalisation from the cell surface (Figure 3B).

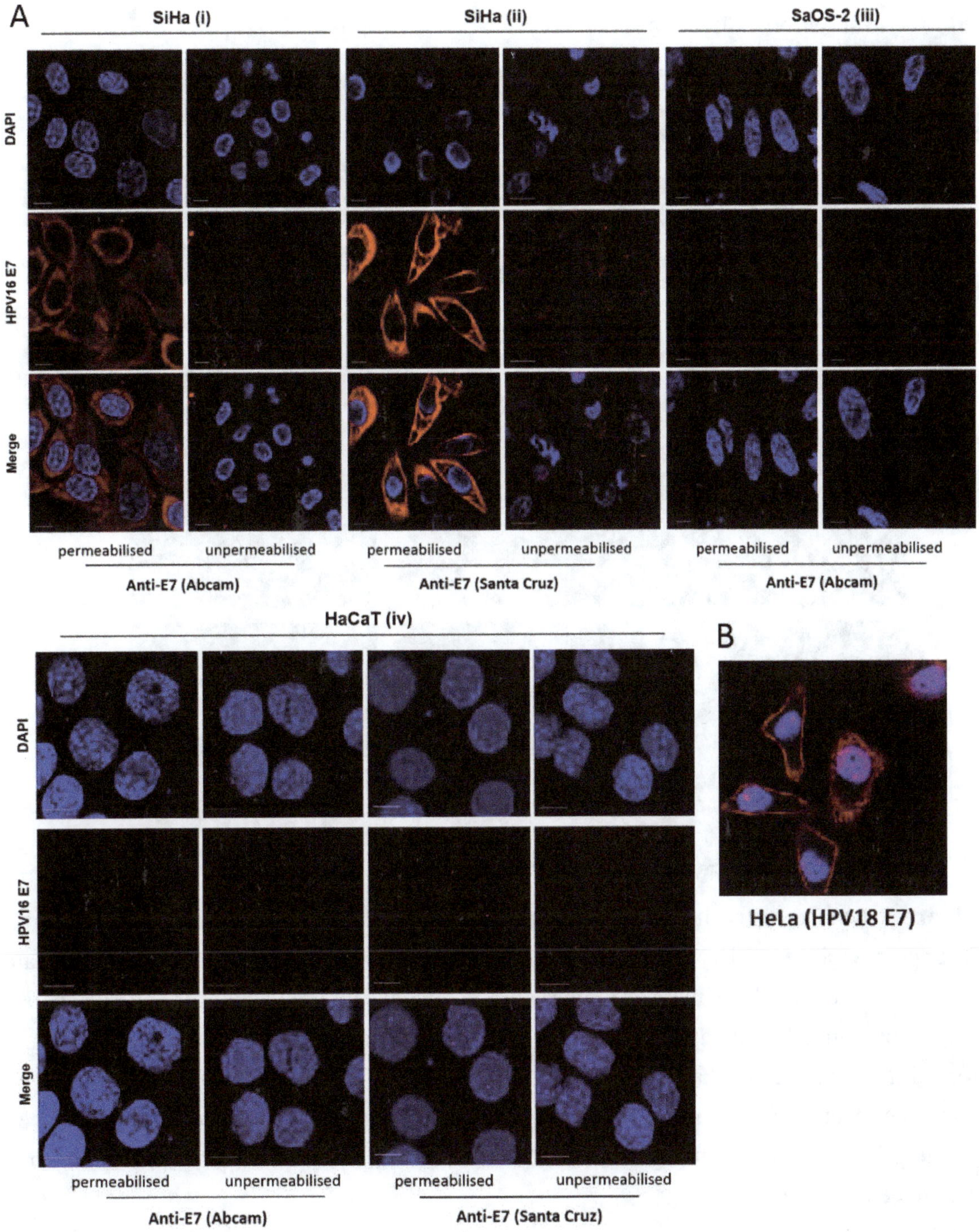

Figure 2. E7 distributes to the plasma membrane of HPV-transformed cells. (**A**) HPV16 E7+ SiHa cells (i and ii) and SaOS-2 cells (iii) HaCaT cells (iv) (as negative controls, containing no E7) were fixed, permeabilised and incubated with antibodies recognising full-length HPV16 E7 (i) and (iii) and residues 35–56 (ii). A comparable group of live cells was incubated with these antibodies in parallel. Cells were fixed and stained with AlexaFluor568 anti-mouse antibodies. Fluorescent imaging was performed using either a Zeiss LSM700 or LSM510 inverted microscope. The scale bar = 10 μm. Representative images are shown; (**B**) HeLa cells were fixed, permeabilised and labelled with anti-HPV18 E7 antibodies, which recognise residues 36–70, followed by staining with AlexaFluor594 goat anti-mouse IgG.

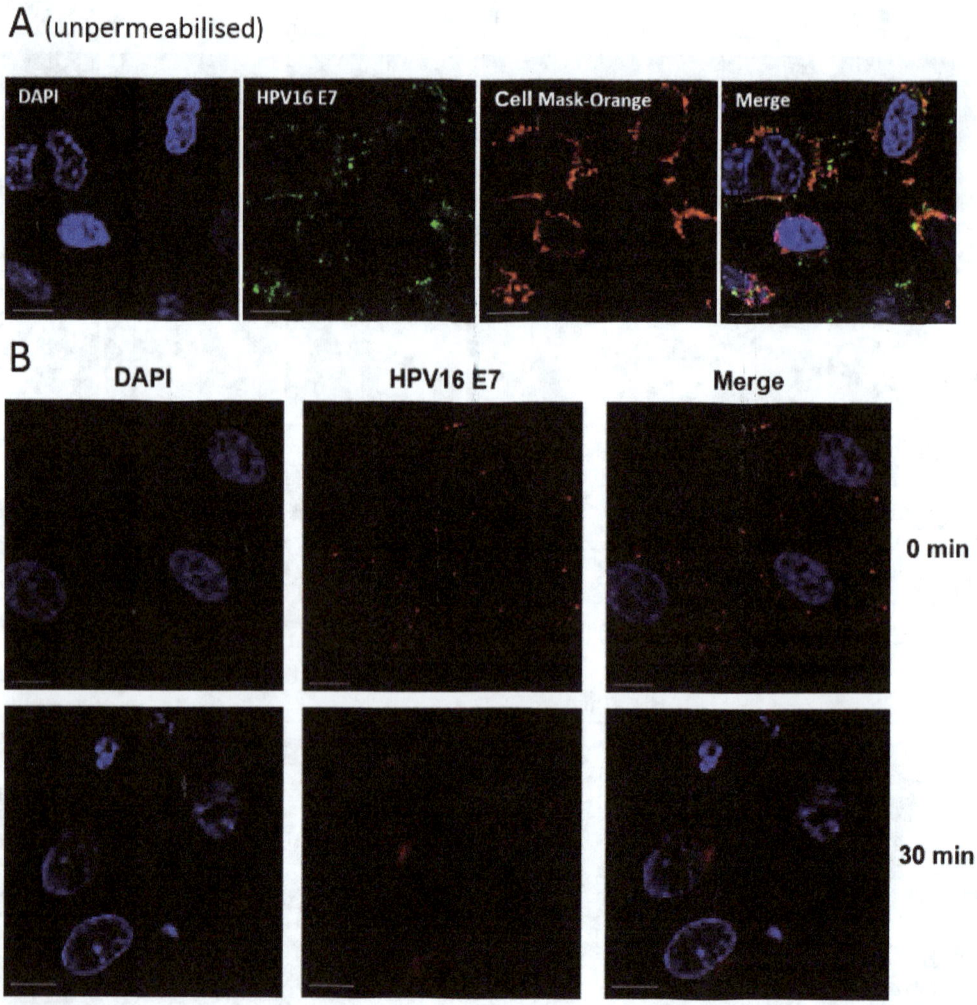

Figure 3. (**A**) Co-distribution of E7 with the cell membrane marker CellMask Orange (red) in unpermeabilised SiHa cells. Live cells were dual-stained with anti-E7 (Abcam) and CellMask Orange; (**B**) Time and temperature-dependent internalisation of cell surface E7, chased by anti-E7 antibody (Abcam). SiHa cells were incubated with the anti-E7 antibody for 1 h at 4 °C and incubated at 37 °C for 30 min to allow E7 internalisation. Cells were fixed, permeabilised and stained with AlexaFluor568 anti-mouse antibodies. Fluorescent imaging was performed using either a Zeiss LSM700 or LSM510 inverted microscope. The scale bar = 10 μm.

3.3. Aptamers Localise to Early/Late Endosomes upon Transfection

The internalisation of ligands, extracellular molecules, plasma membrane proteins and lipids commonly occur by endocytosis. Typically, endocytosed cargo is delivered to early endosomal compartments, followed by transit to the late endosomes/lysosomes for degradation, to the trans-Golgi network (TGN) or recycling endosomes in order to return the cargo back to the plasma membrane, reviewed in [35]. However, little is known about the sub-cellular localisation of RNA molecules after uptake.

To investigate uptake of RNA aptamers in E7-expressing cells, we utilised chemically-synthesised, model aptamers (*i.e.*, not selected to bind to E7), labelled with Cy3 [26,31] and assessed their transit into cellular compartments at defined time points post-incubation. Counting the number of aptamer-postive cells revealed a transfection efficiency of 87% (n = 90). At 3 h post-transfection, co-localisation with EEA1 demonstrated that the cy3-labelled aptamer 21-2 predominantly localised to early endosomes (63.3%, Figure 4A,C). However, in cells transfected for 6 h, this co-localisation was reduced and the aptamer was localised to both early and late endosomes/lysosomes (45.5% and 33.2% respectively, Figure 4B,C). A second aptamer, Cy3-labelled 47tr, displayed a similar pattern of distribution to Cy3 21-2 in SiHa cells (data not shown). Taken together these data suggest that RNA aptamers are targeted to early/late endosomal/lysosomal pathways following cell entry. However, the fate of these aptamers at later time points is currently unknown.

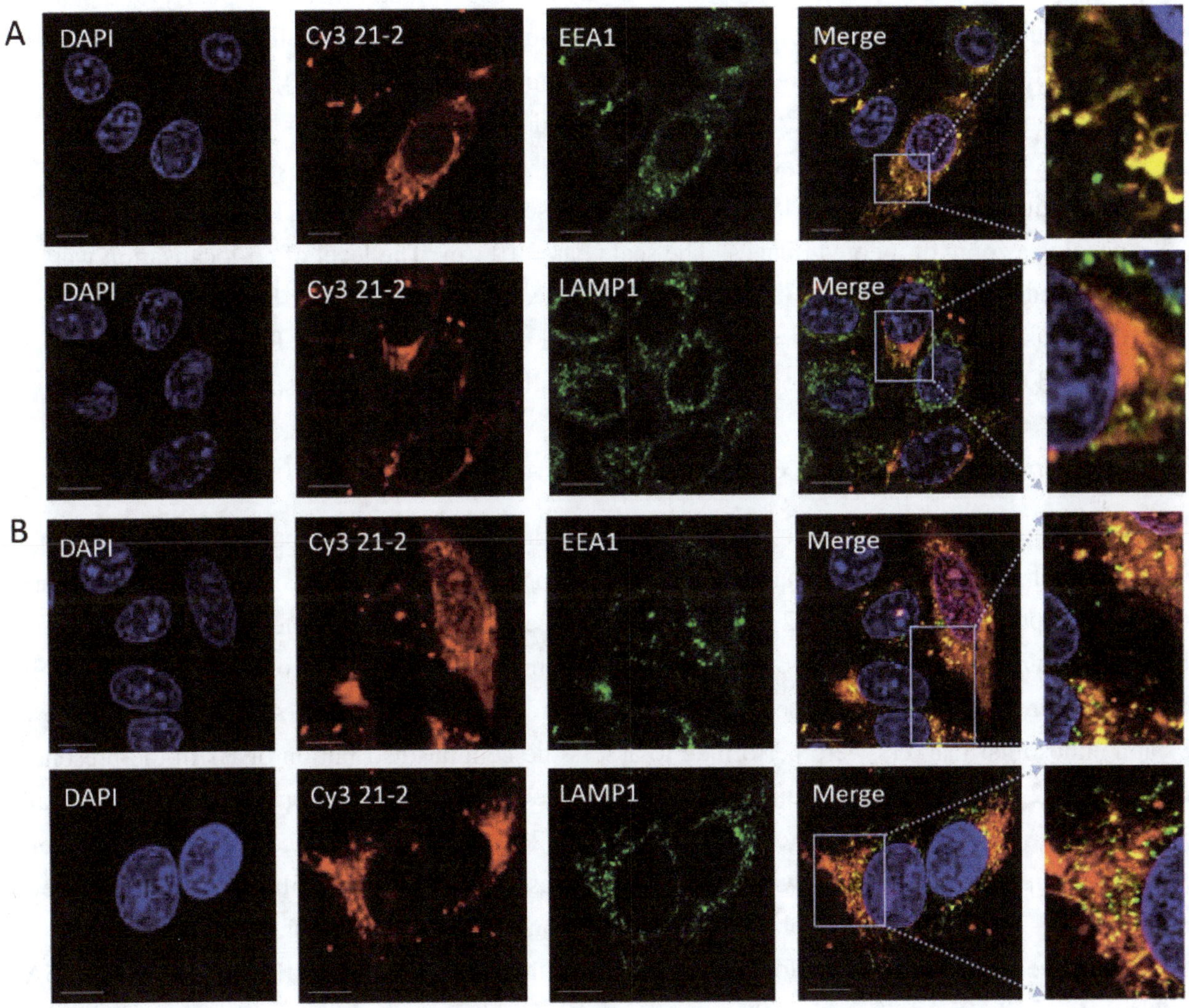

Figure 4. *Cont.*

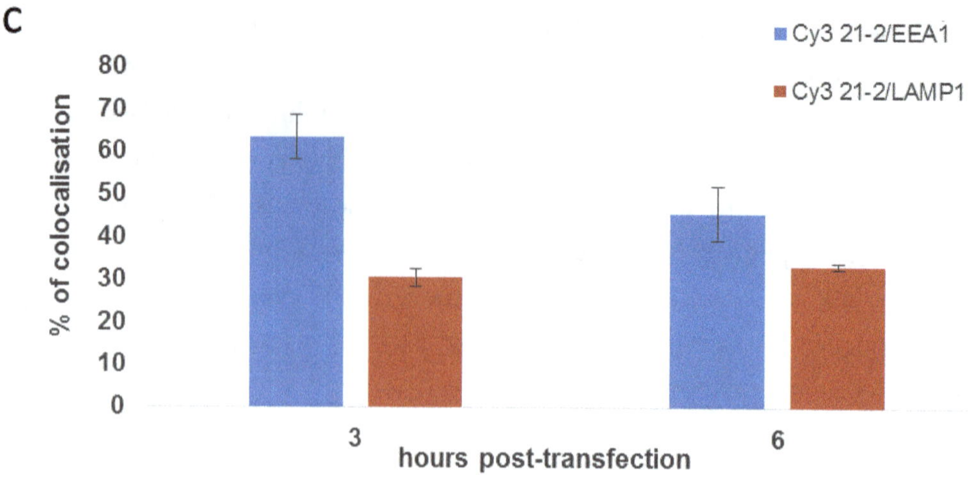

Figure 4. A model aptamer (aptamer 21-2) localises predominantly in early and late endosomes in SiHa cells following Oligofectamine transfection. Cells were transfected with 80 nM Cy3-labelled 21-2 using Oligofectamine. At 3 (Panel (**A**)) or 6 h (Panel (**B**)) post-transfection, cells were fixed, permeabilised and incubated with primary antibodies anti-EEA1 or anti-LAMP1 (staining early and late endosomes, respectively) prior to incubation with AlexaFluor488 goat anti-rabbit secondary antibody. The right hand side panel is a zoom of merged images. The scale bar = 10 μm. The level of co-localisation was analysed by Bitplane:Imeris image analysis software (Panel (**C**)). For EEA1 and LAMP1 colocalisation respectively, $n = 8$ and 29 at 3 h and $n = 30$ and 19 at 6 h. Red, green and blue are Cy3 (21-2), FITC (early or late endosomes) and DAPI (nucleus), respectively.

3.4. Localisation of E7 in Cellular Compartments upon Aptamer Transfection

We have previously shown that aptamer A2 can reduce E7 levels [24] but the mechanism of this effect was not addressed. Given our finding that E7 can distribute to the plasma membrane (Figures 2 and 3) we hypothesised that the A2 aptamer may bind cell surface E7, and mediate E7 degradation via the endosomal/lysosomal pathways. As labelling of A2 may have effects on conformation and therefore function, indirect methods were used to evaluate the effects of A2 on E7. Co-localisation studies with E7 and endosomal markers were performed to assess the cellular distribution of E7 in the presence or absence of A2 and the control aptamer, SF1. Cells were fixed 16 h post-transfection, in order to allow time for any A2-mediated effects to become apparent [24]. It should be noted that we were unable to quantitate transfection efficiency with A2 or SF1. These aptamers are similar in size, but somewhat larger than 21-2. It is therefore likely that the transfection will be less efficient.

We observed only minimal co-localisation of E7 with the endosomal marker EEA1 (Figure 5A,C) with values of 12.6%, 13.0% and 16.0% for mock-, A2- and SF1-treated SiHa cells, respectively. There were no statistical significant differences between the three treatments. It should be noted that these data were collected at a later timepoint than the data shown in Figure 3, as we aimed to allow time for A2-mediated effects on E7 to become apparent. It is therefore possible that co-localisation between E7 and endosomal markers may have been evident at earlier times post-transfection. Co-localisation with LAMP1 (Figure 5B,C) was low and very similar for the three treatments (ranged between 2.0% and 2.5%, not significant. The level of colocalisation between the autophagosomal marker LC3 (Figure 6A,C) and

E7 also showed no difference between the three treatments (12.7%, 10.2%, 11.6%). In contrast, there was an increased co-localisation of E7 with the ER marker, calreticulin, upon transfection with A2 (Figure 6B,C). Co-localisation in mock- and SF1-treated cells was 15.1% and 15.1%, but significantly higher at 32.3% in A2-transfected cells ($p \leq 0.01$). Taken together, these data suggest that A2 perturbs normal E7 trafficking and cellular distribution through enhancing E7 ER retention following E7 binding.

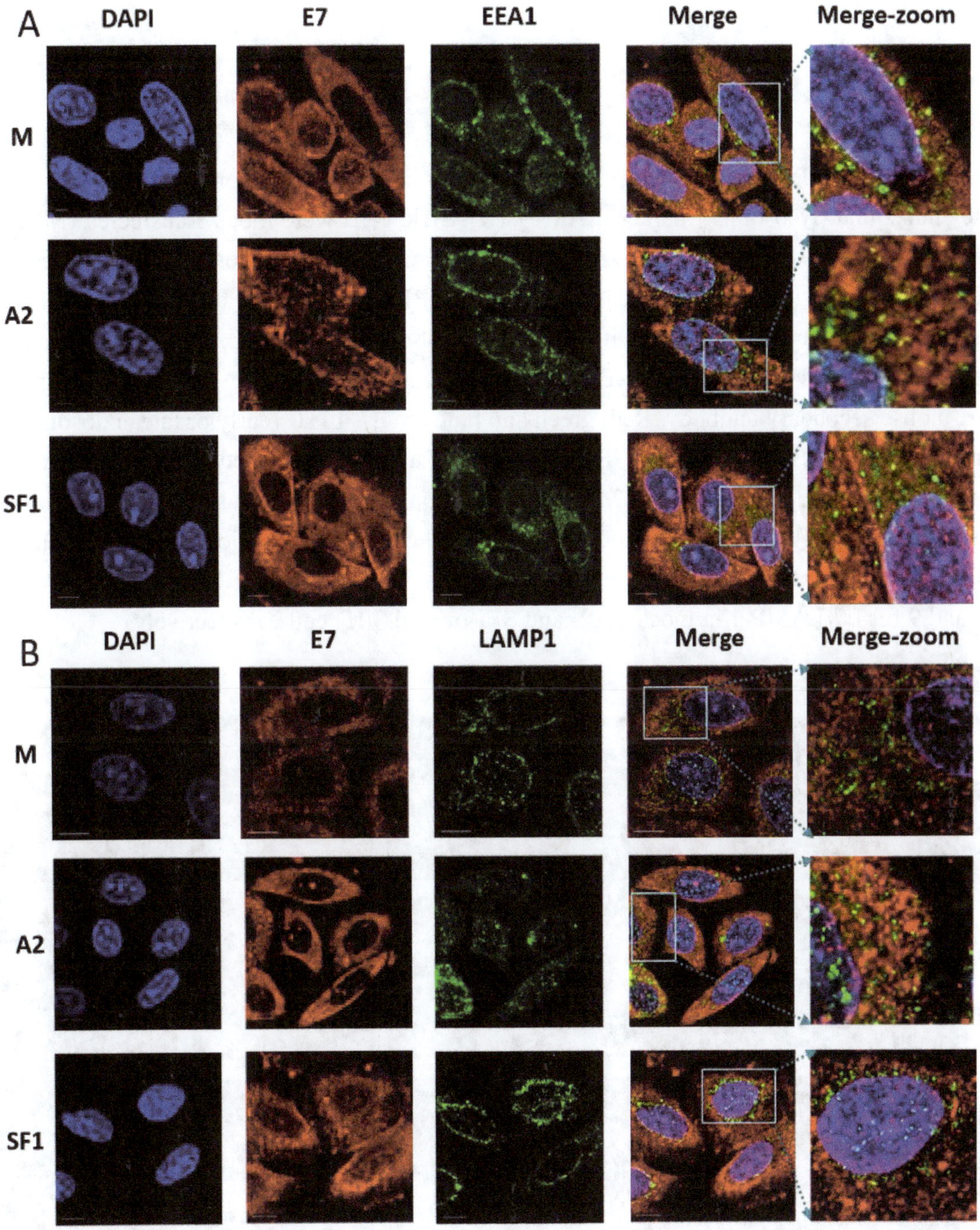

Figure 5. *Cont.*

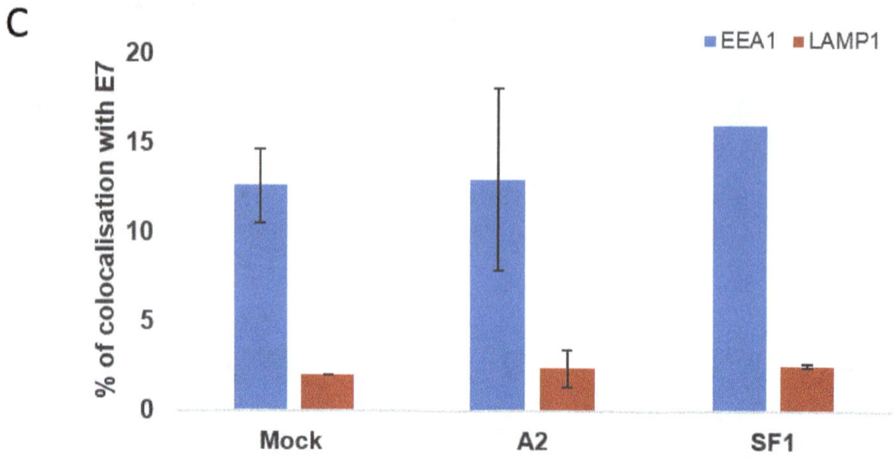

Figure 5. E7 does not co-localise with the early endosomal marker, EEA1 (**A**) or the late endosomal (lysosomal) marker, LAMP1 (**B**). SiHa cells were mock-transfected (M) or transfected with 100 nM A2 or SF1 using Oligofectamine. At 14 h post-transfection, cells were co-stained with either anti-EEA1 or anti-LAMP1 (staining early and late endosomes, respectively) prior to incubation with AlexaFluor488 goat anti-rabbit secondary antibody. Cells were then incubated with anti-E7 antibody (Abcam) followed by AlexaFluor568 rabbit anti-mouse secondary antibody. Red, green and blue are E7, FITC (early or late endosomes) and DAPI (nucleus), respectively. The last panel is a zoom of merged images. The scale bar = 10 μm. E7/EEA1 and E7/LAMP1 colocalisation were analysed using Bitplane:Imeris image analysis software based on the calculation of Pearson's correlation coefficient values and presented as percentage co-localisation (**C**). n = 27, 23 and 4 for E7/EEA1 and n = 12, 24 and 9 for E7/LAMP-1 in mock-, A2- and SFI-treated SiHa cells, respectively.

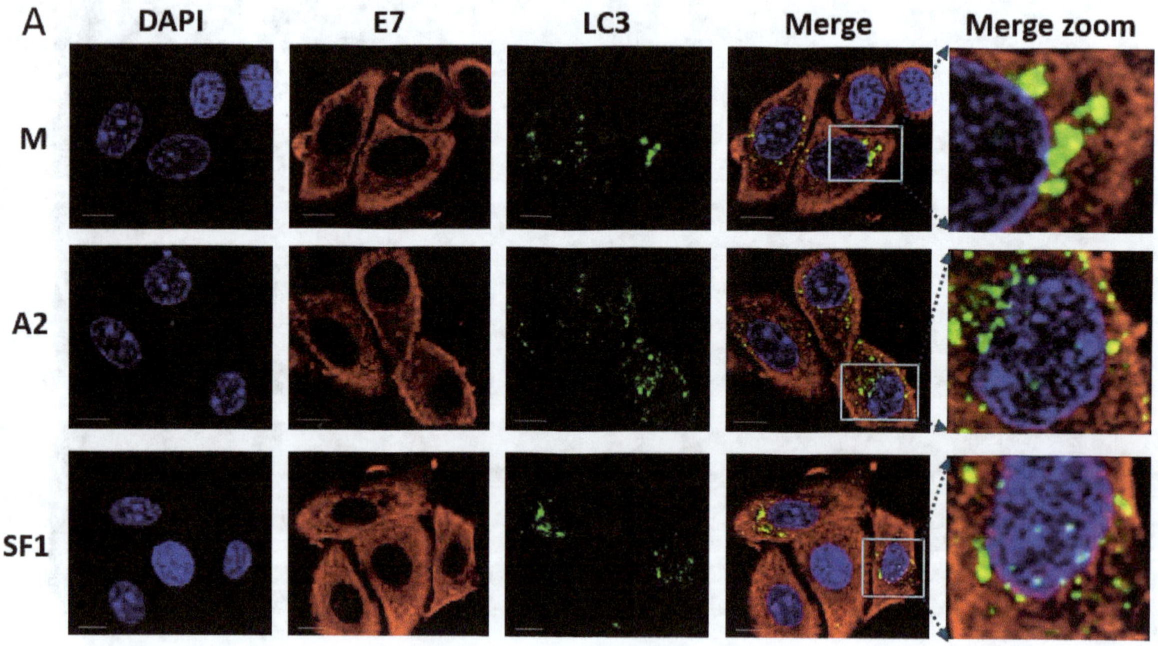

Figure 6. *Cont.*

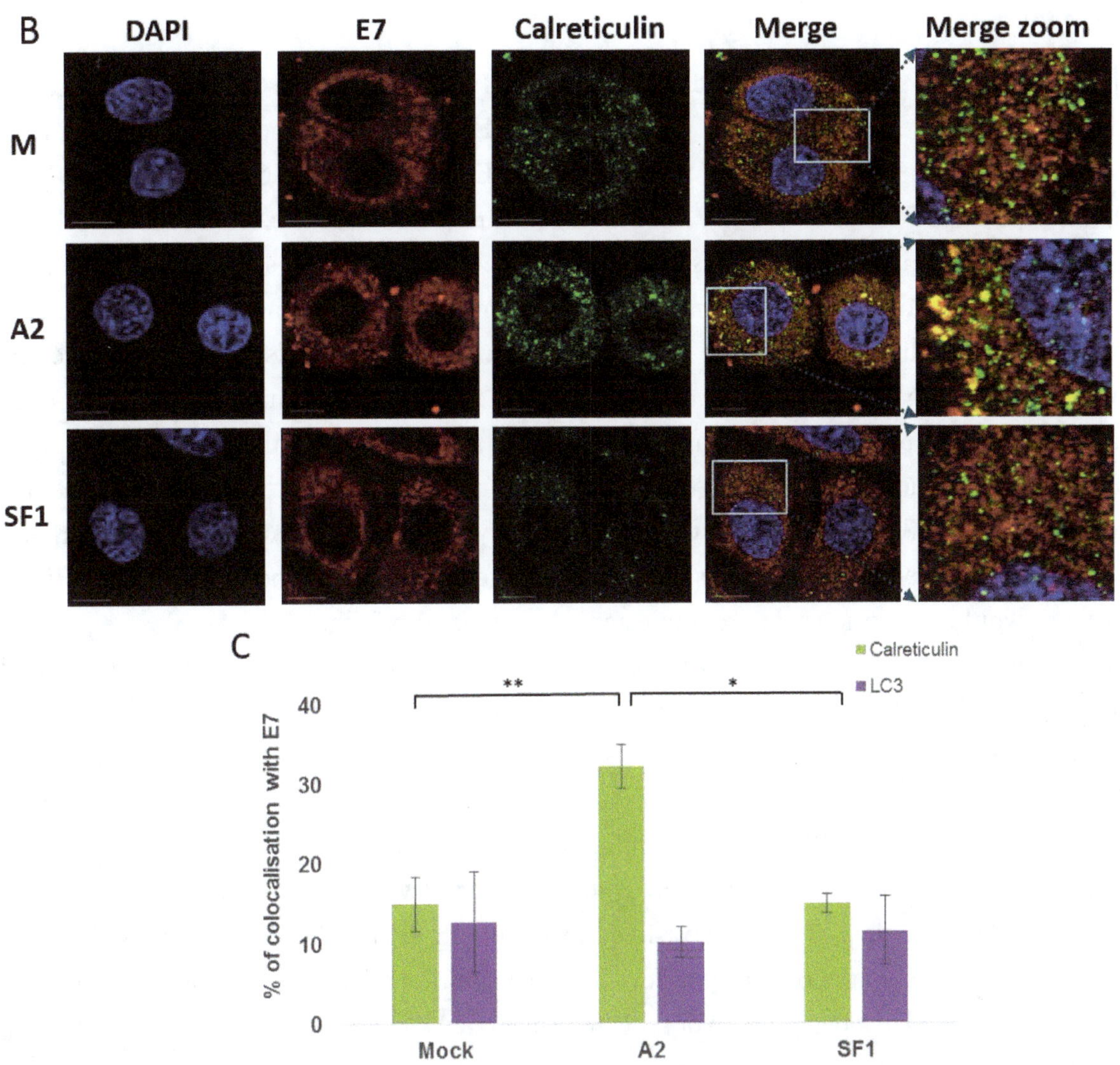

Figure 6. E7 does not co-localise with an autophagosome marker, LC3 (**A**) but appears to co-localise with endoplasmic reticulum marker calreticulin (**B**) in the presence of A2. SiHa cells were mock-transfected (M) or transfected with 100 nM A2 or SF1 using Oligofectamine. At 14 h post-transfection, cells were co-stained with anti-E7 (Abcam) and either anti-LC3 (an autophagosomal marker) or anti-calreticulin (an ER marker) prior to incubation with either AlexaFluor568 rabbit anti-mouse or AlexaFluor488 goat anti-rabbit secondary antibodies. Red, Green and Blue are E7, FITC (LC3, autophagosome) and DAPI (nucleus), respectively. The last panel is a zoom of merged images. The scale bar = 10 μm. E7/LC3 and E7/calreticulin colocalisation was analysed using Bitplane:Imeris image analysis software based on the calculation of Pearson's correlation coefficient values and presented as percentage co-localisation (**C**). n = 21, 23 and 17 for E7/LC3 and n = 19, 39 and 20 for E7/calreticulin with mock-, A2- and SFI-treatment, respectively. * $p \leq 0.0005$, ** $p \leq 0.002$.

4. Discussion

This work is the first to describe the localisation of E7 to the plasma membrane and to propose a mechanism for E7 degradation in the presence of the E7-specific aptamer, A2. Three independent antibodies recognising full-length HPV16 E7, HPV16 E7 residues 35–56 and HPV18 E7 residues 36–70 were employed to show that E7 distributed to the plasma membrane. It is therefore likely that the N-terminal region of E7 is accessible and extracellularly-exposed since we could detect E7 in unpermeabilised SiHa cells. We were unable to produce membrane fractions that were completely free of cytoplasmic contamination, therefore were unable to confirm E7 localisation by cell fractionation. However, the data above, together with the ability of E7 to undergo internalisation and removal from the plasma membrane provide compelling evidence for membrane localisation. It should be noted that the amount of membrane-associated E7 is relatively low and this could explain why this has not been detected previously [13,36]. The level of cell confluency could also be a factor [18]. Although the data with HPV18 is preliminary, it is possible that this effect may be common across other HPV types. Further work would be necessary in order to establish whether this is the case.

We have previously reported that transfection of CaSki cells with the aptamer A2 resulted in a decrease of E7 levels with an accompanying increase in pRb, which was suggested as the reason behind the apoptotic effects of A2 observed in HPV-transformed cells [24]. The loss of E7 in A2-transfected cells was previously suggested to be due to the inability of A2-bound E7 to interact with its major cellular partners including pRb, thus remaining unfolded which could lead to destabilisation and degradation [24]. The proteasome/ubiquitin system is primarily responsible for clearance of cellular misfolded/unfolded proteins. E7 is a short-lived protein with a half-life of 30–40 min [13], allowing detection of protein accumulation within a few hours of addition of MG132. Consistent with previous studies [37], we showed that degradation of E7 can be mediated by 26S proteasomes as MG132 treatment resulted in the accumulation of E7. However, in the presence A2, E7 accumulation was much less evident. Given this data, we propose an alternative non-proteasomal mechanism for aptamer-mediated E7 degradation.

Studies with a control, labelled aptamer revealed that this molecule localised to both early and late endosomes. Localisation to early endosomes was particularly striking at early timepoints post-transfection (3 h). It is interesting to note that the reduction in co-localisation seen after 6 h did not correlate with an increase in co-localisation with the late endosomal marker. Further time points might be useful, however, this could be indicative of escape of aptamers from the endocytic pathway. Whilst there is a paucity of data on the sub-cellular localisation of aptamers, transfection of siRNAs using cationic lipids, nanoparticles or cell-type-specific delivery reagents have shown that siRNAs are trafficked to the endosomal pathway (early and then late endosomes), reviewed in [38]. It is clear that such siRNA molecules must escape the endosomal pathway to function, and the observation led to a hypothesis for A2-mediated activity. E7 on the cell surface could be internalised along with the bound aptamer during transfection, resulting in its accumulation in endosomes and then late endosomes/lysosomes for degradation. In order to investigate this hypothesis, HPV16+ SiHa cells were co-stained with E7 and several endosomal markers in the presence and absence of A2. We found no evidence of E7 accumulation in lysosomes or autophagosomes in aptamer-transfected or mock-transfected SiHa cells after 14 h. However, E7 localisation in the ER (using calreticulin as a marker) increased in cells transfected with A2. Interestingly, E7 localisation to the ER has been demonstrated previously in CaSki cells (using calnexin as a marker) [39]. These authors also noted localisation to the Golgi, we have not investigated whether A2 has any effect here. Our data suggest that a possible conformational change of E7, mediated by A2 binding, leads to an accumulation in the ER. This would be predicted to perturb normal biosynthetic delivery of E7 to the plasma membrane or other organelles (Figure 7). As E7 does not possess common peptide ER retention motifs such as [K/H]DEL, KKXXX, KXKXXX and PL[Y/F][F/Y]XXN, it is likely that A2 binding prevents correct E7 folding/oligomerisationleading to its accumulation in an unfolded/aberrant state. This accumulation of unfolded E7 and subsequent stimulation of related stress responses may contribute to the stimulation of apoptosis previously observed in HPV+ cells [24,40–42]. Future work (including the use of specific inhibitors) would be necessary to validate this model.

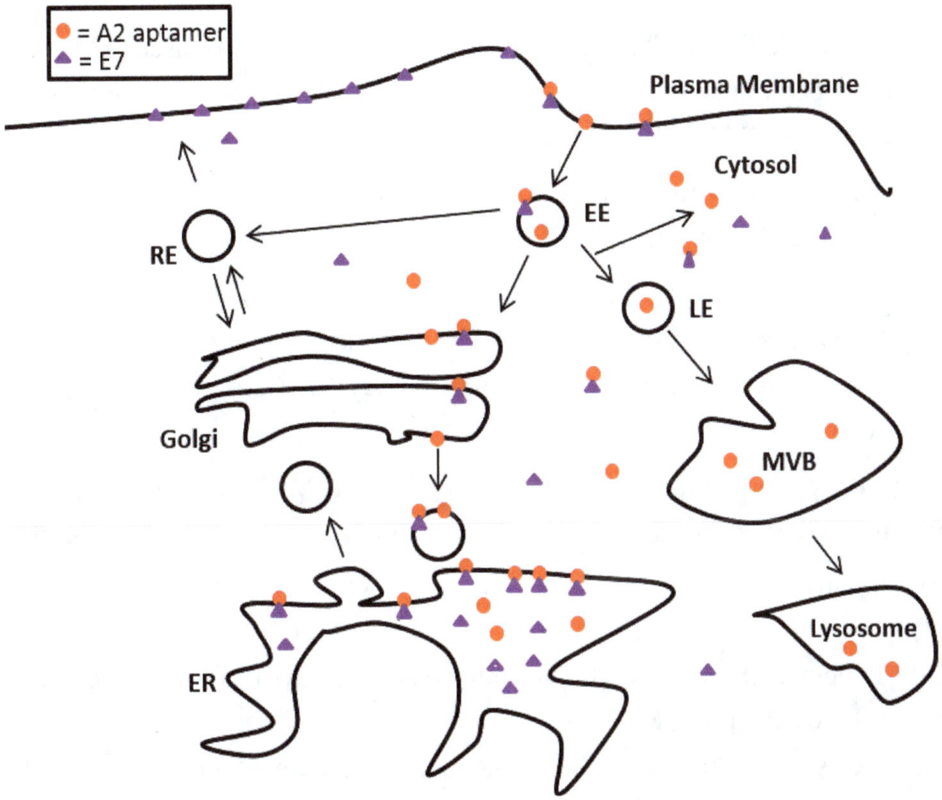

Figure 7. A2 can enter the cells alone or via the endosomal system. Upon contact with E7; either at the plasma membrane or intracellularly, A2 enhances E7 retention in the ER. This would be predicted to reduce E7 delivery to the plasma membrane via its normal biosynthetic route. ER: endoplasmic reticulum, EE: early endosome, LE: late endosome, MVB: multivesicular bodies, RE: recycling endosome.

5. Conclusions

In summary, the data reported here demonstrate the utility of RNA aptamers as molecular tools to aid our understanding of the cellular function of the HPV E7 oncoprotein.

Acknowledgments

O.C. would like to thank to the Turkish Ministry of National Education for funding. We also thank all members of the Stonehouse, Blair and Mankouri groups for helpful discussions.

Author Contributions

All authors contributed to manuscript preparation. O.C., C.N. and H.G. generated experimental data. J.M., G.E.B. and N.J.S. contributed to experimental design and data analysis.

References

1. PaVE: Papilloma Virus Genome Database. Available online: http://pave.niaid.nih.gov/#home (accessed on 23 June 2015).
2. Bernard, H.U.; Burk, R.D.; Chen, Z.; van Doorslaer, K.; zur Hausen, H.; de Villiers, E.M. Classification of papillomaviruses (PVs) based on 189 PV types and proposal of taxonomic amendments. *Virology* **2010**, *401*, 70–79. [CrossRef] [PubMed]
3. Zur Hausen, H. Papillomaviruses in the causation of human cancers—A brief historical account. *Virology* **2009**, *384*, 260–265. [CrossRef] [PubMed]
4. Naucler, P.; Mabota da Costa, F.; da Costa, J.L.; Ljungberg, O.; Bugalho, A.; Dillner, J. Human papillomavirus type-specific risk of cervical cancer in a population with high human immunodeficiency virus prevalence: Case-control study. *J. Gen. Virol.* **2011**, *92*, 2784–2791. [CrossRef] [PubMed]
5. Bosch, F.X.; Lorincz, A.; Muñoz, N.; Meijer, C.J.; Shah, K.V. The causal relation between human papillomavirus and cervical cancer. *J. Clin. Pathol.* **2002**, *55*, 244–265. [CrossRef] [PubMed]
6. Human papillomavirus vaccines: WHO position paper, October 2014-Recommendations. *Vaccine*. [CrossRef]
7. McLaughlin-Drubin, M.E.; Munger, K. The human papillomavirus E7 oncoprotein. *Virology* **2009**, *384*, 335–344. [CrossRef] [PubMed]
8. Liu, X.; Clements, A.; Zhao, K.; Marmorstein, R. Structure of the human Papillomavirus E7 oncoprotein and its mechanism for inactivation of the retinoblastoma tumor suppressor. *J. Biol. Chem.* **2006**, *281*, 578–586. [CrossRef] [PubMed]
9. Ohlenschlager, O.; Seiboth, T.; Zengerling, H.; Briese, L.; Marchanka, A.; Ramachandran, R.; Baum, M.; Korbas, M.; Meyer-Klaucke, W.; Dürst, M.; *et al.* Solution structure of the partially folded high-risk human papilloma virus 45 oncoprotein E7. *Oncogene* **2006**, *25*, 5953–5959. [CrossRef]
10. McIntyre, M.C.; Frattini, M.G.; Grossman, S.R.; Laimins, L.A. Human papillomavirus type 18 E7 protein requires intact Cys-X-X-Cys motifs for zinc binding, dimerization, and transformation but not for Rb binding. *J. Virol.* **1993**, *67*, 3142–3150. [PubMed]
11. Clements, A.; Johnston, K.; Mazzarelli, J.M.; Ricciardi, R.P.; Marmorstein, R. Oligomerization properties of the viral oncoproteins adenovirus E1A and human papillomavirus E7 and their

complexes with the retinoblastoma protein. *Biochemistry* **2000**, *39*, 16033–16045. [CrossRef] [PubMed]

12. Alonso, L.G.; García-Alai, M.M.; Smal, C.; Centeno, J.M.; Iacono, R.; Castaño, E.; Gualfetti, P.; de Prat-Gay, G. The HPV16 E7 viral oncoprotein self-assembles into defined spherical oligomers. *Biochemistry* **2004**, *43*, 3310–3317. [CrossRef] [PubMed]
13. Smotkin, D.; Wettstein, F.O. The major human papillomavirus protein in cervical cancers is a cytoplasmic phosphoprotein. *J. Virol.* **1987**, *61*, 1686–1689. [PubMed]
14. Smith-McCune, K.; Kalman, D.; Robbins, C.; Shivakumar, S.; Yuschenkoff, L.; Bishop, J.M. Intranuclear localization of human papillomavirus 16 E7 during transformation and preferential binding of E7 to the Rb family member p130. *Proc. Natl. Acad. Sci. USA* **1999**, *96*, 6999–7004. [CrossRef] [PubMed]
15. Zatsepina, O.; Braspenning, J.; Robberson, D.; Hajibagheri, M.A.; Blight, K.J.; Ely, S.; Hibma, M.; Spitkovsky, D.; Trendelenburg, M.; Crawford, L.; *et al.* The human papillomavirus type 16 E7 protein is associated with the nucleolus in mammalian and yeast cells. *Oncogene* **1997**, *14*, 1137–1145. [CrossRef] [PubMed]
16. Dantur, K.; Alonso, L.; Castaño, E.; Morelli, L.; Centeno-Crowley, J.M.; Vighi, S.; de Prat-Gay, G. Cytosolic accumulation of HPV16 E7 oligomers supports different transformation routes for the prototypic viral oncoprotein: The amyloid-cancer connection. *Int. J. Cancer* **2009**, *125*, 1902–1911. [CrossRef] [PubMed]
17. Knapp, A.A.; McManus, P.M.; Bockstall, K.; Moroianu, J. Identification of the nuclear localization and export signals of high risk HPV16 E7 oncoprotein. *Virology* **2009**, *383*, 60–68. [CrossRef] [PubMed]
18. Laurson, J.; Raj, K. Localisation of human papillomavirus 16 E7 oncoprotein changes with cell confluence. *PLoS ONE* **2011**, *6*, e21501. [CrossRef] [PubMed]
19. Tuerk, C.; Gold, L. Systematic evolution of ligands by exponential enrichment: RNA ligands to bacteriophage T4 DNA polymerase. *Science* **1990**, *249*, 505–510. [CrossRef] [PubMed]
20. Keefe, A.D.; Cload, S.T. SELEX with modified nucleotides. *Curr. Opin. Chem. Biol.* **2008**, *12*, 448–456. [CrossRef] [PubMed]
21. Blind, M.; Blank, M. Aptamer Selection Technology and Recent Advances. *Mol. Ther. Nucleic Acids* **2015**, *4*, e223. [CrossRef]
22. Belyaeva, T.A.; Nicol, C.; Cesur, O.; Travé, G.; Blair, G.E.; Stonehouse, N.J. An RNA Aptamer Targets the PDZ-Binding Motif of the HPV16 E6 Oncoprotein. *Cancers* **2014**, *6*, 1553–1569. [CrossRef] [PubMed]
23. Nicol, C.; Bunka, D.H.; Blair, G.E.; Stonehouse, N.J. Effects of single nucleotide changes on the binding and activity of RNA aptamers to human papillomavirus 16 E7 oncoprotein. *Biochem. Biophys. Res. Commun.* **2011**, *405*, 417–421. [CrossRef] [PubMed]
24. Nicol, C.; Cesur, Ö.; Forrest, S.; Belyaeva, T.A.; Bunka, D.H.; Blair, G.E.; Stonehouse, N.J. An RNA aptamer provides a novel approach for the induction of apoptosis by targeting the HPV16 E7 oncoprotein. *PLoS ONE* **2013**, *8*, e64781. [CrossRef] [PubMed]
25. Ellingham, M.; Bunka, D.H.; Rowlands, D.J.; Stonehouse, N.J. Selection and characterization of RNA aptamers to the RNA-dependent RNA polymerase from foot-and-mouth disease virus. *RNA*

2006, *12*, 1970–1979. [CrossRef] [PubMed]

26. Forrest, S.; Lear, Z.; Herod, M.R.; Ryan, M.; Rowlands, D.J.; Stonehouse, N.J. Inhibition of the foot-and-mouth disease virus subgenomic replicon by RNA aptamers. *J. Gen. Virol.* **2014**, *95*, 2649–2657. [CrossRef] [PubMed]
27. Bellecave, P.; Cazenave, C.; Rumi, J.; Staedel, C.; Cosnefroy, O.; Andreola, M.L.; Ventura, M.; Tarrago-Litvak, L.; Astier-Gin, T. Inhibition of hepatitis C virus (HCV) RNA polymerase by DNA aptamers: Mechanism of inhibition of in vitro RNA synthesis and effect on HCV-infected cells. *Antimicrob. Agents Chemother.* **2008**, *52*, 2097–2110. [CrossRef] [PubMed]
28. Biroccio, A.; Hamm, J.; Incitti, I.; De Francesco, R.; Tomei, L. Selection of RNA aptamers that are specific and high-affinity ligands of the hepatitis C virus RNA-dependent RNA polymerase. *J. Virol.* **2002**, *76*, 3688–3696. [CrossRef] [PubMed]
29. Bates, P.J.; Kahlon, J.B.; Thomas, S.D.; Trent, J.O.; Miller, D.M. Antiproliferative activity of G-rich oligonucleotides correlates with protein binding. *J. Biol. Chem.* **1999**, *274*, 26369–26377. [CrossRef] [PubMed]
30. Sayyed, S.G.; Hägele, H.; Kulkarni, O.P.; Endlich, K.; Segerer, S.; Eulberg, D.; Klussmann, S.; Anders, H.J. Podocytes produce homeostatic chemokine stromal cell-derived factor-1/CXCL12, which contributes to glomerulosclerosis, podocyte loss and albuminuria in a mouse model of type 2 diabetes. *Diabetologia* **2009**, *52*, 2445–2454. [CrossRef] [PubMed]
31. Doble, R.; McDermott, M.F.; Cesur, O.; Stonehouse, N.J.; Wittmann, M. IL-17A RNA aptamer: Possible therapeutic potential in some cells, more than we bargained for in others? *J. Investig. Dermatol.* **2014**, *134*, 852–855. [CrossRef] [PubMed]
32. Nafissi, N.; Alqawlaq, S.; Lee, E.A.; Foldvari, M.; Spagnuolo, P.A.; Slavcev, R.A. DNA ministrings: Highly safe and effective gene delivery vectors. *Mol. Ther. Nucleic Acids* **2014**, *3*, e165. [CrossRef] [PubMed]
33. Rossignol, J.F.; La Frazia, S.; Chiappa, L.; Ciucci, A.; Santoro, M.G. Thiazolides, a new class of anti-influenza molecules targeting viral hemagglutinin at the post-translational level. *J. Biol. Chem.* **2009**, *284*, 29798–29808. [CrossRef] [PubMed]
34. Mankouri, J.; Taneja, T.K.; Smith, A.J.; Ponnambalam, S.; Sivaprasadarao, A. Kir6.2 mutations causing neonatal diabetes prevent endocytosis of ATP-sensitive potassium channels. *EMBO J.* **2006**, *25*, 4142–4151. [CrossRef] [PubMed]
35. Grant, B.D.; Donaldson, J.G. Pathways and mechanisms of endocytic recycling. *Nat. Rev. Mol. Cell Biol.* **2009**, *10*, 597–608. [CrossRef] [PubMed]
36. Greenfield, I.; Nickerson, J.; Penman, S.; Stanley, M. Human papillomavirus 16 E7 protein is associated with the nuclear matrix. *Proc. Natl. Acad. Sci. USA* **1991**, *88*, 11217–11221. [CrossRef] [PubMed]
37. Reinstein, E.; Scheffner, M.; Oren, M.; Ciechanover, A.; Schwartz, A. Degradation of the E7 human papillomavirus oncoprotein by the ubiquitin-proteasome system: Targeting via ubiquitination of the N-terminal residue. *Oncogene* **2000**, *19*, 5944–5950. [CrossRef] [PubMed]
38. Dominska, M.; Dykxhoorn, D.M. Breaking down the barriers: siRNA delivery and endosome escape. *J. Cell Sci.* **2010**, *123*, 1183–1189. [CrossRef] [PubMed]
39. Valdovinos-Torres, H.; Orozco-Morales, M.; Pedroza-Saavedra, A.; Padilla-Noriega, L.;

Esquivel-Guadarrama, F.; Gutierrez-Xicotencatl, L. Different Isoforms of HPV-16 E7 Protein are Present in Cytoplasm and Nucleus. *Open Virol. J.* **2008**, *2*, 15–23. [CrossRef] [PubMed]

40. Casagrande, R.; Stern, P.; Diehn, M.; Shamu, C.; Osario, M.; Zúñiga, M.; Brown, P.O.; Ploegh, H. Degradation of proteins from the ER of S. cerevisiae requires an intact unfolded protein response pathway. *Mol. Cell* **2000**, *5*, 729–735. [CrossRef]
41. Liu, C.Y.; Kaufman, R.J. The unfolded protein response. *J. Cell Sci.* **2003**, *116*, 1861–1862. [CrossRef] [PubMed]
42. Travers, K.J.; Patil, C.K.; Wodicka, L.; Lockhart, D.J.; Weissman, J.S.; Walter, P. Functional and genomic analyses reveal an essential coordination between the unfolded protein response and ER-associated degradation. *Cell* **2000**, *101*, 249–258. [CrossRef]

6

Papillomavirus Infectious Pathways: A Comparison of Systems

Jennifer Biryukov and Craig Meyers *

Department of Microbiology and Immunology, The Pennsylvania State University, 500 University Drive, Hershey, PA 17033, USA; E-Mail: jhopkins@hmc.psu.edu

* Author to whom correspondence should be addressed; E-Mail: cmm10@psu.edu;

Academic Editor: Joanna Parish

Abstract: The HPV viral lifecycle is tightly linked to the host cell differentiation, causing difficulty in growing virions in culture. A system that bypasses the need for differentiating epithelium has allowed for generation of recombinant particles, such as virus-like particles (VLPs), pseudovirions (PsV), and quasivirions (QV). Much of the research looking at the HPV life cycle, infectivity, and structure has been generated utilizing recombinant particles. While recombinant particles have proven to be invaluable, allowing for a rapid progression of the HPV field, there are some significant differences between recombinant particles and native virions and very few comparative studies using native virions to confirm results are done. This review serves to address the conflicting data in the HPV field regarding native virions and recombinant particles.

Keywords: human papillomavirus (HPV); virus; native virions (NV); virus-like particles (VLPs); pseudovirions (PsV); quasivirions (QV)

---

1. Introduction

Human papillomaviruses are the etiologic agent of cervical cancer and other anogenital and oral cancers [1–4]. To date, over 150 types have been identified. Cervical cancer is the third most common cancer in women worldwide, causing a quarter of a million deaths per year [5]. All HPV types replicate within epithelium, however, they are subdivided based on their ability to infect either mucosal or cutaneous keratinocytes. HPVs that infect mucosal keratinocytes are further sub-divided into low-risk and high-risk types. Low-risk HPVs cause benign lesions such as condylomas or warts while high-risk types cause malignant neoplasms such as cervical cancer [6,7]. The most significant risk of developing cervical cancer is infection with a high-risk type. High-risk types such as HPV16, HPV18, HPV31, HPV45, and HPV58 have a strong link with malignant progression [6–8].

HPV virions consist of an icosahedral capsid containing histone-associated dsDNA. The viral genome is circular and approximately 8000 bp in length. There is an average of 8 open reading frames (ORFs), which are divided into early and late gene expression classes. HPV replication is tightly linked to the differentiation program of host epithelial cells. Infection occurs in basal epithelial cells via microabrasions. Once infected, early non-structural proteins involved in activities such as genome maintenance and transcription activation are expressed. As the daughter cells divide and become increasingly differentiated in the suprabasal layers, viral genomes are amplified, the late structural proteins are expressed, and new virions assembled [9–13].

Because the HPV life cycle is tightly linked to the host cell differentiation, the virus has been hard to grow in culture. Therefore, systems to create viral particles bypassing epithelial differentiation were developed. Recent research studying the HPV life cycle including infectivity, transmission, and viral structure predominantly relies on the use of recombinant papillomavirus particles. These recombinant particles such as virus-like particles (VLPs), pseudovirions (PsVs), and quasivirions (QVs) all bypass the need for stratifying and differentiating human epithelium. While data collected using recombinant particles has allowed for a rapid progression of the field of HPV research, there are few comparative studies utilizing native virions produced in organotypic raft culture, xenografts, or native tissue to confirm results in the context of stratifying and differentiating human epithelial tissue.

Table 1. A comparison of the advantages and disadvantages of the different types of papillomavirus particles.

<table>
<tr><th>HPV Particle Type</th><th>Method of Production</th><th>Particle and System Advantages</th><th>Particle and System Disadvantages</th></tr>
<tr><td>Native Virions</td><td>Organotypic raft culture system</td><td>Contains the full HPV capsid as well as full HPV genome
Assembles and matures over a period of 10–20 days in tissue</td><td>Expensive
Slow production time</td></tr>
<tr><td>Virus Like Particles (VLPs)</td><td>Transfection based system</td><td>Quick and inexpensive particle production</td><td rowspan="3">Codon modification of L1 and L2 is necessary for production
Over-expression system
Particles produced in non-relevant cell lines
Particle assembly within 48 hours
Maturation occurs overnight
Deletion of in frame methionines upstream of the consensus methionine in L1
VLPs contain no genomes, which may alter particle structure</td></tr>
<tr><td>Pseudovirions (PsVs)</td><td>Transfection based system</td><td>Quick and inexpensive particle production
Ability to track cellular infectivity</td></tr>
<tr><td>Quasivirions (QVs)</td><td>Transfection based system</td><td>Quick and inexpensive particle production
Contains L1, L2, and a full HPV genome
Closest to NVs—retains majority of cell surface exposed conformational epitopes</td></tr>
</table>

The main focus of this review will be to compare native virions produced in stratifying epithelium to recombinant particles (Table 1). All aspects of the viral life cycle including particle synthesis, maturation, attachment/entry, and infectivity will be evaluated. While much of the data generated utilizing recombinant particles has served to advance the field, there are many instances of conflicting results when compared to data generated utilizing native virions. A fraction of the conflicting data is likely due to utilization of different cell lines, particle maturation, and the multiplicity of infection used. Additionally, much of the research has been done using recombinant HPV16 with the assumption that what holds true for one HPV type is true for all HPV types. However, some recent data suggests that this may not be the case [14,15]. We hope to highlight not only the necessity for confirmatory studies but also the importance of studying more than one HPV type.

2. Papillomavirus Particle Production

Organotypic raft culture is the only system outside of the xenograft system that allows for the production of infectious HPV in its natural environment, a differentiating epithelium [9,16–18]. This *in vitro* system preserves the molecular events that occur during differentiation with the convenience of not having to use animals such as in the xenograft system. In the organotypic system, human keratinocytes that stably maintain HPV viral genomes are grown above a dermal equivalent made of fibroblast cells embedded in a collagen matrix. Keratinocytes grow at the air liquid interface and are fed via diffusion from cell culture media below the dermal equivalent [9]. After a period of 10–20 days, tissue is harvested and homogenized to generate a virus stock (Figure 1). This system allows for the study of genetic mutants in the natural life cycle as genomes can be mutated, electroporated into keratinocytes, and grown in raft culture for the production of mutant virions. One drawback to using this system is the increased cost for virion production. Additionally, instead of producing particles in a matter of days, the raft culture system takes 3–4 weeks. Overall, this system allows researchers to examine, temporally and spatially, all parts of the viral life cycle including viral genome amplification, late gene expression, virion assembly, maturation, and infectivity.

The increased cost and technical challenges associated with acquiring virions from either an *in vivo* or *in vitro* system created a need for the development of the recombinant system (Figure 2). The basis of recombinant particle production comes from the fact that expression of either L1 alone or L1 and L2 together results in the self-assembly of proteins into viral capsids called VLPs [19–25]. For production of PsVs, in addition to the capsid proteins, a reporter plasmid encoding GFP or other reporter is co-transfected to function as a mock genome. These particles allow for researchers to easily track cellular infectivity [26,27]. Finally, when the full HPV genome is transfected into cells along with expression vectors for the capsid proteins, the particles are called QVs [26,27]. VLPs, PsVs, and QVs are assembled over a period of 48 h in monolayer culture and do not go through the natural maturation process. QVs represent the closest resembling recombinant particle to native virions, resembling NVs when compared by cryoelectron microscopy. The QV particles also retain the majority of surface exposed conformational dependent epitopes [28–32]. It is unclear if there are any structural differences between recombinant particles and NVs that might affect the biology of the virus. Due to the ease and low cost of production, recombinant particles remain the main tool used to study HPV structure, assembly, entry, and infectivity.

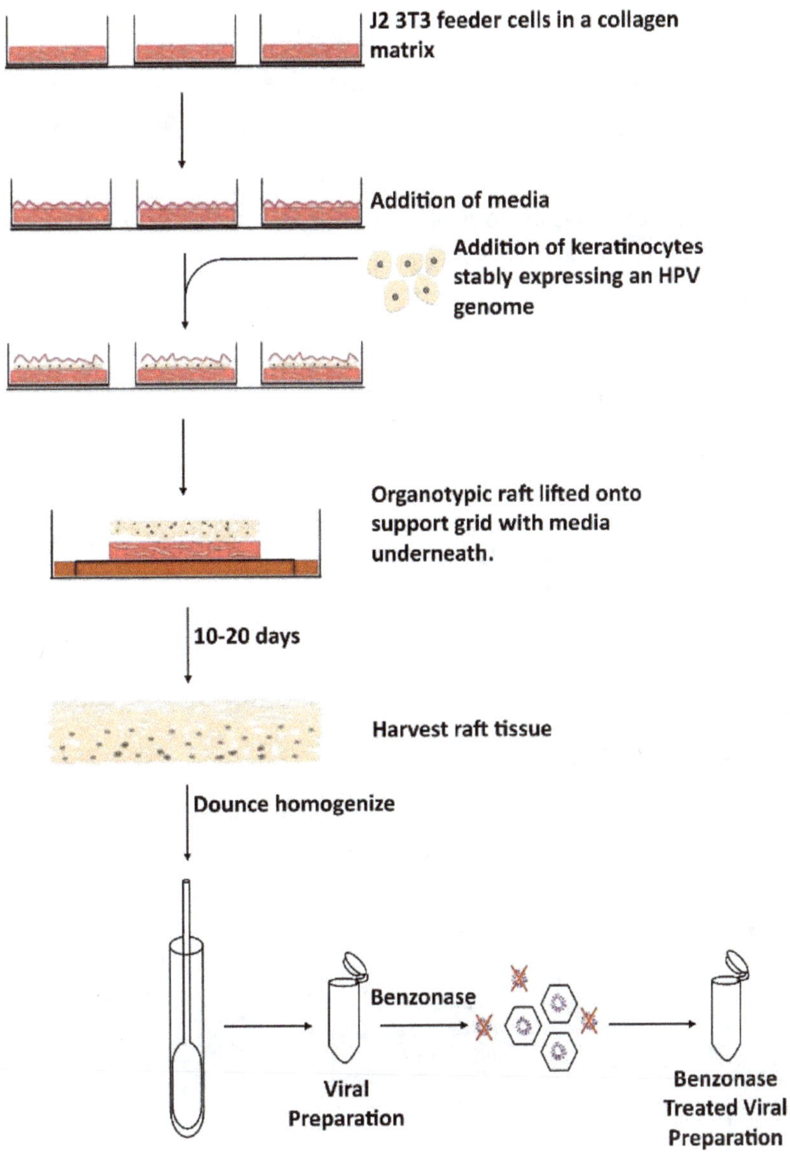

Figure 1. Schematic of native HPV virion production. HPV-positive cells are seeded on top of collagen plugs comprised of collagen and J2 3T3 feeder cells. Once the cells are have grown to confluence, the plugs are lifted onto a support grid. The rafts are then fed via diffusion from media underneath the grid. After 10–20 days, the tissue is harvested, homogenized, and benzonase treated to get a final viral preparation.

While the use of recombinant particles allows for rapid collection of data, there are some caveats to this system of particle production that should be considered. The first being that expression plasmids utilized to synthesize L1 and L2 have been codon optimized to remove rare codons and negate any possible limitations in protein expression [33,34]. While this does not change the protein sequence, this can affect the speed at which proteins are translated, leading to an increased chance of errors in the final amino acid sequence, or could affect protein folding [35]. Additionally, expression of proteins in non-keratinocytes, and especially in prokaryotic cells, could lead to a change in the post translational modifications in the protein. When comparing HPV6b L1 produced using a recombinant baculovirus in Sf9 insect cells or using a recombinant vaccinia virus in kidney cells, differing post-translation modifications were observed. Specifically, L1 produced in the Sf9 cells presented with several post-translationally modified variants, both threonine and serine residues were phosphorylated compared to just serine residues in the L1 produced in the kidney cells, and Sf9 produced L1 incorporated with both mannose and galactose whereas kidney cell produced L1 incorporated with only galactose [36]. While there are likely differences, studies to look at the differences in post-translational modifications between raft-culture derived virions and recombinant particles have not been done and the possibility of these differences should be kept in mind when drawing conclusions from experiments.

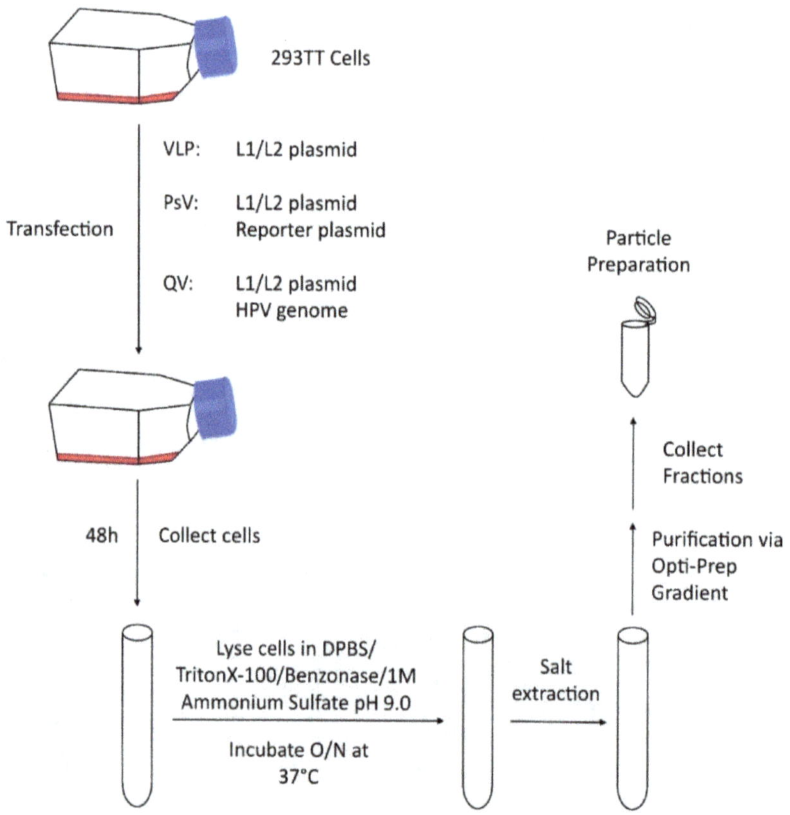

Figure 2. Schematic of recombinant HPV particle production. 293TT cells are transfected with a L1/L2 plasmid (VLPs), a L1/L2 plasmid and a reporter plasmid (PsVs), or a L1/L2 plasmid and a full HPV genome (QVs). Forty-eight hours post transfection, cells are harvested, lysed, and incubated at 37 °C overnight in the presence of cell lysate. Particles are then purified on a gradient.

In the recombinant particle system, the L1 in all recombinant particles begins at a consensus methionine that was found when aligning the L1 N-terminal open reading frame (ORF) of many papillomaviruses. However, some HPV types, such as HPV16 and HPV18 actually have upstream, in frame, methionines that allow for the production of more than one L1 species. Specifically, HPV16 has one upstream methionine that allows for production of an L1 26 amino acids longer then L1 started at the consensus methionine and HPV18 has two upstream methionines enabling production of L1 proteins that are 61 and 26 amino acids longer then the L1 produced from the consensus methionine. These methionines were removed from the expression plasmids utilized in the recombinant system because only production of L1 from the consensus methionine allowed for efficient expression of L1 and production of particles [37]. A HPV18 NV 35 amino acid deletion mutant, deleting the region from the upstream methionine to the consensus methionine, was produced and tested for neutralization with two conformational dependent antibodies created using HPV18 VLPs—H18.K2 and H18.J4. The deletion mutant loses the ability to be neutralized with the H18.K2 antibody but is still neutralized by the conformation dependent H18.J4 antibody. The H18.K2 antibody was produced against VLPs, and therefore, the binding site cannot be contained in the 35 upstream amino acids. This suggests that the 35 upstream amino acids induce structural changes within the HPV18 capsid. When HPV16 virions produced in organotypic raft culture are run on an SDS-PAGE gel, two bands for L1 can be detected on the western blot [38–41]. In contrast, western blots of HPV16 QV appear to only have one form of L1 incorporated into virions, as only one band is visible [38]. This suggests both a potential conformational and structural difference between capsids produced in differentiated epithelium compared to those produced in monolayer cells. While the ability to quickly and easily produce infectious recombinant particles allows for quick experimentation, it is becoming clear that any important results generated should be verified utilizing native particles derived from differentiating epithelium.

3. Maturation and Assembly of Viral Particles

During the process of developing into fully infectious virions, many viruses undergo structural changes, called maturation [42,43]. In the raft culture system, virions mature over a period of 10–20 days within the tissue. In contrast, recombinant particles are matured over a period of 24 h after they are released from cells. After 10 days in foreskin epithelial raft culture, encapsidated and infectious virions are present, however, given another 10 days (20-day tissue) the virions are more mature as displayed by an increase in stability, defined by an enhanced resistance to stress imposed by fractionation in an ultracentrifuge [38]. This is similar to what has been seen for PsVs, with mature capsids having an increased stability [44]. Matured PsVs have also been shown to have an increased resistance to trypsin digestion and chemical reduction, as well as a more ordered structure when viewed by transmission electron microscopy (TEM) [44]. In addition to a more stable and mature phenotype, 20-day native virions were twice as infectious as 10-day virions and had an increased sensitivity to antibody neutralization by both L1 and L2 antibodies [38]. Both immature and mature PsV capsids were equally neutralized by many L1 and L2 antibodies [44]. This suggests that, for NV, the particles may be changing their exposure of key epitopes during the assembly and maturation process.

Analysis of both 10-day and 20-day tissue sections show a difference in virion localization with 10-day virions predominantly localized in the nuclei of suprabasal cells and 20-day virions being found mainly in the cornified layers of the epithelium. Human epithelium has a natural redox gradient with the lower part of the tissue being a reducing environment and the upper layers being an oxidizing environment [38]. This natural redox gradient coincides with the location of immature and mature virions, leading to the conclusion that virion maturation occurs when virions move from a reducing environment to an oxidizing environment. When an oxidizing agent, oxidized glutathione (GSSG) was added to the tissue during virion production, 10-day virions exhibited increased maturation [38,45]. This suggests that movement to an oxidizing environment induces changes in the viral capsid, converting it to a more stable and mature phenotype. PsVs are matured in an oxidizing environment in the presence of cellular lysate after being released from cells. Incubation of particles with cellular lysate, but not clarified lysate produced more mature particles, indicating that currently unknown cellular factors, the same of which are presumably present in tissue, are required for maturation as well [46].

While not absolutely essential for particle formation, a series of disulfide bonds in L1 and L2 molecules form both intra- and interpentameric interactions, stabilizing particles and making them more resistant to environmental influences from nucleases and proteases [44,47]. Within the epithelium, disulfide bond formation is thought to happen slowly during virion maturation in an oxidizing environment [38,44,47,48]. There are 12 conserved cysteine residues across L1 from multiple HPV types [48]. Evaluation of bovine papillomavirus (BPV) via cryoelectron microscopy showed that two separate disulfide bonds are present. However, only one of these is conserved among the human papillomaviruses [49]. Native and recombinant particles have both been reported to contain disulfide bonds. In HPV16, the disulfide bonding occurs at C175 and C428, forming an interpentameric bond between two neighboring capsomeres [50]. Based on mass spectrometry data for HPV18 VLPs, the homologous cysteines that participate in disulfide bonding are C175 and C429. Additionally, both genetic and biochemical analysis of HPV16 and HPV33 PsVs have shown the importance of these conserved cysteines in the structural integrity of the particles as mutation of the cysteines in HPV16 PsV prevents maturation of the particles [44,48]. Mutation and analysis of all 12 conserved cysteines in HPV16 VLPs identified three cysteines potentially involved in disulfide bonding—C175, C185, and C428. Mutation of C428 was especially detrimental to the capsid formation as only capsomeres were visible by EM. The C175S mutation produced tube like structures and the C185S mutation made smaller capsids [48]. These cysteine mutations were also evaluated in the context of NVs grown in differentiating epithelium [45]. Only the C175S mutation severely reduced production of infectious virions in both 10-day and 20-day tissue while C428S, C185S, and the C175S, C185S double mutation only affected 20-day virions. In contrast to the C428S PsV mutant, particle formation was observed for the C428S NV mutant. This suggests that in the context of differentiating epithelium, these cysteines are important for the formation of mature NV. Other conserved cysteines in HPV16 that do not play a role in interpentameric disulfide bonding were also evaluated. In HPV16 VLPs, cysteine to serine mutations of C161, C229, and C379, produced particles with a high susceptibility to tryptic proteolysis [48]. The same cysteine to serine substitutions in HPV16 NV hindered the accumulation of endonuclease resistant genomes in a stratifying epithelium with only the C229S mutant forming non-infectious virions. This suggests that these cysteines may be involved in forming transient disulfide bonds early in the assembly process to guide the capsid to its mature form [51]. Determining the precise roles of these cysteines in the HPV capsid may lead to be much better understanding of HPV capsid stability.

In addition to disulfide bonds in L1, L2 plays an important role in capsid formation and stabilization. L2 forms heterotypic interactions with L1 on the inside of the capsid as well as homotypic interactions with other L2 molecules. When L1 disulfide bonds were unable to form, L1 only capsomeres did not assemble into capsids. However when L2 was present, VLPs were formed [52]. Within the L2 terminus exists two highly conserved cysteines which, when mutated in PsVs, leads to production of non-infectious particles [53,54]. The importance of the L2 cysteines in particle formation was evaluated in the context of NVs produced in differentiating epithelium [55]. In contrast to previous studies using HPV16 PsV and QV, when one or both of the cysteines were mutated, infectious NVs were produced in both 10-day and 20-day tissue [53,54]. Evaluation of the mutant virions produced compared to wild-type showed that the mutants were more infectious but less stable. This could be due to enhanced presentation of a favored binding site on the capsid or a more effective release of viral genomes after host entry due to reduced capsid stability [53]. These L2 cysteines are in close proximity of the proposed external loop, which has been implicated as a feasible candidate for a cross neutralizing epitope across many HPV types for vaccine development. This loop is likely exposed in the final stages of virion maturation as only 20-day virions more efficiently neutralized with the L2 specific antibody RG-1 [38]. Other antibodies targeting this loop also only efficiently neutralized 20-day virions [38,39]. This data provides evidence for the importance of L2 in capsid stability and highlights a significant structural difference between virions assembled in monolayer *vs.* differentiating epithelium.

One of the remaining unknowns of HPV assembly and structure is the concentration of L2 in the viral capsid. L1 itself is able to self-assemble into capsids, however, including L2 into recombinant particles has been shown to increase yield, capsid stability, DNA encapsidation, and infectivity of particles [31,39,52,56–58]. Cryoelectron microscopy of native BPV1 suggests that there are 12 copies of L2 per capsid—one at the center of each of the pentameric capsomeres [59]. However SDS-PAGE analysis from native HPV1 particles, co-immunoprecipitation of HPV11 L1 pentamers with L2, as well as cryoelectron microscopy of HPV16 PsV suggests that up to 72 copies of L2 are present with one being at the center of each capsomere [59,60]. In the natural system, there is regulation as to the quantity of L1 and L2 produced. However, in an over expression system such as the ones used to produce recombinant particles, there would be no regulation of protein production and thus the ratio of L1 and L2 available for particle formation is likely skewed. This could allow for additional L2 to be incorporated into recombinant particles. Additional studies to identify the number of copies of L2 in native particles need to be done.

Organotypic raft culture allows for the generation of not only single base mutant virions but also for the generation of chimeric HPVs composed of different components of different HPV types in the natural environment of differentiating tissue. This whole gene replacement method has aimed at highlighting areas of conservation among different HPV types via complementation experiments. A chimeric virus, named HPV18/16, was created with the L1 and L2 ORF of HPV16 swapped into HPV18 in place of HPV18 L1 and L2 [61]. Substitution of both late gene ORFs did not affect viral genome maintenance in cells and raft cultures were found to have late gene functions such as capsid gene expression and virion morphogenesis. Additionally, chimeric virions purified from raft culture were able to infect keratinocytes [61]. As expected, the chimeric HPV18/16 was unable to be neutralized by HPV18 polyclonal antiserum but was neutralized by a HPV16 polyclonal antiserum. Additional chimeras created by swapping the L1s and L2s of more genetically diverse HPV types such as HPV45, 39, 31, 33, 11, 6b, 1a, CRPV, and BPV1 were also engineered. All the chimeras produced infectious virions, however, titers were much lower then those of wild-type HPV18 [62]. These data demonstrate that there are conserved biological functions between different HPV types. Similar studies illustrate that both capsid proteins play a role in the structure of each other and that this can ultimately affect the overall conformation and behavior of the virion [62,63]. Obviously, both L1 and L2 play an integral role in the biology of HPV.

In addition to L1 and L2, a variety of components comprise the viral capsid including viral DNA and histones. There are other possible viral and cellular components that either directly or indirectly affect the final structure and/or yield of capsids. These components could include HPV early proteins such as E2, E4, E5, and E7 or cellular proteins such as chaperones or karyopherins. There are undoubtedly unknown viral and/or cellular factors necessary for the assembly of native virions. These proteins could act by direction of proper subcellular localization, initial interaction of capsid proteins, mediation of the correct temporal formation of disulfide bonds, and regulation of capsid protein expression.

4. Attachment and Internalization

Our current understanding of the PV infection strategy proposes that, via microabrasions, virus particles gain access to the basal cells as well as the basement membrane. Utilizing recombinant particles, most papillomaviruses have been observed to infect cells by first binding to a glycosaminoglycan (GAG), heparan sulfate (HS), via L1 on either the basement membrane or the cell surface [64–67]. This binding event induces a conformational change allowing for the L2 N-terminus to be cleaved by a proprotein convertase (PC) such as furin or PC5/6 [68,69]. Additionally, these conformational changes may allow for interactions with secondary HS sites on the capsid, transfer the virion to an uptake receptor or receptor complex, and allow for exposure of hidden epitopes that may be important for the interaction with other cellular proteins in the entry process [69–71]. The involvement of GAGs as an attachment receptor was first demonstrated utilizing HPV11 L1 only VLPs and HaCaT cells. Not only was HPV shown to bind, but experiments suggested that L1 interactions with GAGs were GAG type specific [72]. Shortly thereafter, dependence on HS engagement was shown for both HPV16 and HPV33 PsVs [66]. However, in contrast to what was seen for HPV11 VLPs, both HPV16 and HPV33 PsV attachment was to a different subset of GAG molecules. This suggests either a difference between VLPs and PsVs or a difference between HPV types. While primary attachment to heparan sulfate proteoglycans (HSPGs) has been suggested to be a universal step for all PVs, noticeably, tissue derived HPV31 NV and HPV16 NV attachment to and infection of human keratinocytes was shown to be able to occur in the absence of HSPGs [15,73]. HPV31 NV infection of HaCaT cells, n-TERT-1 cells, and primary keratinocytes was unable to be blocked by exogenous heparin competition and could not be blocked by the enzymatic removal of cell surface HS. However, infection of Cos-7 cells and transformed C-33A cells was efficiently blocked by both methods [73]. These data indicate that the virus may use more than one receptor and/or entry pathway to enter a host cell depending on the cell type [73]. It is interesting to note that contradictory findings were observed for HPV31, where HPV31 NV was not dependent on HSPG for attachment, and HPV31 PsV was shown to be dependent on HS for attachment and infection of cells [67]. To complicate the story more, a recent report suggests that both HPV16 and HPV31 PsV attachment and infection can be independent of HSPGs if the non-HSPG molecule laminin-332 is present on the cell surface [14]. Possible explanations for these contradictions include the HPV type being studied, a possible structural variation between NV and PsV due to differences in maturation and assembly, and the cell types being utilized.

Due to minor structural differences between different virus types, it is possible that initial attachment to and interaction with the ECM and cell surface might be HPV type specific. Though the L1 protein displays overall sequence homology and structural conformation, both structural diversity and conformational differences in the loop structures of the pentamer surface have been demonstrated for HPV types 11, 16, 18 and 35 [74]. It is feasible that minor structural differences might have an impact on receptor engagement, including binding to attachment receptors as well as putative entry receptors.

In a study looking at VLP binding for four different HPV types to the ECM and cell surface, some diversity was demonstrated [75]. Two more recent studies, one utilizing native virions [15] and one utilizing PsVs [14] also found HPV type dependent differences in ECM and cell surface binding. It is likely that slightly varying structures of different HPV types facilitate a preferred attachment to a specific GAG/GAG modification, laminin-332, or other unidentified receptors to initially bind to cells and trigger subsequent entry events. For the closely related polyomavirus, different types have been shown to utilize different receptors for infection [76–78]. Thus, a general hypothesis for attachment that encompasses all HPV types is not probable.

The entry process for HPV is slow, with cell surface events such as interaction with several receptors and conformational changes thought to be responsible [79,80]. HPV16 PsV and HPV18 PsV infection have been reported to have an average entry half time of 12 h in HaCaT cells [66,81]. Similarly, entry time for HPV31 NV as well as HPV31 QV was reported to be slow with a half time of about 14 h. In contrast, HPV16 QV was comparably rapid with an average entry half time of only 4 h in HaCaT cells [82]. This data suggests differences in HPV infections to be both HPV type and model system dependent. Several reports suggest that post engagement with cell surface HSPGs, HPV16 PsV particles require interaction with one or more non-HSPG receptors for internalization [69,81,83]. Post-attachment, there is initial co-localization of capsids with HSPGs on the cell surface. However, this co-localization is lost as the particles are internalized into intracellular vesicles, suggesting that particles have been transferred to a non-HSPG receptor [81]. Also giving strong evidence for the existence of other receptors is that furin pre-cleaved virions can bind to and infect HSPG negative cells [83]. Using biochemical inhibitors of endocytosis, it was suggested that HPV16 PsV and HPV58 PsV were internalized via clathrin-mediated endocytosis in COS-7 cells, while HPV31 PsV internalization was dependent on caveolae [84]. This is in contrast to a more recent study whereby HPV31 PsV was also reported to use clathrin mediated endocytosis in both COS-7 and 293TT cells [85]. When utilizing QV, caveolae mediated entry was demonstrated for HPV31 QV and HPV16 QV entry was again suggested to be mediated by clathrin coated pits [82]. HPV16 PsV infection has also been shown to be dependent on entry via caveolin-1 followed by particles trafficking to the ER upon entering cells [86,87]. In another system, this time using dominant negative inhibitors and siRNA knockdown in HeLa, 293TT, and HaCaT cells, the entry pathway of HPV16, HPV18, and HPV31 PsVs was described as a "clatharin, caveolin, lipid raft, flotillin, cholesterol, and dynamin independent mechanism distinct from macropinocytosis" [88,89]. The pathway was defined by a requirement for actin polymerization and tetraspanin microdomains with all particles trafficking to the late endosomal compartment with similar kinetics [89]. Taking into account the multiple HPV types studied, the virus system and cell type utilized, as well as the experimental approach taken, multiple pathways have been identified as playing a role in HPV entry. Considering the number of diverse HPV types, their virus tropisms, and the various HPV related diseases, it is possible that there is both overlapping and non-overlapping receptor usage that could feasibly shunt different HPV types into different entry pathways depending on cell type. It is also important to consider that when attachment assays are done utilizing recombinant particles, often a high multiplicity of infection (MOI) is used—typically in the thousands—which could be shunting particles into cells via pathways the virus would not typically use. In contrast, work with native virions typically uses MOIs of less than 100. Side-by-side comparisons should be done prior to making broad conclusions regarding the mechanism used for infectious entry. A more detailed analysis of the various HPV types using PsV, QV, and NV in relevant keratinocyte cell lines as well as in primary keratinocytes would both show similarities and highlight differences between the types that would help settle the growing amount of conflicting data in the literature.

To date, a multitude of receptors have been identified as potential primary and secondary HPV internalization receptors. One of the first identified was α6-integrin, an epithelial adhesion protein [90]. An α6-integrin specific monoclonal antibody was able to block HPV6b L1 only VLP binding to the cell surface by 60%. Additionally, HPV16 L1 only VLP binding correlated with α6-integrin in a study of 10 different cell lines [91]. However, cells deficient in α6-integrin can bind HPV16 L1 only VLPs and HPV11 NV infects α6-integrin negative cells at levels similar to an α6-integrin expressing cells [92]. In contrast to what is seen for VLPs, β4-integrin along with α6-integrin processing was found to be essential for infection of HaCaT cells with HPV16 PsV [93]. While it appears not to be absolutely essential for all HPV types, α6-integrin may contribute to infection efficiency, especially with its involvement in the Ras/MAPK and PI3K intracellular signaling pathways that are activated upon binding, which may function to create a more proliferative cellular environment to support infection [94]. A role for growth factor receptors (GFRs), both epidermal growth factor receptor (EGFR) and keratinocyte growth factor receptor (KGFR), has also been suggested [95]. Though not yet demonstrated, it is proposed that a HPV-HSPG complex binds directly to GFRs. While blocking EGFR inhibits infection of HaCaT cells with both HPV16 PsV, HPV31 PsV and HPV31 QV, the actual role for EGFR has yet to be determined [88,95]. It is possible that EGFR is directly involved in entry or it is possible that EGFR is activated and involved only in a signaling cascade. Another candidate, Annexin-A2 is a calcium and phospholipid binding protein that is expressed on the cell surface as a part of a heterotetramer, A2t, consisting of two Annexin-A2 monomers associated with a S100A10 dimer [96]. Both HPV16 VLPs and HPV16 PsVs directly interact with A2t, as shown by co-immunoprecipitation. Knockdown of Annexin-A2 by shRNA yields a significant decrease in internalization by HPV16 VLPs and infection by 16 PsV. Further, mutation of a site in L1 shown to be important for A2t binding reduces both binding and infection of HPV16 PsV [97]. HPV16 PsV is still able to infect Annexin-A2 deficient HepG2 cells, suggesting the use of an alternative infectious pathway [98]. While it will be important to discover the internalization receptor(s) for HPV, there is again a necessity for the consideration of HPV type, viral system, and cell line being utilized.

5. Subsequent Steps in HPV Infection

After endocytosis, acidification of the endosomal lumen allows for disassembly of the viral capsid and cellular sorting allows for transport to the nucleus where viral replication occurs [28,65,88,99,100]. Much of the L1 is dissociated from the L2-DNA complex with the help of cyclophillins [101]. Utilizing both HaCaT and HeLa cells, it has been shown that the L1-L2-DNA complex then travels to the Golgi via the retromer, a complex involved in transport of cellular cargo from the endosome to the Golgi [102–107]. This retrograde trafficking is required for HPV infection and HPV16 L2 has been shown to bind directly to the retromer to mediate escape from the endosome [103,108]. Utilizing BPV PsV, Syntaxin 18, which mediates trafficking of vesicles between the ER and the Golgi apparatus, has also been implicated in playing a role in trafficking the L2-DNA complex to the nucleus [109,110]. The

L2-DNA complex then travels through the ER, requiring γ-secretase [87]. Inhibition of γ-secretase blocks infection of HPV after endosomal exit but prior to arrival in the Golgi [87]. Two separate HPV entry siRNA screens have identified ER components that are enriched during entry [102,103]. Additionally, both knockdown of specific ER proteins and use of chemical inhibitors of ER function inhibit HPV infection [102,111]. However, there are conflicting studies regarding ER co-localization with one study reporting co-localization of HPV with ER markers during infection [86] and the other failing to observe ER co-localization [104]. Finally, the L2-DNA complex trafficks to the nucleus, gaining entry during nuclear envelope breakdown during mitosis [27,102,112]. The L2 minor protein is essential for infection, as it facilitates transport of the HPV genome to the nucleus. Specifically, a transmembrane domain along with three GxxxG motifs within L2 have been shown to be essential for infectivity [113]. Much of the research looking at viral infection has been done utilizing PsV, which harbors a non-viral pseudogenome. While this allows for a much faster method of screening, results should be confirmed utilizing native virions.

In a natural infection, HPV infects keratinocytes. However, experiments *in vitro* rarely utilize primary keratinocytes. This is in part due to the extremely low infection efficiency of recombinant particles in primary cells [83]. Conversely, native virions infect primary cells quite well. HPV31 and HPV45 have been shown to infect primary cells just as efficiently as HaCaT cells and HPV16 infects primary cells with a greater efficiency compared to HaCaT cells [15]. HPV18 infects primary cells, however, with lower efficiency compared to HaCaT cell infection. This could be due to a difference in the expression of attachment or internalization receptors present on primary cells compared to other cells. Much of the data for HPV attachment and infection, whether using recombinant particles or native virions, is done in a variety of cell lines including, but not limited to, HaCaT cells, HeLa cells, 293TT cells, and CHO cells. The lack of utilizing a consistent cell line between experiments is likely responsible for some of the conflicting data when looking at both attachment and infectivity.

Of equal importance when looking at infection is the ability to look at virus neutralization. This is especially important due to the use of VLPs in the HPV vaccine that is now being administered to prevent infection. Almost all of the antibodies generated for HPV have been made using recombinant particles. Many of these antibodies generated, such as H16.V5 and H16.E70, have been shown to neutralize both recombinant particles and native virions [16,32,114,115]. However, some antibodies shown to be highly effective in neutralizing recombinant particles, such as H16.U4, have no neutralizing capabilities against native virions [32]. Also of significance are studies highlighting the mechanisms with which different antibodies neutralize particles. For example, H16.V5 and H16.E70 allow attachment of particles to the cell surface but blocks association with the ECM as well as internalization. H16.U4, however, prevented binding to the cell surface but not to the ECM [115]. These neutralization studies again highlight the probable structural differences between recombinant particles and native virions and the importance of confirming data using native virions.

6. Translational Research

There are two approved vaccines against the high-risk HPV types HPV16 and HPV18—Gardasil and Cervarix. Gardasil also provides protection against low-risk HPV types HPV6 and HPV11. These vaccines, however, are not efficiently cross protective against other high-risk HPV types. Therefore, another HPV vaccine, Gardasil 9 was recently approved that, in addition to the four types of HPV previously mentioned also provides protection against high-risk types HPV31, HPV33, HPV45, HP52, and HPV58. While these vaccines have been shown to be highly effective at preventing infection and the development of lesions, their high cost limits their use in developing countries. Additionally, the vaccine rate is low in some developed countries. Thus, the development of less expensive microbicides that would offer protection against a multitude of HPV types would offer women an additional protection against contracting HPV infection.

Due to the importance of GAGs, specifically HS, in HPV attachment to and infection of host cells, agents targeting GAGs are of great interest. Both high molecular weight sulfated or sulfonated polysaccharides and polymers such as cellulose sulfate, dextran sulfate, and polystyrene sulfonate showed microbicidal activity against BPV1 in mouse cells and HPV11 and HPV40 in human A431 cells without showing cellular toxicity [116]. More recently, Carrageenan, a highly sulfated polysaccharide derived from red algae, was identified in an *in vitro* screen of compounds that may effectively block infection by high-risk HPV types [117]. In this study, PsVs were used to determine whether there was a block in infection. However, when tested with NV, carrageenan failed to inhibit infection by HPV16 at concentrations up to 100 μg/mL. In contrast, significant levels of inhibition were observed at concentrations as low as 1 μg/mL for native HPV18. The IC_{50} for carrageenan inhibition of various HPV PsV types was in the ng/mL range [117]. In contrast, utilizing similar titers of NV, infection with HPV18 took at least 10 μg/mL of carrageenan for 50% inhibition and HPV16 was not inhibited. HPV31 NV was also found to be sensitive to inhibition by carrageenan and HPV45 showed no dose-dependent decrease in infection in the presence of carrageenan [15]. These results suggest that not only is there a difference in resistance and susceptibility of NV and PsV to the effects of carrageenan, but that different HPV types are very selective in their requirements for the type of GAG required for infection. Virion attachment to the cell surface in the presence of carrageenan was then analyzed. Attachment of HPV16 NV to the cell surface was unaffected in the presence of carrageenan. Conversely, HPV18 NV attachment was completely ablated in the presence of carrageenan. Additionally, HPV31 NV attachment was slightly reduced, whereas HPV45 attachment was not significantly reduced [15]. Taken together, these data suggest that when testing microbicides, confirmation of data utilizing native virions is essential. In addition, confirmation of results utilizing multiple HPV types should be done, as these data again confirm that not every HPV type behaves in the same manner.

Preventing the incidence of HPV infection through the use of vaccinations and microbicides is invaluable. Of equal importance is the use of chemical disinfectants to keep surfaces and medical equipment free of virions that could be spread between patients. Determining the efficacy of chemical disinfectants against HPV is important because it includes real world scenarios of disinfection protocols on equipment in hospital settings that are possibly contaminated with HPV. Currently, what little information that is available on HPV disinfection has been based mainly on studies from surrogate viruses, such as hepatitis B virus (HBV), which were deemed, without experimental evidence, to have similar resistance to HPV. Additionally, the United States Centers for Disease Control and Prevention (CDC) currently acknowledges the lack of research regarding effective HPV disinfectants [118]. Disinfectant information from studies that have included HPV has all been acquired utilizing recombinant HPV particles. Until recently, no studies had been done using native virions and there existed no functional assays to determine HPVs susceptibility to clinical disinfectants. A recent study tested the susceptibility of both HPV16 recombinant particles (QV) and native HPV16 grown in organotypic raft culture to a variety of common clinical disinfectants. Viral particles were incubated with common clinical disinfectants such as isopropanol, ethanol, triple phenolic, paracetic acid silver-based disinfectant (PAA), gluteraldehyde, hypochlorite, and ortho-phthalaldehyde. The disinfectant was then washed away and virus was incubated with cells to determine its ability to infect cells compared to untreated virus. HPV16 QV and HPV16 NV had some similarities in their resistance/susceptibility profiles to the disinfectants tested. Both types of particles were resistant to gluteraldehyde and ortho-phthalaldehyde and both were susceptible to hypochlorite and high concentration PAA. Of importance, however, HPV16 QV was also susceptible to isopropanol, triple phenolic, and a lower concentration of PAA [119]. This study highlights the necessity of utilizing native HPV particles when investigating clinical aspects of viral infection and transmission.

7. Concluding Remarks

Taken together, all of the data has provided great insight into the structure of HPV as well as the method of binding to, entering, and infecting cells. The use of recombinant particle technology is invaluable, as it allows for rapid data generation in studies looking at multiple parts of the HPV life cycle. However, as this review points out, there are some significant differences between native virions and recombinant particles that necessitate conformational studies utilizing native virions.

Acknowledgments

This work was supported by a PHS grant for the National Institute of Allergy and Infectious Disease (RO1AI57988). Jennifer Biryukov is supported by a grant from the National Cancer Institute (U01CA179724-02).

Author Contributions

Jennifer Biryukov and Craig Meyers discussed the manuscript content and illustrations. Jennifer Biryukov wrote the review.

References

1. Zur Hausen, H. Papillomaviruses in the causation of human cancers—A brief historical account. *Virology* **2009**, *384*, 260–265.
2. Syrjanen, S.; Lodi, G.; von Bültzingslöwen, I.; Aliko, A.; Arduino, P.; Campisi, G.; Challacombe, S.; Ficarra, G.; Flaitz, C.; Zhou, H.M.; *et al.* Human papillomaviruses in oral carcinoma and oral potentially malignant disorders: A systematic review. *Oral Dis.* **2011**, *17*, S58–S72. [CrossRef] [PubMed]

3. D'Souza, G.; Kreimer, A.R.; Viscidi, R.; Pawlita, M.; Fakhry, C.; Koch, W.M.; Westra, W.H.; Gillison, M.L. Case-control study of human papillomavirus and oropharyngeal cancer. *N. Engl. J. Med.* **2007**, *356*, 1944–1956. [CrossRef] [PubMed]
4. Schiffman, M.; Kjaer, S.K. Chapter 2: Natural history of anogenital human papillomavirus infection and neoplasia. *J. Natl. Cancer Inst. Monogr.* **2003**, *31*, 14–19. [CrossRef] [PubMed]
5. Arbyn, M.; Castellsagué, X.; de Sanjosé, S.; Bruni, L.; Saraiya, M.; Bray, F.; Ferlay, J. Worldwide burden of cervical cancer in 2008. *Ann. Oncol.* **2011**, *22*, 2675–2686. [CrossRef] [PubMed]
6. De Villiers, E.M.; Fauquet, C.; Broker, T.R.; Bernard, H.U.; zur Hausen, H. Classification of papillomaviruses. *Virology* **2004**, *324*, 17–27. [CrossRef] [PubMed]
7. Longworth, M.S.; Laimins, L.A. Pathogenesis of human papillomaviruses in differentiating epithelia. *Microbiol. Mol. Biol. Rev.* **2004**, *68*, 362–372. [CrossRef] [PubMed]
8. Madsen, B.S.; Jensen, H.L.; van den Brule, A.J.; Wohlfahrt, J.; Frisch, M. Risk factors for invasive squamous cell carcinoma of the vulva and vagina—Population-based case-control study in Denmark. *Int. J. Cancer* **2008**, *122*, 2827–2834. [CrossRef] [PubMed]
9. Meyers, C.; Frattini, M.G.; Hudson, J.B.; Laimins, L.A. Biosynthesis of human papillomavirus from a continuous cell line upon epithelial differentiation. *Science* **1992**, *257*, 971–973. [CrossRef] [PubMed]
10. Hummel, M.; Hudson, J.B.; Laimins, L.A. Differentiation-induced and constitutive transcription of human papillomavirus type 31b in cell lines containing viral episomes. *J. Virol.* **1992**, *66*, 6070–6080. [PubMed]
11. Bedell, M.A.; Hudson, J.B.; Golub, T.R.; Turyk, M.E.; Hosken, M.; Wilbanks, G.D.; Laimins, L.A. Amplification of human papillomavirus genomes *in vitro* is dependent on epithelial differentiation. *J. Virol.* **1991**, *65*, 2254–2260. [PubMed]
12. Grassmann, K.; Rapp, B.; Maschek, H.; Petry, K.U.; Iftner, T. Identification of a differentiation-inducible promoter in the E7 open reading frame of human papillomavirus type 16 (HPV-16) in raft cultures of a new cell line containing high copy numbers of episomal HPV-16 DNA. *J. Virol.* **1996**, *70*, 2339–2349. [PubMed]
13. Ozbun, M.A.; Meyers, C. Characterization of late gene transcripts expressed during vegetative replication of human papillomavirus type 31b. *J. Virol.* **1997**, *71*, 5161–5172. [PubMed]
14. Richards, K.F.; Mukherjee, S.; Bienkowska-Haba, M.; Pang, J.; Sapp, M. Human papillomavirus species-specific interaction with the basement membrane-resident non-heparan sulfate receptor. *Viruses* **2014**, *6*, 4856–4879. [CrossRef] [PubMed]
15. Cruz, L.; Meyers, C. Differential dependence on host cell glycosaminoglycans for infection of epithelial cells by high-risk HPV types. *PLoS ONE* **2013**, *8*, e68379. [CrossRef] [PubMed]
16. McLaughlin-Drubin, M.E.; Christensen, N.D.; Meyers, C. Propagation, infection, and neutralization of authentic HPV16 virus. *Virology* **2004**, *322*, 213–219. [CrossRef] [PubMed]
17. McLaughlin-Drubin, M.E.; Wilson, S.; Mullikin, B.; Suzich, J.; Meyers, C. Human papillomavirus type 45 propagation, infection, and neutralization. *Virology* **2003**, *312*, 1–7. [CrossRef]
18. Meyers, C.; Mayer, T.J.; Ozbun, M.A. Synthesis of infectious human papillomavirus type 18 in differentiating epithelium transfected with viral DNA. *J. Virol.* **1997**, *71*, 7381–7386. [PubMed]

19. Kirnbauer, R.; Booy, F.; Cheng, N.; Lowy, D.R.; Schiller, J.T. Papillomavirus L1 major capsid protein self-assembles into virus-like particles that are highly immunogenic. *Proc. Natl. Acad. Sci. USA* **1992**, *89*, 12180–12184. [CrossRef] [PubMed]
20. Kirnbauer, R.; Taub, J.; Greenstone, H.; Roden, R.; Dürst, M.; Gissmann, L.; Lowy, D.R.; Schiller, J.T. Efficient self-assembly of human papillomavirus type 16 L1 and L1-L2 into virus-like particles. *J. Virol.* **1993**, *67*, 6929–6936. [PubMed]
21. Rose, R.C.; Bonnez, W.; Reichman, R.C.; Garcea, R.L. Expression of human papillomavirus type 11 L1 protein in insect cells: *In vivo* and *in vitro* assembly of viruslike particles. *J. Virol.* **1993**, *67*, 1936–1944. [PubMed]
22. Hagensee, M.E.; Yaegashi, N.; Galloway, D.A. Self-assembly of human papillomavirus type 1 capsids by expression of the L1 protein alone or by coexpression of the L1 and L2 capsid proteins. *J. Virol.* **1993**, *67*, 315–322. [PubMed]
23. Hagensee, M.E.; Olson, N.H.; Baker, T.S.; Galloway, D.A. Three-dimensional structure of vaccinia virus-produced human papillomavirus type 1 capsids. *J. Virol.* **1994**, *68*, 4503–4505. [PubMed]
24. Chen, X.S.; Garcea, R.L.; Goldberg, I.; Casini, G.; Harrison, S.C. Structure of small virus-like particles assembled from the L1 protein of human papillomavirus 16. *Mol. Cell* **2000**, *5*, 557–567. [CrossRef]
25. Zhang, W.; Carmichael, J.; Ferguson, J.; Inglis, S.; Ashrafian, H.; Stanley, M. Expression of human papillomavirus type 16 L1 protein in *Escherichia coli*: Denaturation, renaturation, and self-assembly of virus-like particles *in vitro*. *Virology* **1998**, *243*, 423–431. [CrossRef] [PubMed]
26. Culp, T.D.; Christensen, N.D. Kinetics of *in vitro* adsorption and entry of papillomavirus virions. *Virology* **2004**, *319*, 152–161. [CrossRef] [PubMed]
27. Pyeon, D.; Lambert, P.F.; Ahlquist, P. Production of infectious human papillomavirus independently of viral replication and epithelial cell differentiation. *Proc. Natl. Acad. Sci. USA* **2005**, *102*, 9311–9316. [CrossRef] [PubMed]
28. Day, P.M.; Lowy, D.R.; Schiller, J.T. Papillomaviruses infect cells via a clathrin-dependent pathway. *Virology* **2003**, *307*, 1–11. [CrossRef]
29. Embers, M.E.; Budgeon, L.R.; Culp, T.D.; Reed, C.A.; Pickel, M.D.; Christensen, N.D. Differential antibody responses to a distinct region of human papillomavirus minor capsid proteins. *Vaccine* **2004**, *22*, 670–680. [CrossRef] [PubMed]
30. Gambhira, R.; Karanam, B.; Jagu, S.; Roberts, J.N.; Buck, C.B.; Bossis, I.; Alphs, H.; Culp, T.; Christensen, N.D.; Roden, R.B. A protective and broadly cross-neutralizing epitope of human papillomavirus L2. *J. Virol.* **2007**, *81*, 13927–13931. [CrossRef] [PubMed]
31. Buck, C.B.; Cheng, N.; Thompson, C.D.; Lowy, D.R.; Steven, A.C.; Schiller, J.T.; Trus, B.L. Arrangement of L2 within the papillomavirus capsid. *J. Virol.* **2008**, *82*, 5190–5197. [CrossRef] [PubMed]
32. White, W.I.; Wilson, S.D.; Parmer-Hill, F.J.; Woods, R.M.; Ghim, S.; Hewitt, L.A.; Goldman, D.M.; Burke, S.J.; Jerson, A.B.; Koening, S.; *et al.* Characterization of a major neutralizing epitope on human papillomavirus type 16 L1. *J. Virol.* **1999**, *73*, 4882–4889. [PubMed]

33. Zhou, J.; Liu, W.J.; Peng, S.W.; Sun, X.Y.; Frazer, I. Papillomavirus capsid protein expression level depends on the match between codon usage and tRNA availability. *J. Virol.* **1999**, *73*, 4972–4982. [PubMed]
34. Leder, C.; Kleinschmidt, J.A.; Wiethe, C.; Müller, M. Enhancement of capsid gene expression: Preparing the human papillomavirus type 16 major structural gene L1 for DNA vaccination purposes. *J. Virol.* **2001**, *75*, 9201–9209. [CrossRef] [PubMed]
35. Spencer, P.S.; Barral, J.M. Genetic code redundancy and its influence on the encoded polypeptides. *Comput. Struct. Biotechnol. J.* **2012**, *1*, e201204006. [CrossRef] [PubMed]
36. Fang, N.X.; Frazer, I.H.; Fernando, G.J. Differences in the post-translational modifications of human papillomavirus type 6b major capsid protein expressed from a baculovirus system compared with a vaccinia virus system. *Biotechnol. Appl. Biochem.* **2000**, *32*, 27–33. [CrossRef] [PubMed]
37. Zhou, J.; Sun, X.Y.; Stenzel, D.J.; Frazer, I.H. Expression of vaccinia recombinant HPV 16 L1 and L2 ORF proteins in epithelial cells is sufficient for assembly of HPV virion-like particles. *Virology* **1991**, *185*, 251–257. [CrossRef]
38. Conway, M.J.; Alam, S.; Ryndock, E.J.; Cruz, L.; Christensen, N.D.; Roden, R.B.; Meyers, C. Tissue-spanning redox gradient-dependent assembly of native human papillomavirus type 16 virions. *J. Virol.* **2009**, *83*, 10515–10526. [CrossRef] [PubMed]
39. Holmgren, S.C.; Patterson, N.A.; Ozbun, M.A.; Lambert, P.F. The minor capsid protein L2 contributes to two steps in the human papillomavirus type 31 life cycle. *J. Virol.* **2005**, *79*, 3938–3948. [CrossRef] [PubMed]
40. Fey, S.J.; Nielsen, T.; Vetner, M.; Storgaard, L.; Smed, V.; Larsen, P.M. Demonstration of *in vitro* synthesis of human papilloma viral proteins from hand and foot warts. *J. Investig. Dermatol.* **1989**, *92*, 817–824. [CrossRef] [PubMed]
41. Larsen, P.M.; Storgaard, L.; Fey, S.J. Proteins present in bovine papillomavirus particles. *J. Virol.* **1987**, *61*, 3596–3601. [PubMed]
42. Joshi, A.; Nagashima, K.; Freed, E.O. Mutation of dileucine-like motifs in the human immunodeficiency virus type 1 capsid disrupts virus assembly, gag-gag interactions, gag-membrane binding, and virion maturation. *J. Virol.* **2006**, *80*, 7939–7951. [CrossRef] [PubMed]
43. Perez-Berna, A.J.; Ortega-Esteban, A.; Menéndez-Conejero, R.; Winkler, D.C.; Menéndez, M.; Steven, A.C.; Flint, S.J.; de Pablo, P.J.; San Martín, C. The role of capsid maturation on adenovirus priming for sequential uncoating. *J. Biol. Chem.* **2012**, *287*, 31582–31595. [CrossRef] [PubMed]
44. Buck, C.B.; Thompson, C.D.; Pang, Y.Y.; Lowy, D.R.; Schiller, J.T. Maturation of papillomavirus capsids. *J. Virol.* **2005**, *79*, 2839–2846. [CrossRef] [PubMed]
45. Conway, M.J.; Cruz, L.; Alam, S.; Christensen, N.D.; Meyers, C. Differentiation-dependent interpentameric disulfide bond stabilizes native human papillomavirus type 16. *PLoS ONE* **2011**, *6*, e22427. [CrossRef] [PubMed]
46. Cardone, G.; Moyer, A.L.; Cheng, N.; Thompson, C.D.; Dvoretzky, I.; Lowy, D.R.; Schiller, J.T.; Steven, A.C.; Buck, C.B.; Trus, B.L. Maturation of the human papillomavirus 16 capsid. *MBio* **2014**, *5*, e01104-14. [CrossRef] [PubMed]

47. Fligge, C.; Schäfer, F.; Selinka, H.C.; Sapp, C.; Sapp, M. DNA-induced structural changes in the papillomavirus capsid. *J. Virol.* **2001**, *75*, 7727–7731. [CrossRef] [PubMed]
48. Ishii, Y.; Tanaka, K.; Kanda, T. Mutational analysis of human papillomavirus type 16 major capsid protein L1: The cysteines affecting the intermolecular bonding and structure of L1-capsids. *Virology* **2003**, *308*, 128–136. [CrossRef]
49. Wolf, M.; Garcea, R.L.; Grigorieff, N.; Harrison, S.C. Subunit interactions in bovine papillomavirus. *Proc. Natl. Acad. Sci. USA* **2010**, *107*, 6298–6303. [CrossRef] [PubMed]
50. Modis, Y.; Trus, B.L.; Harrison, S.C. Atomic model of the papillomavirus capsid. *EMBO J.* **2002**, *21*, 4754–4762. [CrossRef] [PubMed]
51. Ryndock, E.J.; Conway, M.J.; Alam, S.; Gul, S.; Murad, S.; Christensen, N.D.; Meyers, C. Roles for human papillomavirus type 16 l1 cysteine residues 161, 229, and 379 in genome encapsidation and capsid stability. *PLoS ONE* **2014**, *9*, e99488. [CrossRef] [PubMed]
52. Ishii, Y.; Ozaki, S.; Tanaka, K.; Kanda, T. Human papillomavirus 16 minor capsid protein L2 helps capsomeres assemble independently of intercapsomeric disulfide bonding. *Virus Genes* **2005**, *31*, 321–328. [CrossRef] [PubMed]
53. Campos, S.K.; Ozbun, M.A. Two highly conserved cysteine residues in HPV16 L2 form an intramolecular disulfide bond and are critical for infectivity in human keratinocytes. *PLoS ONE* **2009**, *4*, e4463. [CrossRef] [PubMed]
54. Gambhira, R.; Jagu, S.; Karanam, B.; Day, P.M.; Roden, R. Role of L2 cysteines in papillomavirus infection and neutralization. *Virol. J.* **2009**, *6*, e176. [CrossRef] [PubMed]
55. Conway, M.J.; Alam, S.; Christensen, N.D.; Meyers, C. Overlapping and independent structural roles for human papillomavirus type 16 L2 conserved cysteines. *Virology* **2009**, *393*, 295–303. [CrossRef] [PubMed]
56. Kondo, K.; Ishii, Y.; Ochi, H.; Matsumoto, T.; Yoshikawa, H.; Kanda, T. Neutralization of HPV16, 18, 31, and 58 pseudovirions with antisera induced by immunizing rabbits with synthetic peptides representing segments of the HPV16 minor capsid protein L2 surface region. *Virology* **2007**, *358*, 266–272. [CrossRef] [PubMed]
57. Roden, R.B.; Greenstone, H.L.; Kirnbauer, R.; Booy, F.P.; Jessie, J.; Lowy, D.R.; Schiller, J.T. *In vitro* generation and type-specific neutralization of a human papillomavirus type 16 virion pseudotype. *J. Virol.* **1996**, *70*, 5875–5883. [PubMed]
58. Zhao, K.N.; Sun, X.Y.; Frazer, I.H.; Zhou, J. DNA packaging by L1 and L2 capsid proteins of bovine papillomavirus type 1. *Virology* **1998**, *243*, 482–491. [CrossRef] [PubMed]
59. Trus, B.L.; Roden, R.B.; Greenstone, H.L.; Vrhel, M.; Schiller, J.T.; Booy, F.P. Novel structural features of bovine papillomavirus capsid revealed by a three-dimensional reconstruction to 9 Å resolution. *Nat. Struct. Biol.* **1997**, *4*, 413–420. [CrossRef] [PubMed]
60. Doorbar, J.; Gallimore, P.H. Identification of proteins encoded by the L1 and L2 open reading frames of human papillomavirus 1a. *J. Virol.* **1987**, *61*, 2793–2799. [PubMed]
61. Meyers, C.; Bromberg-White, J.L.; Zhang, J.; Kaupas, M.E.; Bryan, J.T.; Lowe, R.S.; Jansen, K.U. Infectious virions produced from a human papillomavirus type 18/16 genomic DNA chimera. *J. Virol.* **2002**, *76*, 4723–4733. [CrossRef] [PubMed]

62. Bowser, B.S.; Chen, H.S.; Conway, M.J.; Christensen, N.D.; Meyers, C. Human papillomavirus type 18 chimeras containing the L2/L1 capsid genes from evolutionarily diverse papillomavirus types generate infectious virus. *Virus Res.* **2011**, *160*, 246–255. [CrossRef] [PubMed]
63. Chen, H.S.; Conway, M.J.; Christensen, N.D.; Alam, S.; Meyers, C. Papillomavirus capsid proteins mutually impact structure. *Virology* **2011**, *412*, 378–383. [CrossRef] [PubMed]
64. Kines, R.C.; Thompson, C.D.; Lowy, D.R.; Schiller, J.T.; Day, P.M. The initial steps leading to papillomavirus infection occur on the basement membrane prior to cell surface binding. *Proc. Natl. Acad. Sci. USA* **2009**, *106*, 20458–20463. [CrossRef] [PubMed]
65. Sapp, M.; Bienkowska-Haba, M. Viral entry mechanisms: Human papillomavirus and a long journey from extracellular matrix to the nucleus. *FEBS J.* **2009**, *276*, 7206–7216. [CrossRef] [PubMed]
66. Giroglou, T.; Florin, L.; Schäfer, F.; Streeck, R.E.; Sapp, M. Human papillomavirus infection requires cell surface heparan sulfate. *J. Virol.* **2001**, *75*, 1565–1570. [CrossRef] [PubMed]
67. Johnson, K.M.; Kines, R.C.; Roberts, J.N.; Lowy, D.R.; Schiller, J.T.; Day, P.M. Role of heparan sulfate in attachment to and infection of the murine female genital tract by human papillomavirus. *J. Virol.* **2009**, *83*, 2067–2074. [CrossRef] [PubMed]
68. Richards, R.M.; Lowy, D.R.; Schiller, J.T.; Day, P.M. Cleavage of the papillomavirus minor capsid protein, L2, at a furin consensus site is necessary for infection. *Proc. Natl. Acad. Sci. USA* **2006**, *103*, 1522–1527. [CrossRef] [PubMed]
69. Day, P.M.; Gambhira, R.; Roden, R.B.; Lowy, D.R.; Schiller, J.T. Mechanisms of human papillomavirus type 16 neutralization by 12 cross-neutralizing and 11 type-specific antibodies. *J. Virol.* **2008**, *82*, 4638–4646. [CrossRef] [PubMed]
70. Knappe, M.; Bodevin, S.; Selinka, H.C.; Spillmann, D.; Streeck, R.E.; Chen, X.S.; Lindahl, U.; Sapp, M. Surface-exposed amino acid residues of HPV16 L1 protein mediating interaction with cell surface heparan sulfate. *J. Biol. Chem.* **2007**, *282*, 27913–27922. [CrossRef] [PubMed]
71. Kumar, A.; Jacob, T.; Abban, C.Y.; Meneses, P.I. Intermediate heparan sulfate binding during HPV-16 infection in HaCaTs. *Am. J. Ther.* **2014**, *21*, 331–342. [CrossRef] [PubMed]
72. Joyce, J.G.; Tung, J.S.; Przysiecki, C.T.; Cook, J.C.; Lehman, E.D.; Sands, J.A.; Jansen, K.U.; Keller, P.M. The L1 major capsid protein of human papillomavirus type 11 recombinant virus-like particles interacts with heparin and cell-surface glycosaminoglycans on human keratinocytes. *J. Biol. Chem.* **1999**, *274*, 5810–5822. [CrossRef] [PubMed]
73. Patterson, N.A.; Smith, J.L.; Ozbun, M.A. Human papillomavirus type 31b infection of human keratinocytes does not require heparan sulfate. *J. Virol.* **2005**, *79*, 6838–6847. [CrossRef] [PubMed]
74. Bishop, B.; Dasgupta, J.; Klein, M.; Garcea, R.L.; Christensen, N.D.; Zhao, R.; Chen, X.S. Crystal structures of four types of human papillomavirus L1 capsid proteins: Understanding the specificity of neutralizing monoclonal antibodies. *J. Biol. Chem.* **2007**, *282*, 31803–31811. [CrossRef] [PubMed]
75. Broutian, T.R.; Brendle, S.A.; Christensen, N.D. Differential binding patterns to host cells associated with particles of several human alphapapillomavirus types. *J. Gen. Virol.* **2010**, *91*, 531–540. [CrossRef] [PubMed]

76. Sapp, M.; Day, P.M. Structure, attachment and entry of polyoma- and papillomaviruses. *Virology* **2009**, *384*, 400–409. [CrossRef] [PubMed]
77. Bauer, P.H.; Cui, C.; Liu, W.R.; Stehle, T.; Harrison, S.C.; DeCaprio, J.A.; Benjamin, T.L. Discrimination between sialic acid-containing receptors and pseudoreceptors regulates polyomavirus spread in the mouse. *J. Virol.* **1999**, *73*, 5826–5832. [CrossRef] [PubMed]
78. Neu, U.; Maginnis, M.S.; Palma, A.S.; Ströh, L.J.; Nelson, C.D.; Feizi, T.; Atwood, W.J.; Stehle, T. Structure-function analysis of the human JC polyomavirus establishes the LSTc pentasaccharide as a functional receptor motif. *Cell Host Microbe* **2010**, *8*, 309–319. [CrossRef] [PubMed]
79. Horvath, C.A.; Boulet, G.A.; Renoux, V.M.; Delvenne, P.O.; Bogers, J.P. Mechanisms of cell entry by human papillomaviruses: An overview. *Virol. J.* **2010**, *7*, e11. [CrossRef] [PubMed]
80. Spoden, G.; Freitag, K.; Husmann, M.; Boller, K.; Sapp, M.; Lambert, C.; Florin, L. Clathrin- and caveolin-independent entry of human papillomavirus type 16—Involvement of tetraspanin-enriched microdomains (TEMs). *PLoS ONE* **2008**, *3*, e3313. [CrossRef] [PubMed]
81. Selinka, H.C.; Florin, L.; Patel, H.D.; Freitag, K.; Schmidtke, M.; Makarov, V.A.; Sapp, M. Inhibition of transfer to secondary receptors by heparan sulfate-binding drug or antibody induces noninfectious uptake of human papillomavirus. *J. Virol.* **2007**, *81*, 10970–10980. [CrossRef] [PubMed]
82. Smith, J.L.; Campos, S.K.; Ozbun, M.A. Human papillomavirus type 31 uses a caveolin 1- and dynamin 2-mediated entry pathway for infection of human keratinocytes. *J. Virol.* **2007**, *81*, 9922–9931. [CrossRef] [PubMed]
83. Day, P.M.; Lowy, D.R.; Schiller, J.T. Heparan sulfate-independent cell binding and infection with furin-precleaved papillomavirus capsids. *J. Virol.* **2008**, *82*, 12565–12568. [CrossRef] [PubMed]
84. Bousarghin, L.; Touzé, A.; Sizaret, P.Y.; Coursaget, P. Human papillomavirus types 16, 31, and 58 use different endocytosis pathways to enter cells. *J. Virol.* **2003**, *77*, 3846–3850. [CrossRef] [PubMed]
85. Hindmarsh, P.L.; Laimins, L.A. Mechanisms regulating expression of the HPV 31 L1 and L2 capsid proteins and pseudovirion entry. *Virol. J.* **2007**, *4*, e19. [CrossRef] [PubMed]
86. Laniosz, V.; Dabydeen, S.A.; Havens, M.A.; Meneses, P.I. Human papillomavirus type 16 infection of human keratinocytes requires clathrin and caveolin-1 and is brefeldin a sensitive. *J. Virol.* **2009**, *83*, 8221–8232. [CrossRef] [PubMed]
87. Zhang, W.; Kazakov, T.; Popa, A.; DiMaio, D. Vesicular trafficking of incoming human papillomavirus 16 to the Golgi apparatus and endoplasmic reticulum requires gamma-secretase activity. *MBio* **2014**, *5*, e01777-14. [CrossRef] [PubMed]
88. Schelhaas, M.; Shah, B.; Holzer, M.; Blattmann, P.; Kühling, L.; Day, P.M.; Schiller, J.T.; Helenius, A. Entry of human papillomavirus type 16 by actin-dependent, clathrin- and lipid raft-independent endocytosis. *PLoS Pathog.* **2012**, *8*, e1002657. [CrossRef] [PubMed]
89. Spoden, G.; Kühling, L.; Cordes, N.; Frenzel, B.; Sapp, M.; Boller, K.; Florin, L.; Schelhaas, M. Human papillomavirus types 16, 18, and 31 share similar endocytic requirements for entry. *J. Virol.* **2013**, *87*, 7765–7773. [CrossRef] [PubMed]
90. Evander, M.; Frazer, I.H.; Payne, E.; Qi, Y.M.; Hengst, K.; McMillan, N.A. Identification of

the alpha6 integrin as a candidate receptor for papillomaviruses. *J. Virol.* **1997**, *71*, 2449–2456. [PubMed]

91. Yoon, C.S.; Kim, K.D.; Park, S.N.; Cheong, S.W. Alpha(6) integrin is the main receptor of human papillomavirus type 16 VLP. *Biochem. Biophys. Res. Commun.* **2001**, *283*, 668–673. [CrossRef] [PubMed]
92. Sibbet, G.; Romero-Graillet, C.; Meneguzzi, G.; Campo, M.S. Alpha6 integrin is not the obligatory cell receptor for bovine papillomavirus type 4. *J. Gen. Virol.* **2000**, *81*, 327–334. [PubMed]
93. Aksoy, P.; Abban, C.Y.; Kiyashka, E.; Qiang, W.; Meneses, P.I. HPV16 infection of HaCaTs is dependent on beta4 integrin, and alpha6 integrin processing. *Virology* **2014**, *449*, 45–52. [CrossRef] [PubMed]
94. Fothergill, T.; McMillan, N.A. Papillomavirus virus-like particles activate the PI3-kinase pathway via alpha-6 beta-4 integrin upon binding. *Virology* **2006**, *352*, 319–328. [CrossRef] [PubMed]
95. Surviladze, Z.; Dziduszko, A.; Ozbun, M.A. Essential roles for soluble virion-associated heparan sulfonated proteoglycans and growth factors in human papillomavirus infections. *PLoS Pathog.* **2012**, *8*, e1002519. [CrossRef] [PubMed]
96. Waisman, D.M. Annexin II tetramer: Structure and function. *Mol. Cell. Biochem.* **1995**, *149–150*, 301–322. [CrossRef] [PubMed]
97. Woodham, A.W.; da Silva, D.M.; Skeate, J.G.; Raff, A.B.; Ambroso, M.R.; Brand, H.E.; Isas, J.M.; Langen, R.; Kast, W.M. The S100A10 subunit of the annexin A2 heterotetramer facilitates L2-mediated human papillomavirus infection. *PLoS ONE* **2012**, *7*, e43519. [CrossRef] [PubMed]
98. Raff, A.B.; Woodham, A.W.; Raff, L.M.; Skeate, J.G.; Yan, L.; da Silva, D.M.; Schelhaas, M.; Kast, W.M. The evolving field of human papillomavirus receptor research: A review of binding and entry. *J. Virol.* **2013**, *87*, 6062–6072. [CrossRef] [PubMed]
99. Smith, J.L.; Lidke, D.S.; Ozbun, M.A. Virus activated filopodia promote human papillomavirus type 31 uptake from the extracellular matrix. *Virology* **2008**, *381*, 16–21. [CrossRef] [PubMed]
100. Selinka, H.C.; Giroglou, T.; Sapp, M. Analysis of the infectious entry pathway of human papillomavirus type 33 pseudovirions. *Virology* **2002**, *299*, 279–287. [CrossRef] [PubMed]
101. Bienkowska-Haba, M.; Williams, C.; Kim, S.M.; Garcea, R.L.; Sapp, M. Cyclophilins facilitate dissociation of the human papillomavirus type 16 capsid protein L1 from the L2/DNA complex following virus entry. *J. Virol.* **2012**, *86*, 9875–9887. [CrossRef] [PubMed]
102. Aydin, I.; Weber, S.; Snijder, B.; Samperio Ventayol, P.; Kühbacher, A.; Becker, M.; Day, P.M.; Schiller, J.T.; Kann, M.; Pelkmans, L.; *et al.* Large scale RNAi reveals the requirement of nuclear envelope breakdown for nuclear import of human papillomaviruses. *PLoS Pathog.* **2014**, *10*, e1004162. [CrossRef] [PubMed]
103. Lipovsky, A.; Popa, A.; Pimienta, G.; Wyler, M.; Bhan, A.; Kuruvilla, L.; Guie, M.A.; Poffenberger, A.C.; Nelson, C.D.; Atwood, W.J.; *et al.* Genome-wide siRNA screen identifies the retromer as a cellular entry factor for human papillomavirus. *Proc. Natl. Acad. Sci. USA* **2013**, *110*, 7452–7457. [CrossRef] [PubMed]

104. Day, P.M.; Thompson, C.D.; Schowalter, R.M.; Lowy, D.R.; Schiller, J.T. Identification of a role for the trans-Golgi network in human papillomavirus 16 pseudovirus infection. *J. Virol.* **2013**, *87*, 3862–3870. [CrossRef] [PubMed]
105. DiGiuseppe, S.; Bienkowska-Haba, M.; Hilbig, L.; Sapp, M. The nuclear retention signal of HPV16 L2 protein is essential for incoming viral genome to transverse the trans-Golgi network. *Virology* **2014**, *458–459*, 93–105. [CrossRef] [PubMed]
106. Attar, N.; Cullen, P.J. The retromer complex. *Adv. Enzyme Regul.* **2010**, *50*, 216–236. [CrossRef] [PubMed]
107. Burd, C.; Cullen, P.J. Retromer: A master conductor of endosome sorting. *Cold Spring Harb. Perspect. Biol.* **2014**, *6*, a016774. [CrossRef] [PubMed]
108. Popa, A.; Zhang, W.; Harrison, M.S.; Goodner, K.; Kazakov, T.; Goodwin, E.C.; Lipovsky, A.; Burd, C.G.; DiMaio, D. Direct binding of retromer to human papillomavirus type 16 minor capsid protein L2 mediates endosome exit during viral infection. *PLoS Pathog.* **2015**, *11*, e1004699. [CrossRef] [PubMed]
109. Bossis, I.; Roden, R.B.; Gambhira, R.; Yang, R.; Tagaya, M.; Howley, P.M.; Meneses, P.I. Interaction of tSNARE syntaxin 18 with the papillomavirus minor capsid protein mediates infection. *J. Virol.* **2005**, *79*, 6723–6731. [CrossRef] [PubMed]
110. Laniosz, V.; Nguyen, K.C.; Meneses, P.I. Bovine papillomavirus type 1 infection is mediated by SNARE syntaxin 18. *J. Virol.* **2007**, *81*, 7435–7448. [CrossRef] [PubMed]
111. Campos, S.K.; Chapman, J.A.; Deymier, M.J.; Bronnimann, M.P.; Ozbun, M.A. Opposing effects of bacitracin on human papillomavirus type 16 infection: Enhancement of binding and entry and inhibition of endosomal penetration. *J. Virol.* **2012**, *86*, 4169–4181. [CrossRef] [PubMed]
112. Pyeon, D.; Pearce, S.M.; Lank, S.M.; Ahlquist, P.; Lambert, P.F. Establishment of human papillomavirus infection requires cell cycle progression. *PLoS Pathog.* **2009**, *5*, e1000318. [CrossRef] [PubMed]
113. Bronnimann, M.P.; Chapman, J.A.; Park, C.K.; Campos, S.K. A transmembrane domain and GxxxG motifs within L2 are essential for papillomavirus infection. *J. Virol.* **2013**, *87*, 464–473. [CrossRef] [PubMed]
114. Christensen, N.D.; Cladel, N.M.; Reed, C.A.; Budgeon, L.R.; Embers, M.E.; Skulsky, D.M.; McClements, W.L.; Ludmerer, S.W.; Jansen, K.U. Hybrid papillomavirus L1 molecules assemble into virus-like particles that reconstitute conformational epitopes and induce neutralizing antibodies to distinct HPV types. *Virology* **2001**, *291*, 324–334. [CrossRef] [PubMed]
115. Day, P.M.; Thompson, C.D.; Buck, C.B.; Pang, Y.Y.; Lowy, D.R.; Schiller, J.T. Neutralization of human papillomavirus with monoclonal antibodies reveals different mechanisms of inhibition. *J. Virol.* **2007**, *81*, 8784–8792. [CrossRef] [PubMed]
116. Christensen, N.D.; Reed, C.A.; Culp, T.D.; Hermonat, P.L.; Howett, M.K.; Anderson, R.A.; Zaneveld, L.J. Papillomavirus microbicidal activities of high-molecular-weight cellulose sulfate, dextran sulfate, and polystyrene sulfonate. *Antimicrob. Agents Chemother.* **2001**, *45*, 3427–3432. [CrossRef] [PubMed]
117. Buck, C.B.; Thompson, C.D.; Roberts, J.N.; Müller, M.; Lowy, D.R.; Schiller, J.T. Carrageenan is a potent inhibitor of papillomavirus infection. *PLoS Pathog.* **2006**, *2*, e69. [CrossRef] [PubMed]

118. CDC Guideline for Disinfection and Sterilization in Healthcare Facilities, 2008. Available online: http://www.cdc.gov/hicpac/Disinfection_Sterilization/3_1deLaparoArthro.html (accessed on 13 May 2015).
119. Meyers, J.; Ryndock, E.; Conway, M.J.; Meyers, C.; Robison, R. Susceptibility of high-risk human papillomavirus type 16 to clinical disinfectants. *J. Antimicrob. Chemother.* **2014**, *69*, 1546–1550. [CrossRef] [PubMed]

7

Modulation of DNA Damage and Repair Pathways by Human Tumor Viruses

Robert Hollingworth and Roger J Grand *

School of Cancer Sciences, College of Medicine and Dentistry, University of Birmingham, Birmingham B15 2TT, UK; E-Mail: rxh291@student.bham.ac.uk

* Author to whom correspondence should be addressed; E-Mail: r.j.a.grand@bham.ac.uk;

Academic Editor: Eric O. Freed

Abstract: With between 10% and 15% of human cancers attributable to viral infection, there is great interest, from both a scientific and clinical viewpoint, as to how these pathogens modulate host cell functions. Seven human tumour viruses have been identified as being involved in the development of specific malignancies. It has long been known that the introduction of chromosomal aberrations is a common feature of viral infections. Intensive research over the past two decades has subsequently revealed that viruses specifically interact with cellular mechanisms responsible for the recognition and repair of DNA lesions, collectively known as the DNA damage response (DDR). These interactions can involve activation and deactivation of individual DDR pathways as well as the recruitment of specific proteins to sites of viral replication. Since the DDR has evolved to protect the genome from the accumulation of deleterious mutations, deregulation is inevitably associated with an increased risk of tumour formation. This review summarises the current literature regarding the complex relationship between known human tumour viruses and the DDR and aims to shed light on how these interactions can contribute to genomic instability and ultimately the development of human cancers.

Keywords: DNA damage; DNA repair; human tumour viruses; HPV; MCPyV; HTLV-1; EBV; KSHV; HBV; HCV

---

1. Introduction

Over the past two decades interest in the relationship between viruses and the DNA damage response (DDR) has increased exponentially. For all the commonly studied viruses, at least some investigations have been undertaken into the effect of viral infection, or expression of individual viral genes, on activation of the host DDR. Similarly, the ways in which viruses impinge on pathways responsible for DNA repair have been the subject of multiple investigations. While most attention has focused on DNA viruses [1–3], there is also a growing body of literature concerning both RNA viruses and retroviruses, whose lifecycle includes a DNA intermediate [4–6].

Historically, interest in the relationship between viruses and DNA damage originates from observations made half a century ago, that infection with a number of virus species could lead to extensive chromosomal damage [7]. It was subsequently found that, in the case of adenovirus, herpes simplex virus 1 (HSV-1), and human cytomegalovirus (HCMV), chromosomal breaks induced by viruses frequently occur at specific sites [8]. More recently, as knowledge of the DDR has developed, increasing layers of complexity concerning viral/DDR interactions have been revealed. It is now clear that some aspects of the DDR can represent a potent antiviral defence that may be disabled following entry to the host cell. In other cases, viruses take advantage of DDR activation to modulate the cell cycle while specific proteins are hijacked to aid viral replication.

Over the past few years a number of excellent reviews of the virus/DDR relationship have been published [1,9–11]. Some of these have focused on particular aspects of the DDR whereas others have concentrated on particular viral species. Here we have tried to draw together the relevant published literature specific to viruses associated with human tumours *in vivo*, including relevant RNA viruses as well as those with a DNA genome. Thus we have summarised the literature concerning human papilloma virus (HPV), Merkel cell polyomavirus (MCPyV), human T-cell leukemia virus type 1 (HTLV-1), Epstein-Barr virus (EBV), Kaposi's sarcoma-associated herpesvirus (KSHV), Hepatitis B virus (HBV) and Hepatitis C virus (HCV) (Table 1). By adopting this approach it is hoped that an appreciation can be gained of how the interaction between a virus and the DDR may contribute to its oncogenic potential and, ultimately, to cancer development.

2. Human Tumour Viruses

Human oncogenic viruses have been defined as necessary but not sufficient to initiate cancer. It is now apparent that only in relatively rare cases do oncogenic viruses in isolation give rise to tumours in otherwise healthy individuals. For example, while the majority of the population carries latent persistent EBV infection, EBV-derived tumours are comparatively rare. In the case of KSHV, although most infected individuals remain asymptomatic, when the immune system is incapacitated by HIV, this herpesvirus can induce Kaposi's sarcoma in a significant proportion of patients. In the case of other viruses, which are present in a latent state, it seems that multiple genetic events, often attributable to environmental factors, are required to initiate tumour development. As outlined here, it is probable that genomic instability induced during the viral lifecycle plays a significant role in tumour initiation. Regardless of the mechanisms of tumourigenesis, it is estimated that between 10% and 15%, of human malignancies are attributable to viral infection [12] and viruses are now second only to smoking as a leading cause of theoretically preventable cancer. This review will focus on genetic instability introduced by infection with oncogenic viruses, and how these pathogens subsequently modulate pathways responsible for recognition and repair of DNA damage.

3. The DNA Damage Response (DDR)

The DDR is the response of the cell to lesions in its genome that occur during normal cellular processes or are introduced by exogenous agents. The inability to repair this damage can result in a variety of acquired clinical conditions such as cancer and neurodegeneration [13,14]. In addition, several inherited disorders are associated with defects in genes crucial for proper functioning of the DDR. Here we include a brief outline of a very complex and fast developing area of biological research; mention is made of only a limited number of proteins involved in the DDR which are relevant to the subsequent discussion.

3.1. Sensors and Transducers

The cellular response to DNA damage is primarily regulated by the activities of three phosphatidylinositol 3-kinase-like kinases (PIKKs): ataxia telangiectasia mutated (ATM), ATM and Rad3-related (ATR) and DNA-dependent protein kinase (DNA-PK) [15–17]. ATM and DNA-PK are principally activated in response to double strand breaks (DSBs) while ATR can be activated following stalled replication forks and by DNA lesions that result in persistent single stranded DNA (ssDNA). Subsequent phosphorylation of transducer and effector molecules by these kinases results in cell cycle arrest, DNA repair and, potentially, apoptosis or senescence.

DSBs are recognised by the MRN complex (comprising Mre11, Rad50 and NBS1), which mediates the recruitment and activation of ATM [18–20] (Figure 1). The activation of ATM also requires acetylation by TIP60, and autophosphorylation that results in disassociation of the inactive dimer to an active monomer [21,22]. ATM can phosphorylate a large number of downstream targets that include CHK2 and H2AX. The phosphorylation of histone H2AX (giving rise to γH2AX) at sites of DSBs allows binding of MDC1, which acts as a scaffold for the formation of large protein complexes spreading appreciable distances from the site of the actual break [23]. MDC1 promotes recruitment of ubiquitin ligases, such as RNF8 and RNF168, which in turn facilitate binding of 53BP1 and BRCA1 [24–26]. DSBs also lead to activation of DNA-PK, which is involved in the non-homologous end joining (NHEJ) repair pathway summarised below.

The stalling of replication forks and resection of DSBs can generate stretches of ssDNA that provide a signal for activation of the ATR kinase (Figure 2) [17]. The ssDNA is bound by RPA which recruits ATR via its binding partner ATRIP. The generation of ds/ssDNA junctions can promote loading of the Rad9-Rad1-Hus1 (9-1-1) complex by the Rad17-RFC complex [27]. The recruitment of TOPBP1 then facilitates ATR activation which subsequently phosphorylates CHK1 with the help of the adaptor protein Claspin [28]. The Timeless-Tipin complex also contributes to CHK1 activation by interacting with both RPA and Claspin [29]. Activation of the ATR-CHK1 pathway is able to slow replication by inhibition of replication origin firing and initiate cell cycle check-points by phosphorylation of the Cdc25 phosphatases [17,30].

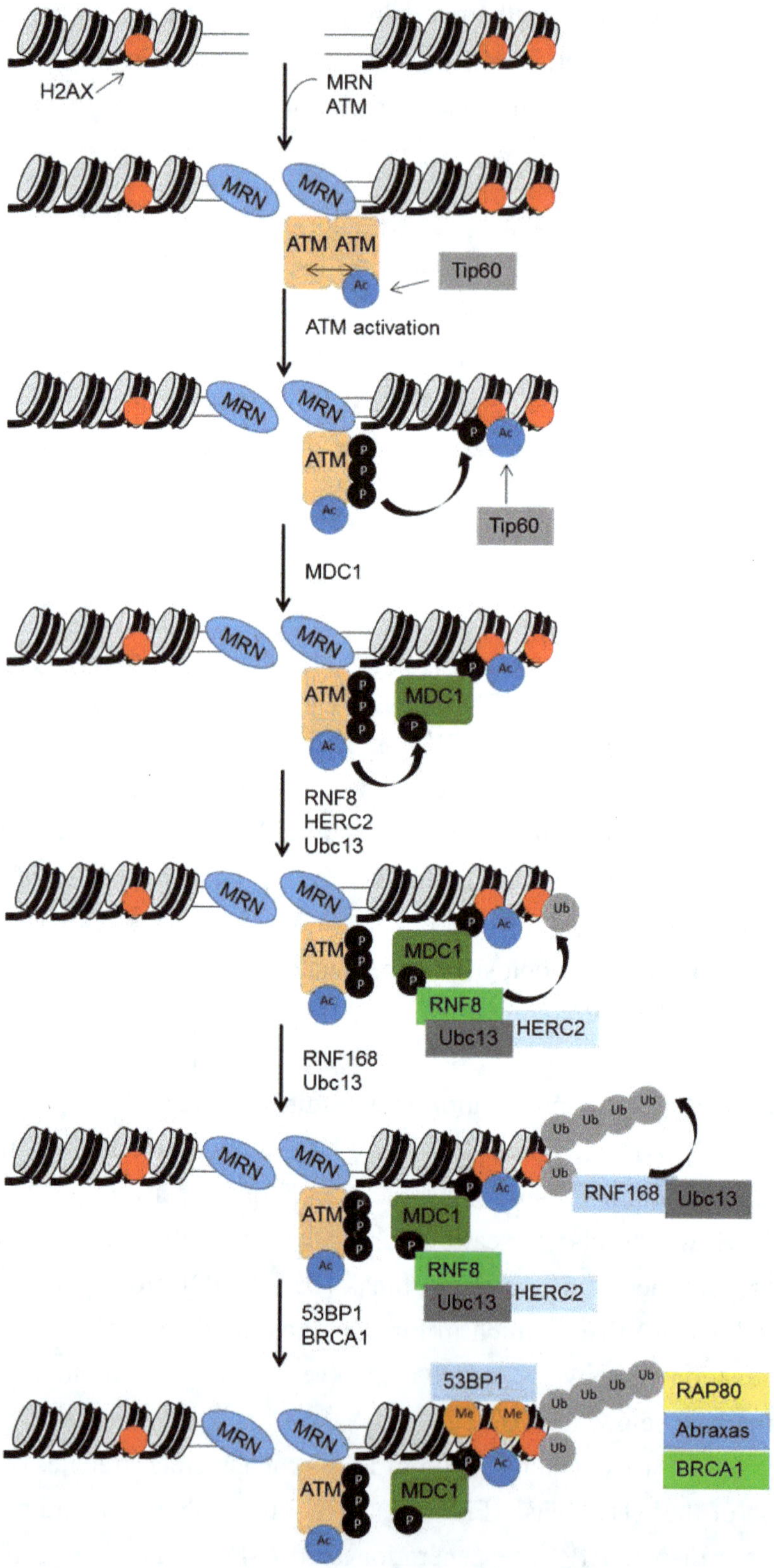

Figure 1. ATM activation in response to DSBs. The MRN complex rapidly migrates to sites of DSBs and, along with the acetyltransferase Tip60, contributes to activation of ATM kinase activity. Phosphorylation of histone H2AX by ATM results in binding of MDC1 which subsequently mediates recruitment of factors, such as 53BP1 and BRCA1, which participate in DSB repair and regulation of cell cycle checkpoints.

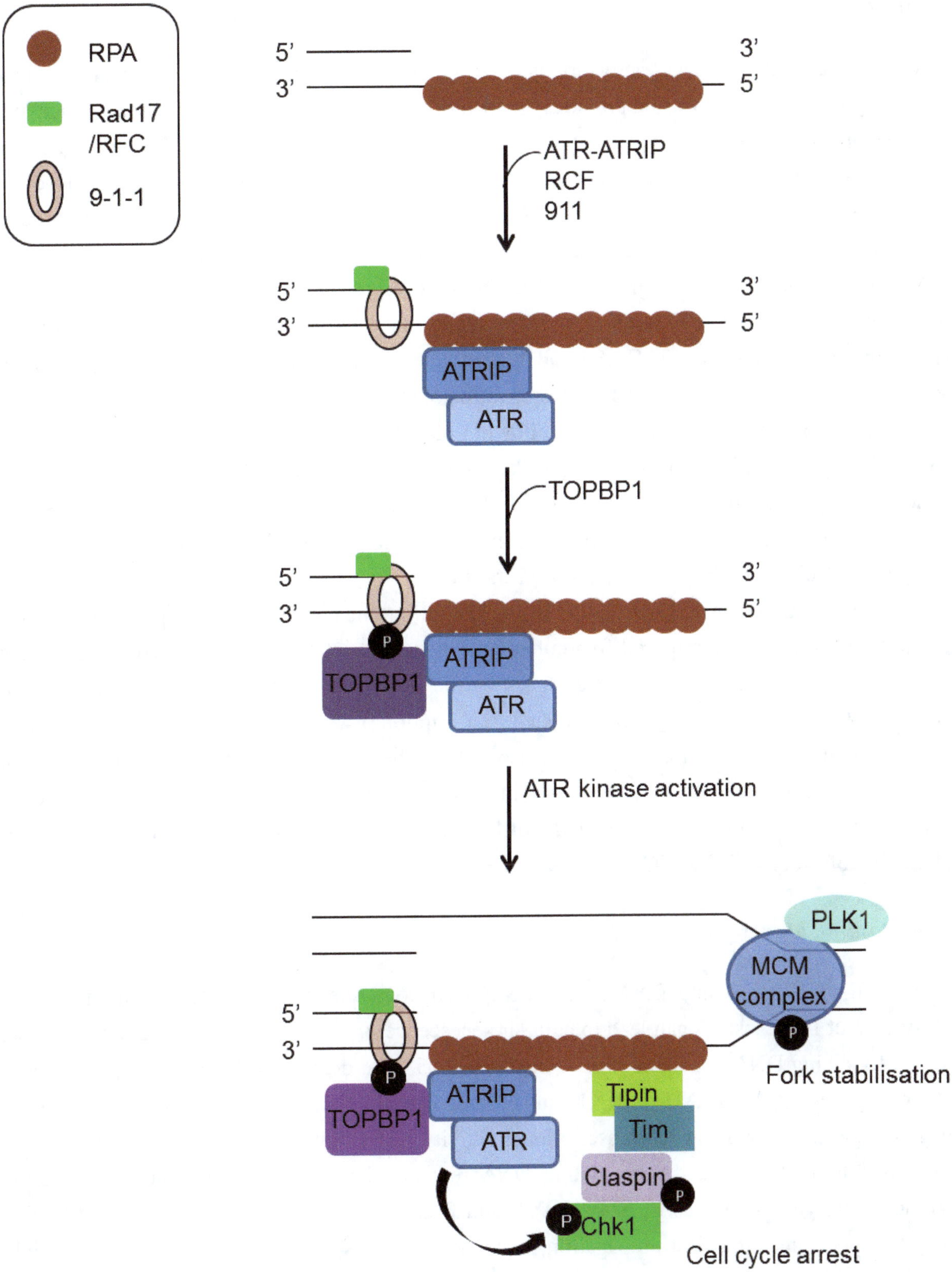

Figure 2. ATR activation in response to stalled replication forks. ATR and ATRIP bind to stretches of ssDNA coated with RPA while the Rad17-RFC complex independently loads the 9-1-1 checkpoint clamp onto ssDNA/dsDNA junctions. Subsequent recruitment of TOPBP1 mediates activation of ATR while Claspin and the Timeless (Tim)/Tipin complex facilitate CHK1 activation.

3.2. Activation of Cell Cycle Checkpoints

A typical consequence of DDR activation is the triggering of cell cycle arrest that prevents replication of potentially mutagenic lesions and provides opportunity for DNA repair [31]. Three major checkpoints are involved in monitoring the integrity of the genome under normal circumstances. The G1/S checkpoint is activated to prevent the initiation of cellular replication in the presence of DNA damage. The intra-S-phase checkpoint can slow or arrest DNA synthesis following replication stress or DNA damage that occurs during DNA replication. Finally, the G2/M checkpoint is activated to ensure that damage incurred during S and G2 is not segregated during mitosis (Figure 3).

Activation of ATM and ATR leads to phosphorylation of CHK1 and CHK2, which in turn regulate downstream targets, such as p53, Cdc25 and Wee1. The phosphorylation of the Cdc25 phosphatases leads to their degradation, which prevents the activation of cyclin-dependent kinases (CDKs) causing cell cycle delay. The key transcriptional target following p53 stabilization is p21, which can impede G1/S transition through inhibition of the cyclin E/Cdk2 complex. The retinoblastoma protein (Rb) also has a key role in cell cycle progression by binding the E2F transcription factors and inhibiting progression into S-phase. In addition, activation of the tyrosine kinase Wee1 following DNA damage leads to inhibition of the cyclin B/Cdk1 complex preventing G2/M transition.

Many viruses have evolved mechanisms of disrupting the G1/S checkpoint to allow S-phase progression, which is often required for replication of their genetic material. The best characterised of these is disassociation of the Rb/E2F complex by the small DNA tumour viruses (adenovirus, HPV, simian virus 40 [SV40]) allowing E2F-mediated transcription of viral genes [32]. Several viruses, such as human immunodeficiency virus (HIV), can also activate the G2/M checkpoint to prevent mitotic entry or to maintain a pseudo S-phase state [33]. This can be achieved via several mechanisms including prevention of nuclear entry of the cyclin B/Cdk1 complex, activation of the ATR-CHK1 pathway or manipulation of Wee1 and Cdc25C activities [33].

3.3. Apoptosis and Senescence

While cell cycle arrest and DNA repair are typical consequences of DDR activation, failure to properly correct DNA lesions can lead to cellular senescence or apoptosis. The activation of apoptotic pathways following DNA damage typically occurs via p53 and defects in this response are associated with tumorigenesis. ATM, ATR, CHK1, and CHK2 can all directly phosphorylate p53 preventing its degradation and increasing its transcriptional activity [34]. While p53 can play a protective role by arresting the cell cycle and upregulating DNA repair pathways, it can also induce transcription of pro-apoptotic genes, such as PUMA, NOXA and BAX [35]. Since apoptosis of the host cell can reduce the opportunity for viral propagation, many viral species have evolved mechanisms to inhibit programmed cell death and promote cellular survival [36]. For example, oncogenic herpesviruses encode homologs of BCL-2, an anti-apoptotic protein that prevents the release of cytochrome c from mitochondria [37,38]. HPV E6 meanwhile promotes the ubiquitination and degradation of p53, as well as other pro-apoptotic proteins, such as BAK, FADD and c-Myc [39,40]. Lymphocytes expressing the HTLV-1 Tax protein have elevated levels of c-FLIP, a protein that can inhibit apoptosis mediated by the CD95 death receptor [41].

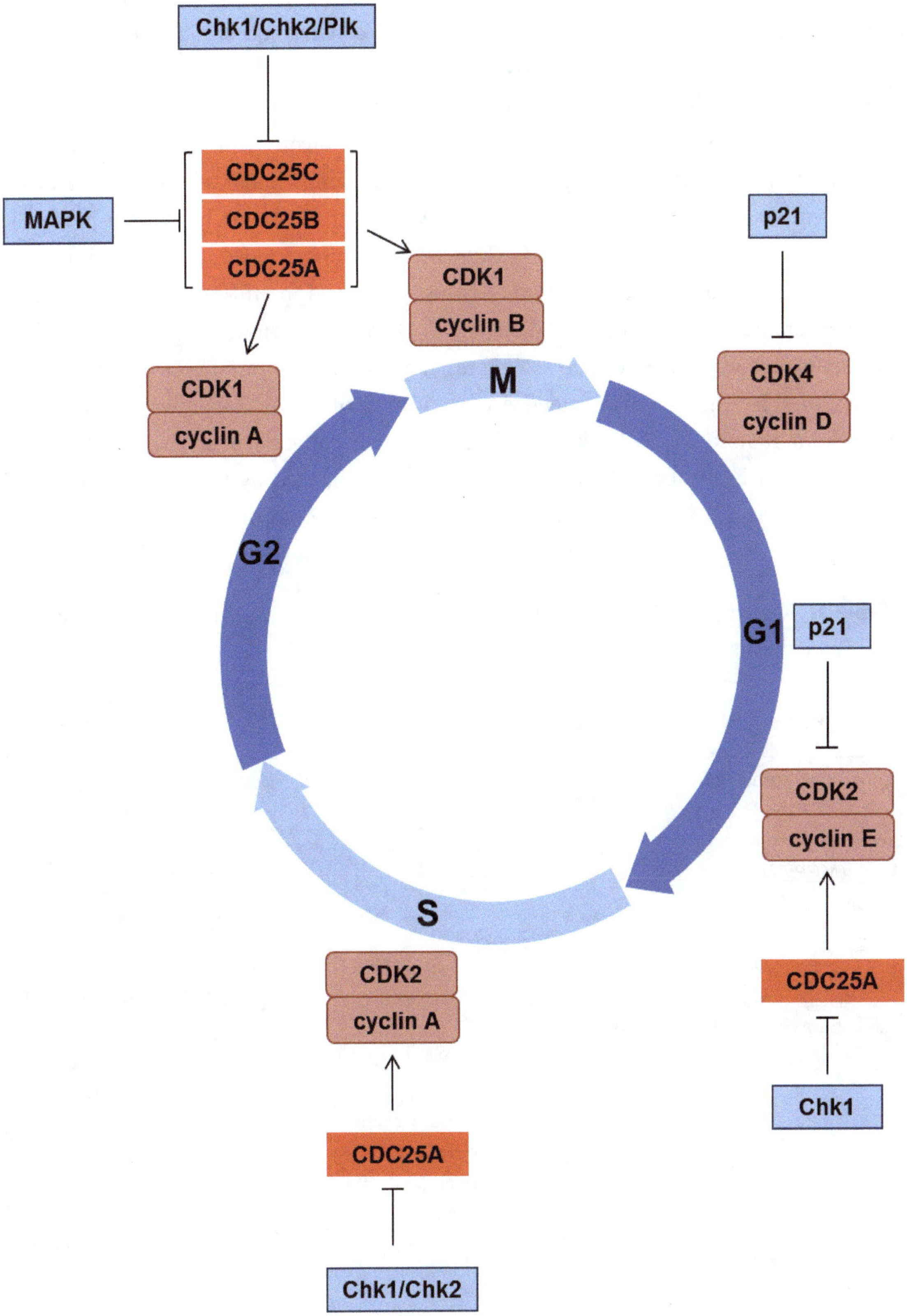

Figure 3. Regulation of the cell cycle by cyclins and CDKs. In response to DNA damage phosphorylation of CHK1 and CHK2 can lead to degradation of Cdc25 phosphatases. Cdc25 degradation inhibits activation of CDKs and delays progression of the cell cycle. Increased expression of p21 by p53 following DNA damage can also mediate cell cycle arrest through inhibition of CDKs.

Persistent activation of the DDR can also lead to cellular senescence whereby the cell remains viable but replicative capacity is lost. A DDR that results in cellular senescence can be triggered by the progressive shortening of telomeres, repetitive DNA sequences that protect chromosome ends, following successive cell divisions [42]. As this provides an important safeguard against malignant proliferation, the interference of tumour viruses with cellular mechanisms involved in the maintenance of telomeres could play a role virally-induced oncogenesis. To promote elongation of telomeres, and thus replicative immortality, viruses can both activate telomerase enzymes and stimulate a more error-prone alteRNAtive lengthening of telomere (ALT) pathway [43]. Cellular proliferation induced by viruses can lead to progressive shortening of telomeres and this has been observed in HPV-associated cervical carcinoma and in hepatocarcinomas containing HBV and HCV [44,45]. To counteract this effect, HPV and HBV oncoproteins have been shown to increase expression and activity of hTERT, the catalytic subunit of telomerase [46,47]. There is also evidence of activation of the ALT pathway in human embryonic fibroblasts immortalized by HPV E6 and E7 and also in endothelial cells immortalised by KSHV vGPCR [48,49]. It is also conceivable that DNA damage induced by viruses could cause irreparable damage to telomeric DNA that, if the senescence response is compromised due to deregulation of cell cycle checkpoints, may lead to telomere dysfunction and genomic instability [43].

Table 1. Known human tumour viruses. *Includes well-characterised proteins rather than an exhaustive list.

Virus	Genome	Viral Oncoproteins *	Associated Cancer
Human papilloma virus (HPV)	dsDNA	E6 and E7	Cervical cancer, penile cancer, anogenital carcinoma, head and neck cancer
Merkel cell polyoma virus (MCPyV)	dsDNA	Large T antigen	Merkel cell carcinoma (MCC)
Human T cell leukaemia virus-1 (HTLV-1)	ssRNA	Tax	Adult T cell leukaemia (ATL)
Epstein Barr virus (EBV)	dsDNA	EBNA2, EBNA3C, LMP-1, LMP-2	Nasopharyngeal carcinoma (NPC), Burkitt's lymphoma, Hodgkin's lymphoma, post-transplant lymphoproliferative disease (PTLD), T cell lymphoma, gastric cancer
Kaposi's sarcoma-associated herpesvirus (KSHV)	dsDNA	LANA, v-cyclin, vGPCR, vIL-6, vBcl-2, vFLIP, Kaposin B	Kaposi's sarcoma (KS), primary effusion lymphoma (PEL), multicentric Castleman's disease (MCD)
Hepatitis B virus (HBV)	ssDNA + ssRNA	HBx	Hepatocellular carcinoma (HCC)
Hepatitis C virus (HCV)	ssRNA	Core, NS3, NS5A	Hepatocellular carcinoma (HCC), B-cell lymphoma

4. DNA Damage Repair Pathways

As DNA lesions can take many forms, multiple DNA repair pathways have evolved to correct specific type of DNA damage. A brief overview of the principle mechanisms of DNA repair pathways are included below. In addition, the interactions between human tumour viruses and key components of these repair pathways are summarised in Table 2.

Table 2. Viral interactions with components of core DNA repair pathways. This list is not exhaustive but includes observations mentioned in this article. VRCs—Viral replication centres.

Repair Pathway	DDR Target Protein	Virus/Viral Protein	REFERENCE
Direct repair	MGMT	HPV E6	[[50]]
Base excision repair (BER)	XRCC1	HPV E6	[[51]]
	ÎŠ polymerase	HTLV-1 Tax	[[52]]
Nucleotide excision repair (GG-NER)	XPC	MCPy LT	[[53]]
	PCNA	HTLV-1 Tax	[[54]]
	DDB1	EBV BPLF1	[[55]]
	TFIIH subunits	HBx	[[56],[57]]
	(XPB, XPD)	HBx	[[58],[59]]
Mismatch repair (MMR)	MSH2, MSH6	KSHV VRCs	[[60]]
	MSH2, MSH6,	HTLV-1 Tax	[[61]]
	MLH1, hPSM2	EBV VRCs	[[62]]
Single strand break repair	PARP-1	KSHV VRCs	[[60]]
	XRCC1	HPV E6	[[51]]
Homologous recombination (HR)		HPV16 E7	[[63]]
	Rad51	EBV VRCs	[[64]]
	BRCA1	HPV31 VRCs	[[65]]
	Rad52	HPV31 VRCs	[[65]]
		HTLV-1 VRCs	[[66]]
		EBV VRCs	[[64]]
Non-homologous end joining (NHEJ)		KSHV VRCs	[[60]]
	DNA-PKcs	HTLV-1 VRCs	[[66]]
	Ku70/Ku80	KSHVorf59	[[67]]
		KSHV VRCs	[[60]]

4.1. Non-Homologues End Joining (NHEJ)

Double-strand breaks in DNA can be repaired by non-homologous end joining (NHEJ) that operates throughout the cell cycle (Figure 4). DNA ends are first recognised and bound by the Ku70/80 heterodimer which recruits the catalytic subunit of DNA-PK (DNA-PKcs) [68,69]. Subsequent phosphorylation by DNA-PK results in its disassociation from the site of damage. End processing involves Artemis, an endonuclease, together with polynucleotide kinase/phosphatase (PNKP), DNA polymerase μ (Pol μ) and DNA polymerase λ (Pol λ). These are required to synthesise complementary nucleotides to fill in single strand overhangs [70]. DNA-PK also facilitates recruitment of the NHEJ ligation complex, comprising DNA Ligase IV, XRCC4 and XLF, which is required for the final joining of the DNA strands [71,72].

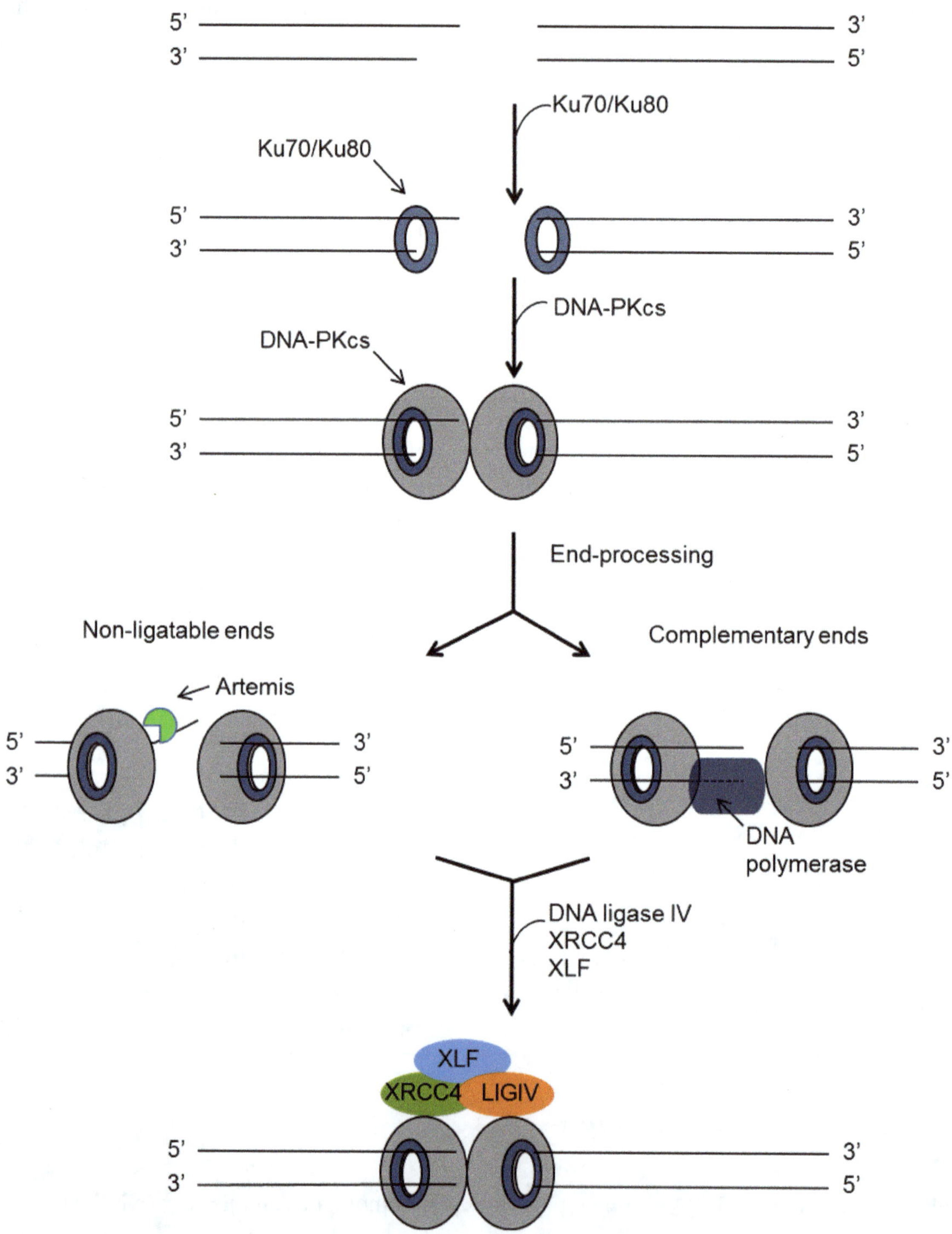

Figure 4. Non-homologous end joining repair of DSBs. Ku70/80 binds to DNA ends and provides a scaffold for the recruitment of additional proteins such as DNA-PKcs. If required, DNA ends may be cleaved by the Artemis nuclease and gaps filled by DNA polymerases. Finally, the ligation complex consisting of XLF, XRCC4 and DNA Ligase IV ligates the DNA ends to complete the repair.

4.2. Homologous Recombination (HR)

Repair of double strand breaks by homologous recombination (HR), which occurs in the S and G2 phases of the cell cycle, is considered more accurate than NHEJ because an undamaged sister chromatid is used as a template (Figure 5). During HR, DNA ends are processed to form 3´ssDNA tails that are bound by RPA. This requires the endonuclease activity of the MRN component Mre11 together with CtIP [73,74]. Additional resection involves the combined activities of exonuclease-1 (EXO1), DNA replication helicase 2 (DNA2) and Bloom Syndrome protein (BLM) [24]. The recombinase Rad51, together with BRCA2 and Rad52, displaces RPA and regions of homology on the sister chromatid are located through the action of Rad52 [70,75,76]. A Rad51 nucleoprotein complex with Rad54 locates homologous regions in the undamaged dsDNA template. Strand invasion which leads to the formation of a displacement loop is followed by DNA synthesis by DNA polymerases such as Pol δ using the homologous DNA as a template. HR can be completed either by the synthesis-dependent strand annealing pathway (SDSA) or the DSBR pathway through a process of "second end capture" facilitated by Rad52 [77]. During SDSA the newly synthesised strand is displaced by RTEL helicase, annealing with single ssDNA on the other side of the break. Second end capture gives rise to double Holliday junctions which are resolved to separate sister chromatids. This resolution requires the endonucleases Mus1/Eme1 and SLX1/SLX4 and the resolvase GEN1 [78].

4.3. Single Strand Break Repair

Single strand breaks (SSBs) are much more common than DSBs although they are often converted to DSBs which are more deleterious to the cell [79]. SSBs can arise from a variety of sources such as the action of reactive oxygen species (ROS) and the erroneous incorporation of ribonucleotides into DNA. They can also arise indirectly during the process of excision repair and as a result of the activity of DNA topoisomerase 1. SSBs are generally recognised by poly (ADP-ribose) polymerase 1 (PARP1), which is activated by DNA strand breaks and then ribosylates both itself and a number of target proteins [80]. Poly (ADP-ribose) chains are rapidly degraded by poly (ADP-ribose) glycohydrolase (PARG) after SSB repair is completed. PARP1 is responsible for recruitment of XRCC1, to the site of damage. This acts as a scaffold for the accumulation of further factors such as polynucleotide kinase/phosphatase (PNKP), aprataxin, and Polβ. Depending on how the SSB has arisen, and therefore the structure of the 3´and 5´DNA ends, different enzymes are involved in processing and repairing the break. For example, PNKP and AP endonuclease 1 (APE1) modify 3´ends whereas 5´termini are substrates for DNA polymerase β [81]. After processing of the damaged termini, gaps in the DNA are filled by Polβ, Polδ and Polε. However, other proteins, such as XRCC1, PARP1, FEN-1 and proliferating cell nuclear antigen (PCNA) may also contribute to this process [79]. As a final step, the DNA is ligated by Ligase 3α (short patch repair) or Ligase 1 (long patch repair) [82–84].

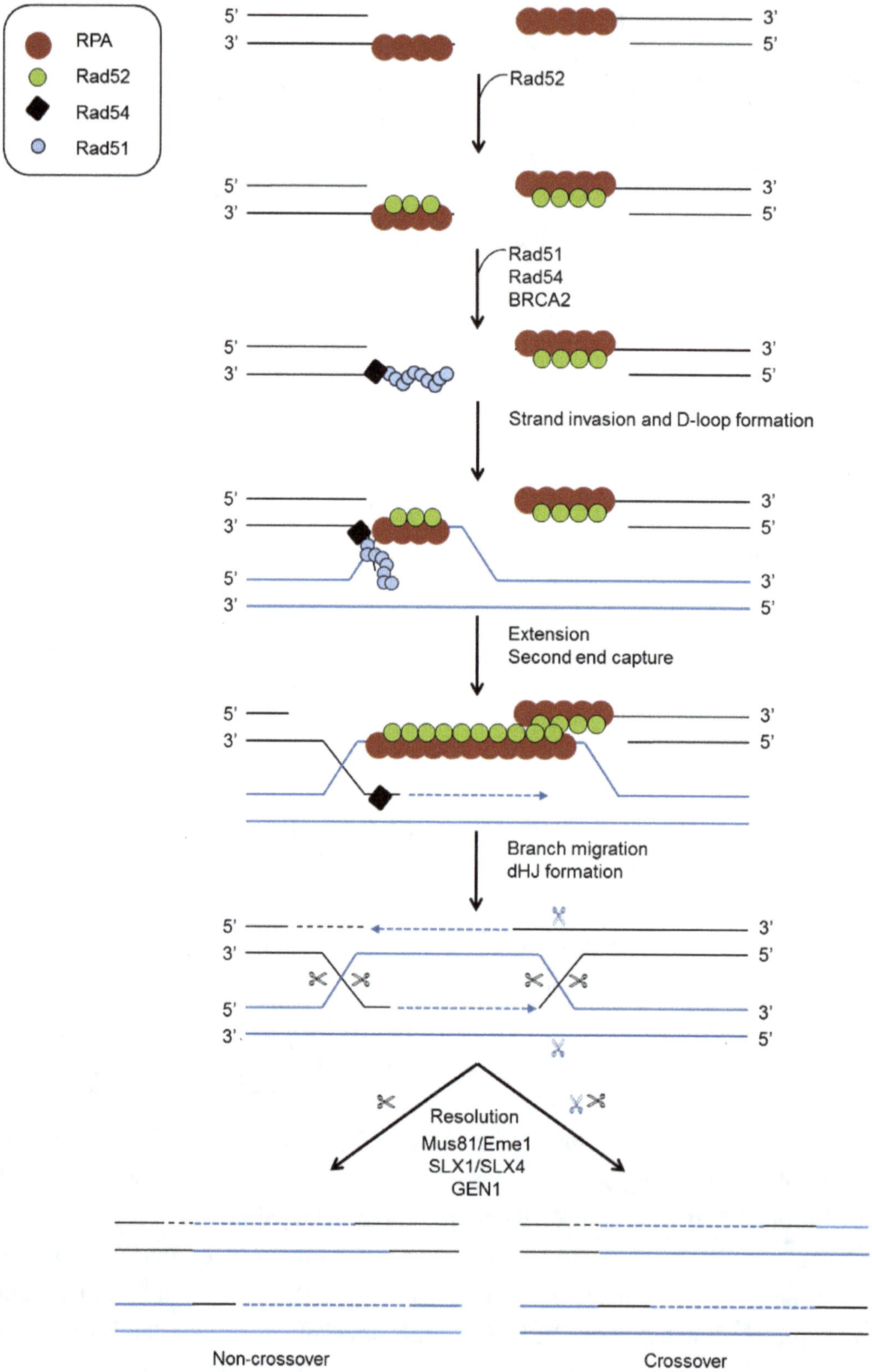

Figure 5. Homologous recombination repair of DBSs. DNA end resection results in ssDNA that is first coated by RPA. Rad51, in conjunction with Rad52 and BRCA2, then displaces RPA. Rad51 and Rad54 catalyse strand invasion and homology search with the undamaged template. Following DNA synthesis via polymerases, the resulting Holliday junctions are resolved.

4.4. Base Excision Repair (BER)

Lesions and mutations, which affect single bases, are removed by the base excision repair pathway (BER). Adducts in DNA tend to occur following exposure to alkylating agents and ROS. Certain modifications, such as O^6-methyl guanine, 1-methyl adenine and 3-methyl cytosine can be repaired directly by alkyltransferases and DNA dioxygenases [85,86]. During BER, damaged DNA bases resulting from single base loss or base oxidation are recognised and removed by one of a number of DNA glycosylases which cleave the bond linking the base to the sugar-phosphate backbone [87]. Removal of the base and end processing by the AP endonuclease 1 (APE1) results in formation of an apyrimidinic/apurinic (AP) site and a SSB. The single nucleotide gap is filled by Polβ and the DNA religated by Ligase 3 and XRCC1 [88]. AlteRNAtive BER pathway components, such as PNKP, may come into play depending on the specific DNA glycosylases involved [89].

4.5. Nucleotide Excision Repair (NER)

Nucleotide excision repair (NER) is used to repair DNA which contains large helix-distorting adducts such as cyclo-butane pyrimidine dimers (CPD) and 6, 4 pyrimidine-pyrimidone photoproducts formed as a result of UV irradiation [90]. Two forms of NER are recognised: global genome NER (GG-NER), which is used to generally repair lesions, and transcription-coupled NER (TC-NER), which is used for repair of transcriptionally active DNA [91]. During GG-NER, lesions are recognised by the Xeroderma-pigmentosum C (XPC)-RAD23B-centrin 2 complex. Recruitment of TFIIH, containing the helicases XPB and XPD and the endonucleases XPG and ERCC1-XPF results in opening of the DNA double helix and cleavage and removal of the aberrant base. The gap is filled by Polδ and PolÉŻ in the presence of PCNA and the DNA is religated by Ligase 1 or Ligase 3 [92]. During TC-NER, the lesion is detected by RNA polymerase II (Pol II) when it becomes stalled during elongation [93]. This results in the recruitment of a large protein complex which includes Cockayne Syndrome proteins, ERCC6 and ERCC8, certain core NER factors as well as TC-NER specific proteins UVSSA, USP7 and HMG14 [91]. Repair then proceeds by a similar mechanism to that of GG-NER.

4.6. Mismatch Repair (MMR)

The mismatch repair (MMR) pathways are activated to deal with DNA base mispairings which arise during DNA replication, generally due to errors of DNA polymerases [94]. Two MMR complexes detect mismatched DNA: MutSα, comprising MSH2 and MSH6, recognises mismatched insertions/deletions 1–2 bases long and MutSβ, comprising MSH2 and MSH3, recognises longer insertion/deletion mispairs [95]. The MutLα-ATPase complex (MLH1 and PMS2) is recruited to the MutSα complex on the mismatched DNA with PCNA and RPA [96]. PMS2 is an endonuclease which, together with EXO1, is required for excision of the mismatched region [97]. The gap is filled by DNA Pol δ using the sister strand as a template and the DNA religated by Ligase 1, together with PCNA [96]. Whilst this simplified account explains MMR *in vitro*, it appears that *in vivo* other chromatin remodelling/modification factors and epigenetic modifications of histones are involved [98].

4.7. *Fanconi Anaemia (FA) Pathway*

The Fanconi anaemia (FA) pathway comprises between 15 and 20 proteins and is activated in response to interstrand cross-links (ICLs) [99,100]. ICLs arise following exposure to chemicals such as cisplatin and mitomycin C and result in the covalent cross linking of two DNA strands, inhibiting transcription and replication. The ICL is recognised by a FA anchor complex containing a number of proteins such as FANCM [99]. Subsequent recruitment of the FA core complex, comprising eight proteins, leads to monoubiquitination of FANCD2 and FANCI. This monoubiquitination results in the recruitment and activation of nucleases, such as FANCP and FANCQ, which cleave the DNA and "unhook" the cross-link. HR proteins are engaged in the later stages of ICL repair to resolve DSBs which are generated [99].

4.8. *DNA Repair Pathways and the Cell Cycle*

Although the DNA repair pathways outlined above have evolved to deal with specific types of DNA damage, their activity can vary significantly during different phases of the cell cycle [101]. As detailed above, DSB repair by HR is restricted to S and G2 phases due to the requirement of a template sister chromatid that allows faithful repair of the damaged region. The other primary DSB repair pathway, NHEJ, can occur throughout the cell cycle but is more prevalent in G1 due to the unavailability of HR. The CtIP protein has been identified as an important factor in stimulating HR since its phosphorylation by CDKs in S and G2 phases promotes its role in the initial resection step of HR [102]. Proteasomal degradation of CtIP in G1 may also contribute to inhibiting HR during this phase [103].

While the principle excision repair pathways can operate throughout the cell cycle, activity can also vary in different phases. For example, MMR is more prevalent during S-phase to correct replication errors while NER plays a key role in G1 to remove bulky lesions that could block DNA polymerases [101,104]. It has also been shown that the activities of key BER enzymes are higher in G1 following IR-induced DNA damage compared with the G2 phase [105]. S-phase is also associated with DNA damage tolerance pathways (DDT) that allow replication to proceed in the presence of unrepaired DNA damage. Lesions can be bypassed in an error-prone manner using specialised translesion synthesis (TLS) DNA polymerases, or more accurately by template switching (TS) which employs the sister chromatid as a template [106]. Since viruses can specifically interact with proteins involved in both DNA repair and cell cycle regulation, it is worthwhile to consider possible cell cycle effects when evaluating the efficiency of DNA repair pathways during viral infection.

The following text summarises the published literature concerning how the pathways detailed above are activated or subverted by viruses known to cause tumours in humans (Table 2).

5. Human Papillomaviruses (HPV)

Human papillomaviruses (HPV) are small double stranded DNA viruses of approximately 8 kb that target the mucosal and cutaneous epithelium. HPV infection is associated with malignancies of the anogenital tract and the oropharynx and is a particular risk factor for the development of cervical cancer [107]. Over 100 HPV strains have been identified although only a limited number have been classified as high-risk based on their potential to cause disease. Among these high risk types, type 16, 18, 31, and 33 are responsible for approximately 90% of all cervical cancers [108].

HPV initially establishes infection in undifferentiated and actively proliferating cells in the basal layer of epithelium where progression of the viral lifecycle is tightly linked to cellular differentiation. In undifferentiated cells, the viral genomes are maintained as extra-chromosomal nuclear episomes, which are replicated in synchrony with cellular DNA. Upon cellular differentiation, the HPV genome is amplified to produce infectious particles and the cell cycle is deregulated to aid viral replication. In HPV-containing cancer cells, the viral episome is often lost and in high grade lesions HPV DNA is typically found integrated into the host genome [109].

The HPV genome can be divided into an early region that comprises six open reading frames (ORFs) designated E1 to E7, a noncoding region and a late region comprising two ORFs, L1 and L2, that transcribe major and minor capsid proteins respectively [110]. The E1 and E2 viral proteins are necessary for initiation of HPV replication while E6 and E7, highly expressed during genome amplification, are the primary oncoproteins required for malignant transformation. E6 and E7 are known to promote degradation of the tumour suppressors, p53 and retinoblastoma protein (pRB) respectively, while disruption of the E2F/RB complex by E7 drives progression of the cell cycle [111,112].

5.1. Activation of the DDR by HPV

Expression of the viral helicase E1 in several high-risk HPV types can induce a DDR that principally comprises activation of the ATM-CHK2 pathway [113–116]. Activation of ATM has been attributed to the induction of DSBs in cellular DNA caused by E1 which specifically requires the ATPase and dsDNA melting activity of the protein [116]. ATM activation by E1 has also been shown to induce cell cycle arrest in S and G2 phases leading to suppression of cell growth [114,116]. Nuclear export of E1 prevents DDR activation and cell cycle arrest in undifferentiated keratinocytes and the formation of a complex with E2 limits DDR activation while E1 is in the nucleus [114]. In several studies a subset of E1-expressing cells were found to contain phosphorylated CHK1 suggesting that HPV may induce cell cycle-dependent activation of the ATR pathway [113,115,117].

While a number of studies have focused on the ability of E1 to induce DNA damage directly, it has also been demonstrated that the coexistence of HPV episomes and integrated HPV DNA in some cells can lead to unscheduled DNA replication and host genomic alterations [117,118]. The re-replication of integrated HPV18 DNA can generate heterogeneous replication intermediates that recruit DNA repair proteins and activate the ATM-CHK2 pathway [117]. In this study, DDR activation was ascribed to the recognition of viral DNA structures rather than the direct induction of DNA damage by viral proteins, although E1 expression was still required to initiate HPV replication.

Expression of E7 has also been shown to cause DNA damage, which can subsequently activate the Fanconi anemia (FA) repair pathway in squamous cell carcinomas (SCCs) [119–121]. FANCD2 foci, a marker of FA activation, have been observed in SSC tissues while FANCD2, FANCD1 and BRCA2 are recruited to chromatin in HPV16 E7-expressing cells [120]. Consequently, expression of E7 in cells deficient in the FA pathway leads to unrepaired DNA damage and increases the risk of genetic instability.

5.2. Involvement of DDR Factors in HPV Replication

Several studies have examined a role for DDR activation and individual DDR proteins in replication of HPV DNA [65,113,115]. It has been suggested that HPV-induced ATM activation and subsequent cell cycle arrest can provide a more suitable environment for viral replication in differentiating cells [113]. ATM inhibition during HPV31 infection was shown to adversely affect late viral genome amplification but not episomal maintenance [113]. In the same study it was demonstrated that CHK2 activity is required for capase activation, which subsequently plays a role in viral replication through cleavage of E1.

Numerous DNA damage and repair proteins have been observed associated with HPV replication centres suggesting a role for these factors in the viral lifecycle. Levels of the DSB markers γH2AX and 53BP1 are elevated in HPV31-positive cells compared with uninfected cells and both can localize to HPV DNA foci along with phosphorylated ATM and CHK2 [65]. In addition, HR factors such as Rad51, BRCA1 and phosphorylated RPA have been seen associated with HPV31 replication centres suggesting that HR may be involved in HPV replication [65]. ATR pathway proteins ATRIP and TOPBP1 have also been observed at HPV18 replication sites [116,117]. TOPBP1 interacts directly with HPV E2 and suppression of this interaction results in an inability of the virus to establish episomes and reduces overall viral DNA replication [122].

5.3. Deregulation of DDR Signalling by E6 and E7

As well as activating the cellular DDR and recruiting DDR factors to replication centres, HPV also interferes with several DNA repair pathways, principally through the actions of E6 and E7. Expression of HPV16 E7 can increase persistence of γH2AX and Rad51 foci following IR-induced DNA damage in head and neck cancer cells [63]. While E7 expression can increase overall levels of the HR protein Rad51, the normal kinetics of DNA repair including the resolution of γH2AX foci are impeded.

E6 from at least three HPV types interacts with XRCC1, a scaffold protein involved in BER, impairing the ability of E6-expressing cells to repair SSBs [51]. E6 also interacts with O^6methylguanine-DNA methyl transferase (MGMT), a protein that protects against harmful mutations by repairing DNA adducts, and promotes its ubiquitin-dependent degradation [50]. Expression of HPV16 E6 was found to interfere with the recovery of fibroblasts from UV radiation by deregulating CHK1 activity [123] while HPV5 and 8 E6 proteins can promote degradation of the histone acetyl transferase p300. Degradation of p300 by E6 was shown to reduce ATR protein levels and subsequently increase thymine dimer persistence and DSB formation following UV exposure [124].

5.4. Summary

HPV activates the ATM pathway primarily through the expression of E1, although other viral proteins as well as viral DNA structures can also simulate DDR signalling. Several components of the ATM and ATR signalling pathways, as well as DNA repair factors, are localised to HPV DNA foci and may contribute to viral replication. Despite the presence of DNA damage, E6 and E7 promote cellular proliferation and survival by deregulating the cell cycle and impairing the apoptotic response.

By driving cellular proliferation in the presence of unrepaired DNA damage and abrogating repair mechanisms, the introduction of genomic instability is an inevitable consequence of the HPV lifecycle that increases the chances of malignant transformation of the host cell. In addition, it has been demonstrated that the introduction of DSBs in cellular DNA leads to an increase in HPV16 integration events [125]. Since viral integration is frequently observed in HPV-related malignancies, it is conceivable that DNA damage induced by HPV proteins can facilitate viral integration which subsequently drives HPV-mediated carcinogenesis [126].

6. Merkel Cell Polyomavirus (MCPyV)

Merkel cell polyomavirus (MCPyV), the most recent human tumour virus to be identified, is responsible for approximately 80% of cases of the aggressive skin cancer known as Merkel cell carcinoma (MCC) [127]. As with other polyomarviruses, MCPyV has a small double-stranded DNA genome divided into early and late coding regions separated by a non-coding control region (NCCR). The early region produces a transcript whose alteRNAtive splicing results in the translation of three proteins; a large T antigen (LT), a small T antigen (sT) and the 57kT antigen. Three capsid proteins, VP1, VP2 and VP3, are encoded by the late region. In MMC tumours positive for MCPyV, the viral genome is integrated prior to clonal expansion of the cancer cells, strongly suggesting a viral driver of oncogenesis [128].

Similar to other polyomarviruses, MCPyV sT is involved in viral replication and targets the protein phosphatase 2A (PP2A). MCPyV sT may also play a role in regulation of the innate immune response and has been implicated in the development and progression of MCC [129,130]. Most attention, however, has focused on the multifunctional LT protein which contributes to initiating replication of the viral genome and also modulates a range of host cellular processes, some of which are analogous to the actions of SV40 LT [131]. In MCPyV-positive MCC, mutations in the carboxy terminus of LT result in production of a truncated LT protein that lacks the helicase activity required for viral replication but retains oncogenic properties, such as an ability to inactivate Rb [131,132]. Since exposure to UV is a known risk factor for the development of MCC and pyrimidine dimer substitutions are common among LT mutations, it is speculated that UV-induced DNA damage plays a role in carcinogenesis [131].

6.1. Activation of the DDR by MCPyV

It has been demonstrated that activation of both the ATM and ATR pathways occurs following MCPyV infection [133]. Activation of both pathways was observed following infection with native MCPyV virions and after viral genomes were directly introduced into cells via transfection. Expression of LT alone led to activation of ATR but not ATM while comet assays revealed that LT expression can cause DNA damage in the host cell. Use of various LT mutants indicated that the C-terminal region of the protein was responsible for both ATR activation and DNA damage. Activation of ATR by LT *C*-terminal region led to p53 phosphorylation, cell cycle arrest and suppression of cellular proliferation. The authors concluded that the C-terminal region of LT can act as a brake on cellular proliferation via DDR activation which offers a possible explanation as to why mutations in this region can contribute to development of MCC.

6.2. Involvement of DDR Factors in MCPyV Replication

It was recently shown that in MCPyV-infected cells, several DDR proteins associated with both the ATM and ATR pathways localise to foci containing MCPyV LT [134].Using immuno-FISH and BrdU staining to visualise viral DNA, it was found that DDR factors including ATR, phosphorylated CHK2, and γH2AX co-localised with LT at sites of active MCPyV replication. This localisation was abolished following introduction of a replication-defective virus or a virus containing a mutated origin of replication. Experiments using DDR kinase inhibitors and small interfering RNA (siRNA) suggested that the ATR kinase is important for efficient viral replication.

6.3. Interference with DNA Repair by LT

It has been demonstrated that MCC cells containing MCPyV have impaired ability to respond to UV-induced DNA damage compared to uninfected MCC cells [53]. These effects were attributed to a defect in the GG-NER pathway, in particular reduced expression of the XPC protein in the MCPyV-positive cells. Ectopic expression of both wild type and mutated LT inhibited G1 arrest following UV exposure but only expression of the mutated protein led to defects in DNA repair. The results suggest that mutated LT could increase genomic instability leading to MCC and provide a possible explanation for the higher incidence of MCC on sun-exposed skin.

6.4. Summary

Similar to SV40 LT [135], expression of MCPyV LT can activate a cellular DDR. But while SV40 LT interferes with downstream activation of p53, the DDR elicited by MCPyV LT leads to cell cycle arrest in a p53-dependent manner. In this way, checkpoint activation may provide selective pressure for generation of the truncated LT protein that fails to activate a growth-suppressive DDR. Truncated LT can also interfere with DNA repair of UV damage that could further contribute to genomic instability and tumorigenesis. During MCPyV infection, DDR factors are localised to sites of viral replication centres while ATR activation plays a positive role in viral replication. It has also been reported that ATM can directly phosphorylate LT although the functional significance of this has yet to be fully determined [136].

Investigations into the interaction between MCPyV and the DDR are clearly at an early stage although findings from closely related polyomarviruses, as well as other tumour viruses, have provided a basis for current research projects. Future studies may uncover how exactly the virus benefits from activation of the DDR and assess the relevant contribution of DDR dysregulation and other factors to the development of MCPyV-associated MCC.

7. Epstein-Barr Virus (EBV)

Epstein–Barr virus (EBV) is a ubiquitous gammaherpesvirus carried by over 90% of the human population [137]. EBV has a dsDNA genome of approximately 170 kbp, primarily targets resting B lymphocytes and epithelial cells and is implicated in the development of human malignancies that include Burkitt's lymphoma, Hodgkin's lymphoma, nasopharyngeal carcinoma and gastric carcinoma [138].

The EBV lifecycle consists of two distinct states: latent infection and lytic replication. Following initial infection, the virus can establish life-long latency in the host where it is typically maintained as an extra-chromosomal episome that is replicated synchronously with cellular DNA by host polymerases. Latency is characterised by the expression of a tightly restricted subset of genes required for viral genome persistence. EBV latency transcripts include three membrane proteins (LMPs), six nuclear proteins (EBNAs), two non-coding RNAs (EBERs) and several microRNAs (miRNAs) [139]. The expression pattern of latent viral genes is variable among EBV-associated tumours and has led to the classification of four latency programmes known as Latency 0, I, II and III [139].

In a subset of cells, EBV can enter the lytic replication programme in which the viral genome can be amplified 100- to 1000-fold. The method of genome replication is distinct from latency in that there is greater requirement for replication proteins encoded by the virus. The immediate–early genes BZLF1 and BRLF1 are expressed first and encode transactivator proteins. These proteins then mediate expression of an ordered cascade of early and late viral genes that culminates in release of progeny virus from the host cell. Proteins expressed in both the latent and lytic stages have unique interactions with the host DDR.

7.1. Genetic Instability Induced by EBV Proteins

Several reports have demonstrated that EBV infection can lead to genetic instability in host cells through the introduction of DNA damage and dysregulation of DNA repair mechanisms. EBV-infected Burkitt's lymphoma cell lines have elevated levels of γH2AX in the absence of exogenous damaging agents as well as an increased number of chromosomal abnormalities [140]. EBV nuclear antigen 1 (EBNA-1), expressed during latency and present in all EBV-associated malignancies, has been shown to induce chromosomal aberrations and DSBs through the production of ROS via NADPH oxidase activation [141,142]. Latent membrane protein 1 (LMP1), known to be essential for EBV-induced transformation of lymphocytes, can induce micronucleus formation and repress DNA repair in epithelial cells [143,144]. It was shown that LMP1 can stimulate the PI3K/Akt pathway resulting in phosphorylation of FOXO3a [144]. FOXO3a phosphorylation causes its retention in the nucleus impairing its ability to activate target genes such as DDB1, a component of the NER pathway.

Several EBV lytic proteins have also been shown to contribute to genetic instability in host cells. In nasopharyngeal carcinoma cells, EBV terminase BALF3 can induce DNA strand breaks and micronuclei formation and recurrent expression leads to tumorigenic features such as enhanced cell migration and invasiveness [145]. The EBV-encoded kinase BGLF4 is also associated with genetic instability [146]. BGLF4 expression leads to DDR activation that interferes with host DNA replication and delays the progression through S-phase [146]. Expression of the EBV DNase BGLF5 in epithelial cells can induce DSBs leading to an increase in microsatellite instability and genetic mutations [147]. BGLF5 expression also results in the down-regulation of several DNA repair genes involved in pathways such as MMR, NER, BER, and HR. Finally, BPLF1, a late tegument protein, deubiquitinates PCNA resulting in reduced recruitment of DNA polymerase η to sites of stalled replication where it would normally play a role in the translesion synthesis (TLS) DNA damage tolerance pathway [55].

7.2. Involvement of DDR Factors in EBV Replication

The role of the DDR proteins in EBV lytic replication has been studied by several research groups although the findings have not always been consistent. During lytic replication in B cells, EBV can elicit an ATM-mediated DDR with phosphorylation of H2AX, CHK2 and p53 observed following induction of the lytic cycle [148]. Phosphorylated ATM, NBS1 and Mre11 were found localised to sites of viral replication while downstream p53 signalling was inhibited. Inhibition of ATM activation by caffeine (a general PIKK inhibitor) during this investigation did not affect production of infectious virus. Two subsequent studies by the same group found that MMR proteins, such as MSH2, MSH6, MLH1, and hPSM2, as well as HR factors, including RPA, Rad51 and Rad52, are also localised to EBV replication compartments [62,64]. The HR factors, as well as PCNA and Mre11, were shown to be loaded onto newly synthesised viral DNA while knockdown of RPA and Rad51 significantly reduced viral replication. These findings point to a key role for individual DNA repair factors and the HR pathway in synthesis of EBV DNA. An interaction has also been reported between the early lytic protein BZLF1 and 53BP1, a protein that usually forms foci at the sites of DSBs [149]. Knockdown of 53BP1 inhibited production of progeny virus indicating that the protein is involved in EBV replication, possibly by protecting exposed DNA ends during genome amplification.

In a mechanism believed to be conserved among herpesviruses, the EBV lytic protein BGLF4 activates the acetyl transferase TIP60, a known regulator of the DDR through acetylation of ATM [150]. This interaction subsequently triggers an ATM-mediated DDR that plays a positive role in lytic replication of EBV. In contrast to previous reports, viral replication was suppressed in a dose-dependent manner following application of a specific ATM inhibitor. A further study provided evidence that ATM activation is required for efficient expression of EBV early lytic genes but not for viral DNA replication [151]. This study presented a model in which cellular stress activates the ATM pathway leading to activation of the EBV early lytic BZLF1 promoter by ATM substrates that can modify viral chromatin. More recently it has been shown that ATM activation during EBV lytic replication leads to phosphorylation of the transcription factor Sp1 [152]. Sp1 is subsequently localised to sites of replicating viral DNA along with other DDR factors associated with the ATM pathway. Phosphorylation of Sp1 was shown to mediate the recruitment of EBV replication proteins to viral DNA, highlighted by the fact that knockdown of Sp1 dramatically suppressed viral replication.

7.3. Dysregulation of Cell Cycle Checkpoints during EBV Infection

It has also been demonstrated that EBV-induced cellular proliferation can activate cell cycle checkpoints that lead to DDR signalling [153,154]. Activation of the ATM-CHK2 pathway has been observed following hyper-proliferation of primary B cells containing EBV [153]. In this context the DDR can act as an anti-tumour barrier as inhibition of ATM and CHK2 significantly increased the efficiency of B cell transformation by EBV. The study also demonstrated that expression of the EBV nuclear antigen 3C (EBNA3C) latent protein could attenuate DDR signalling that would otherwise arrest the growth of EBV-infected cells.

EBNA3C can also interact directly with CHK2 and disrupt the G2/M cell cycle checkpoint induced by treatment with nocodazole which blocks cells in mitosis [155]. The binding of EBNA3C to CHK2 leads to phosphorylation of Cdc25c at Ser^{216}. This causes Cdc25c to be localised to the cytoplasm allowing cyclin B/Cdc2 activation and progression through the G2/M checkpoint. EBNA3C has subsequently been shown to form a complex with H2AX facilitating its degradation via the ubiquitin proteasome pathway [156]. In lymphoblastoid cell lines (LCLs), H2AX knockdown resulted in down-regulation of the tumour suppressor p53 and increased expression of the oncoprotein Bub1. In addition to the actions of EBNA3C, expression of LMP1 in nasopharyngeal epithelial cells impairs the G2 checkpoint through defective CHK1 activation resulting in increased chromosomal instability [157].

Activation of the ATR pathway has also been demonstrated following oncogene-driven cellular replication induced by EBV infection [154]. EBV can interrupt downstream ATR signalling by increasing expression of STAT3, which leads to the loss of Claspin due to caspase 7 activity. Since Claspin is involved in mediating CHK1 phosphorylation by ATR, its loss leads to relaxation of the intra S-phase checkpoint, which would normally act as a barrier against EBV-driven cellular proliferation.

7.4. Summary

Activation of the DDR has been observed in EBV-infected B cells and epithelial cells, during both the latent and lytic stages of the viral lifecycle. The cause of this DDR activation has been ascribed to several sources including the introduction of damage and inhibition of DNA repair, recognition of viral DNA as host cell damaged DNA, and aberrant cellular proliferation induced by viral proteins. In addition, the virus can interfere with cell cycle checkpoints to allow continued cellular proliferation in the presence of DNA damage. EBV also appears to recruit several DDR factors, including HR proteins, to replication sites where they may participate in viral DNA synthesis.

While several studies have noted the activation of ATM following lytic reactivation of EBV, there have been diverging opinions regarding the role of this kinase in viral replication. Contradictory observations could be the result of using different cell types, varying methods of inducing viral replication or the use of non-specific ATM inhibitors. While question marks remain over the role of the DDR during the lytic cycle, it has been shown that DDR factors contribute to viral genome replication during latency. For example, Mre11 and NBS1 are recruited to the origin of plasmid replication (OriP) in S-phase and play a role in maintenance of viral episomes through the formation of recombination junctions [158]. In summary, EBV appears to take advantage of DDR activation and utilise certain DDR proteins while disabling other aspects of the DDR that could lead to growth suppression and apoptosis. In view of the prevalence of EBV infection, the multiple interactions of the virus with the DDR and its ability to damage host cell DNA, it is perhaps surprising that EBV-associated tumours are not more common.

8. Kaposi's Sarcoma Related Virus (KSHV)

Kaposi's sarcoma-associated herpesvirus (KSHV), also known as human herpesvirus 8 (HHV8), is the second gammaherpesvirus after EBV to be identified as a causative agent of human cancers. KSHV can infect and transform endothelial cells leading to the development of the angioproliferative malignancy known as Kaposi's sarcoma [159]. In addition, KSHV is associated with B cell malignancies, primary effusion lymphoma (PEL), and multicentric Castleman's disease (MCD) [160,161]. Despite its association with cancer, KSHV infection is largely asymptomatic, with disease most likely to occur only following suppression of the host immune system.

As with EBV, the KSHV lifecycle is biphasic and consists of latent and lytic stages. KSHV latency-associated nuclear antigen (LANA) is a multifunctional viral protein expressed in all latently infected cells and present in all KSHV-positive KS tumours [162]. LANA plays a vital role in tethering the KSHV episome to host DNA ensuring its distribution to daughter cells following cellular division [163]. LANA can also interact with multiple host cell proteins and has been implicated in tumorigenesis through interference with cellular pathways associated with cell cycle control, apoptosis, gene expression and immune regulation [164]. In contrast to the latent programme, KSHV lytic replication involves expression of a large set of viral genes necessary for production of new infectious progeny. Both latent and lytic genetic programmes have been implicated in the development of KSHV-related malignancies [165].

8.1. DDR Activation during Latent KSHV Infection

KSHV infection induces phosphorylation of H2AX and elevated levels of γH2AX have been observed in latently infected B cells [166,167]. LANA can interact with H2AX at its C terminus leading to formation of γH2AX, which is important for episomal persistence [166]. KSHV infection of primary endothelial cells was shown to result in phosphorylation of H2AX and ATM as early as 30 minutes after viral entry with γH2AX co-localising with viral genomes [167]. Transient phosphorylation of DDR effector kinases CHK1 and CHK2 was observed but downstream phosphorylation of Cdc25c was unaffected. Total H2AX levels also increased during KSHV infection, which was attributed to a decrease in K^{48}-linked polyubiquitination and an increase in K^{63}-linked polyubiquitination. Inhibition of ATM or depletion of H2AX has a negative effect on the ability of the virus to establish latency, suggesting that KSHV may mediate activation of the ATM arm of the DDR while inhibiting downstream signalling.

Ectopic expression of v-Cyclin, a homolog of mammalian D-type cyclins expressed during latency, leads to activation of the ATM pathway and S-phase arrest in endothelial cells [168]. This DDR acts as a block to cellular proliferation and could create selective pressure for the acquisition of mutations that abrogate this barrier while providing a growth advantage to cells defective in DDR components. Expression of v-Cyclin also leads to the introduction of chromosomal instability through disruption of the centrosome cycle resulting in multinucleation and aneuploidy [168–170]. Cells latently infected with KSHV can also bypass a G2/M checkpoint block induced by nocodazole [171]. It was shown that LANA can interact directly with CHK2 leading to activation of the cyclin B/Cdc2 complex that mediates progression through the G2/M checkpoint.

8.2. Involvement of DDR Factors in KSHV Replication

DNA affinity purification combined with mass spectrometry has been used to identify host cell factors that bind to KSHV origins of lytic replication (*ori-Lyt*) [60]. The proteins identified included the MSH2/MSH6 heterodimer involved in MMR and DNA-PKcs, PARP-1, and Ku80/70, all involved in NHEJ. Several of these proteins were also found to localise to viral replication compartments suggesting a role in viral replication. Treatment of KSHV-infected B cells with a PARP-1 inhibitor has been shown to enhance lytic replication but further analysis has also suggested that PARP-1 may play a positive role in replication of viral DNA, although it can negatively regulate late assembly of infectious virions [60,172].

8.3. DDR Activation during Lytic Replication of KSHV

Elevated levels of phosphorylated H2AX have been observed following initiation of KSHV lytic replication [67,173]. This observation has been attributed to the introduction of DSBs in cellular DNA by the viral mRNA export factor orf57 [173]. It was shown that sequestration of the human Transcription and Export complex (hTREX) by orf57 can cause newly transcribed mRNA to form R-loops through annealing to the DNA template strand which in turn leads to formation of DSBs. Another lytic protein, the processivity factor orf59, was shown to interact with Ku70 and Ku80 and impair NHEJ repair of DSBs [67]. Although KSHV lytic replication can activate the DDR, the lytic protein viral interferon regulatory factor 1 (vIRF1) has been shown to interact with ATM and impair DDR activation following etoposide treatment [174]. In addition, vIRF1 can interact with p53 and facilitate its proteasomal degradation.

8.4. Summary

As with EBV, KSHV infection activates the ATM pathway and latently-infected cells display elevated markers of DNA damage and chromosomal aberrations. DDR activation appears to play a positive role in establishing and maintaining latency but does not result in cell cycle arrest or apoptosis that would negatively impact the viral lifecycle. Latent KSHV proteins can also activate the DDR by inducing cellular proliferation while LANA plays a role in abrogating cell cycle checkpoints. KSHV also induces DNA damage during lytic replication and several DDR factors associate with replicating viral DNA.

In both EBV and KSHV, it is problematic to link DNA damage during lytic replication with cellular transformation, since this phase of the viral lifecycle inevitably results in destruction of the host cell. However, several lytic proteins are also expressed briefly following initial viral entry and could conceivably have a detrimental impact on chromosomal stability at an earlier stage of the viral lifecycle [175]. In addition, expression of early lytic proteins during abortive lytic replication of EBV has been linked to the development of lymphomas in mice [176]. Being the most recent human herpesvirus to be identified, there are fewer reports concerning the interaction between KSHV and the DDR compared with other members of the same family. Future studies may focus on identifying a role for DDR activation during lytic replication and the relative contribution of DDR modulation to development of KSHV-related malignancies.

9. Human T-cell Leukemia Virus Type 1 (HTLV-1)

Human T-cell leukemia virus (HTLV-1), the only known human retrovirus that can directly transform human cells, is responsible for the rare and aggressive cancer known as adult T-cell-leukemia/lymphoma (ATL) [177]. HTLV-1 is an enveloped virus with a genome composed of two identicalplus-sense single-stranded RNA molecules that are synthesised into a DNA provirus that integrates into the host genome. Like all retroviruses, the HTLV-1 genome contains gag, pol, and ENV structural genes encompassed by two long terminal repeat (LTR) sequences. Bordering the 3′LTR is the unique pX region that encodes regulatory proteins Tax, Rex, p12, p13, p30, p21, and HTLV-1 basic Zip factor (HBZ) [178].

Like HIV, HTLV-1 predominately targets CD4+ T cells but, while HIV infection can lead to CD4 depletion, HTLV-1-related diseases are characterised by the unregulated proliferation of these lymphocytes. The 40 kDa Tax protein is a transcriptional activator that is essential for viral replication and implicated in HTLV-1-induced cellular transformation [179–181]. Tax can stimulate cellular proliferation and survival through modulation of cell cycle checkpoints, stimulation of the NF-kB pathway and activation of the hTERT promoter in quiescent T cells [182]. In addition, Tax can interfere with tumour suppressor function through the inactivation of p53 [183] and proteasomal degradation of Rb [184]. Tax can also form foci, known as Tax Speckled Structures (TSS) [185] or Tax nuclear bodies [186], in the nuclei of infected cells.

9.1. Genetic Instability in Tax-Expressing Cells

Multiple groups have reported markers of genomic instability in host cells following expression of Tax, characterised by the prevalence of DNA damage markers, formation of micronuclei, and occurrence of aneuploidy [187–189]. Tax was shown to sensitise cells with deleted or mutant p53 to a range of DNA damaging agents including mitomycin C, etoposide and UV light [190]. Expression of Tax can also increase levels of intracellular ROS, DNA damage and the senescence marker SEN1 in both fibroblasts and T cells [191]. All of these markers were reduced following siRNA depletion of Tax or treatment with the ROS scavenger *N*-acetyl-L-cysteine (NAC), indicating that ROS production was the primary source of Tax-induced DNA damage in these cells. Tax has also been shown to impair DNA replication fork progression causing formation of DSBs during S-phase [192]. In the same study, NF-kB activation by Tax also led to DSBs via the production of nitric oxide (NO).

9.2. Interference with DNA Repair by HTLV-1 Proteins

Tax expression has been shown to increase the frequency of mutations in the cellular genome [193]. The random nature of these mutations indicates that this viral protein could interfere with the repair of DNA damage that accumulates during normal cellular processes. Tax has since been shown to interfere directly and indirectly with several different repair pathways that include BER, NER, MMR, NHEJ and HR.

The presence of Tax reduces the expression of human polymerase β, an enzyme involved in BER [52]. Using a range of DNA-damaging agents and a plasmid reactivation assay it was shown that base-excision repair of oxidative damage was the primary repair pathway suppressed in Tax-expressing cells [188]. Tax has also been demonstrated to repress NER through transactivation of PCNA, a cofactor for DNA polymerase δ, that plays a central role in DNA replication and repair [54,194]. In cells containing *wt* p53, Tax has a dose-dependent dual effect on NER [195]. Low levels of Tax stimulated NER through increased transcriptional activity of p53 while high levels of Tax increased p53 levels but functionally inactivated the protein leading to inhibition of p53-dependent NER.Alteredexpression of several MMR genes has also been recorded in primary leukemic cells derived from patients with ATL [61]. Expression of MSH2 and PMS1 was decreased in all cases examined and the reduction in the latter was ascribed to increased methylation of the PMS1 promoter.

Following IR, Tax-expressing cells display defects in the formation of DNA repair foci including disruption of the association between MDC1 and γH2AX and reduced association between ATM and chromatin [196]. As a result of impaired ATM activity, Tax-expressing cells progressed more rapidly into S-phase despite the presence of unrepaired DNA damage. A subsequent study demonstrated that MDC1 is bound by Tax and recruited to nuclear foci that also contain DNA-PK and BRCA1 [66]. Formation of these Tax-containing foci led to a reduction in IR-induced foci containing NBS1 suggesting that viral sequestration of DDR factors impedes their involvement in the normal DDR. Tax has also been found to enhance the expression of the cellular phosphatase WIP1 leading to a reduction in levels of γH2AX following UV radiation [197]. Interference with γH2AX accumulation allows Tax expressing cells to bypass the G1/S checkpoint and enter S-phase with unrepaired DNA damage.

Expression of Tax has been shown to directly induce DSBs during S-phase while NF-kB activation by Tax leads to suppression of HR [189]. Tax also represses transcription of the NHEJ protein Ku80 [198,199]. Reduced Ku80 expression increased the number of unprotected DNA breaks as well as the occurrence of micronuclei and nucleoplasmic bridges in Tax-expressing cells. Although the majority of studies investigating genetic instability during HTLV-1 infection have focused on the activitiesof Tax, there is evidence that HTLV-1 RNA binding protein p30 can also interfere with repair of DSBs [200]. Following DNA damage, p30 alters its distribution from the nucleolus to the nucleoplasm and binds to NBS1 and Rad50, which interferes with the formation of the MRN complex. The disruption of the MRN complex by p30 results in impaired HR during S-phase and facilitates a switch to the more error-prone NHEJ.

9.3. Interaction between Tax and Checkpoint Kinases

Expression of Tax has been shown to induce ATM-CHK2 signalling resulting in the accumulation of cells in the G2 cell cycle phase [201]. Tax can interact directly with CHK2 and, following DDR activation, they, along with 53BP1, have been observed co-localised in nuclear foci [201]. Another study confirmed the interaction between Tax and CHK2 and demonstrated that Tax can also bind to CHK1 [202]. Through this interaction, Tax was shown to inhibit the kinase activity of CHK1 preventing the degradation of Cdc25A and impairing G2 arrest following IR. A subsequent publication attempted to address these contradictory findings by demonstrating that Tax can interact with the kinase domain of CHK2 stimulating oligomerization, autophosphorylation, and stabilisation of the protein [203]. Following IR, Tax sequesters the phosphorylated form of CHK2 within chromatin and impairs its role in the DDR following IR treatment. This study concluded that following Tax expression, CHK2 maintains the ability to orchestrate cell cycle arrest in G2 but is impaired in its role in the DDR following IR. DNA-PK has also been observed associated with nuclear foci containing Tax and CHK2 [204]. Tax can mediate an interaction between DNA-PK and CHK2 leading to increased DNA-PK activity, which impairs the cellular response to IR.

9.4. Summary

Multiple groups have shown that expression of HTLV-1 Tax can cause DNA damage and that this can occur via several mechanisms including the generation of free radicals and interference with DNA replication. There is evidence that at least five key DNA repair pathways are compromised during HTLV infection and that the proper formation of repair complexes is disrupted. In addition, checkpoint kinases are targeted and the virus modulates cell cycle progression to maximise viral replication efficiency.

Following infection, HTLV-1 can enter a long period of asymptomatic latency with only 3%–4% of infected individuals eventually developing ATL [205]. This suggests that cancer development and progression following HTLV-1 infection requires the accumulation of multiple genetic changes [206]. By introducing DNA damage and interfering with repair pathways and cell cycle checkpoints, HTLV-1 can induce cellular proliferation in the presence of genetic aberrations that could ultimately result in cellular transformation.

10. Hepatitis B virus (HBV)

Hepatitis B virus (HBV) is a small enveloped DNA virus with a 3.2 kb genome belonging to the *Hepadnaviridae* family. HBV targets hepatocytes and, while transient infection can cause acute hepatitis, chronic infection is a major risk factor for the development of hepatocellular carcinoma (HCC). The circular HBV genome is partially double stranded and contains four ORFs named S, C, P, and X. The S gene, also known as HBsAg, is divided into Pre-S1, Pre-S2, and S domains and encodes three envelope proteins often referred to as large (L), middle (M), and small (S). The three remaining ORFs encode a DNA polymerase (Pol), a capsid protein (core) and the 154 amino acid X protein (HBx) [207].

HBV has a relatively complex lifecycle that involves reverse transcription. Following entry to the cell, the HBV relaxed circular DNA (rcDNA) is transported to the nucleus where it is converted into covalently closed circular DNA (cccDNA). The cccDNA provides a template for production of viral RNA that is converted by reverse transcriptase to HBV rcDNA in the cytoplasm. Although not an essential step in the viral lifecycle, the HBV genome is often found integrated into the host genome and the process has been proposed to play a role in hepatocarcinogenesis [208].

The multifunctional HBx is involved in viral replication and is implicated in the development of HCC due to its ability to interfere with multiple cellular processes [209]. In the cytoplasm HBx can interact with mitochondria and activate mitogenic signalling cascades [209]. In the nucleus, HBx can influence gene expression through interaction with cellular transcription machinery, although it does not bind DNA directly [210]. HBx can also interact with p53 and impair its transcriptional activation of target genes, thus interfering with its role in apoptotic and DNA repair pathways [211–215].

10.1. Introduction of Oxidative DNA Damage by HBV

Chronic HBV infection can result in increased oxidative stress that has been linked to development of HBV-associated liver disease [216]. Using transgenic mice that expressed the HBV large envelope protein in hepatocytes, it was shown that development of chronic liver disease is associated with an increase in oxidative DNA damage [217]. Mutations in the Pre-S region of the HBV surface antigen (HBsAg) are associated with increased ROS production via endoplasmic reticulum (ER) stress [218,219]. Expression of pre-S mutanT antigens in hepatoma cell lines was shown to cause increased oxidative DNA damage and increase expression of the DNA repair gene ogg1 [218]. However, a subsequent study failed to find a correlation between HBV pre-S mutations and increased oxidative DNA damage in patients with HCC [220].

It has also been demonstrated that DNA damage caused by oxidative stress can promote HBV integration and this has been linked to the development of HCC [221]. Inhibition of PARP-1, involved in SSB repair, also increased the occurrence of HPV genome integration indicating that functional DNA repair pathways, as well as limiting the impact of oxidative DNA damage, may protect against tumour development by restricting viral integration frequency.

10.2. Interference with DNA Repair by HBV

As well as promoting oxidative damage, HBV proteins have been shown to interfere with DNA repair pathways including those associated with processing of ROS-induced DNA lesions. HBx is known to bind to DNA binding protein 1 (DDB1) and the interaction has been shown to be important for HBV replication [56,57,222,223]. As well as being a subunit of an E3 ubiquitin ligase complex, DDB1 also plays a role in both GG-NER and TC-NER by forming complexes with DDB2 and Cockayne syndrome group A protein, respectively [224]. Using a panel of HBx mutants it was shown that, while HBx can impede repair of UV-damage, the interaction between HBx-DDB1 was not absolutely required for this effect [225]. Although it has not been directly linked to impaired NER, the interaction between HBx and DDB1 interferes with normal S-phase progression and increases the incidence of lagging chromosomes during mitosis that can subsequently cause multi-nucleation [226].

HBx, through its interaction with the Sp1 transcription factor, can also reduce expression of the XPD and XPB subunits of the TFIIH transcription factor involved in NER [227]. In addition, HBx has been shown to interact directly with XPD and XPB and sensitise cells to UV-induced DNA damage [58, 59]. The interaction between HBx and p53 has been linked to defects in NER and expression of HBx can inhibit p53-dependent GG-NER in primary mouse hepatocytes [228]. Following UV exposure, levels of HBx and p53 were shown to increase in a hepatocellular carcinoma cell line and both proteins co-localized in the nucleus [229]. The HBx-expressing cells also displayed increased G2/M arrest and apoptosis, as well as a reduced capacity to repair DNA damage compared with controls. HBx expression also impedes the other NER sub-pathway, TC-NER, in both *wt* and p53-null cell lines [215].

Although the majority of studies regarding HBV and DNA repair have focused on the NER pathway, there is also evidence that HBx can interfere with BER. The structure of HBx has been shown to be similar to the human thymine DNA glycosylase (TDG) involved in initiating BER [230]. While the presence of TDG does not affect viral replication, HBx expression strongly supresses BER of G/T mismatches normally initiated by TDG. A more recent study assessed the individual capacity of HBsAg, core protein and HBx to induce DNA damage and interfere with DNA repair [231]. Accumulation of HBsAg was shown to enhance degradation of PML, which led to delayed repair of DSBs and increased resistance to apoptosis following IR. The results also showed that while HBx can induce DNA damage and apoptosis, it did not impede the repair of IR-induced lesions.

10.3. Activation of the ATR Pathway by HBx

HBx expression has been demonstrated to activate the ATR pathway [232–234]. HBV infection can activate the ATR-CHK1 pathway with minimal effect on ATM-CHK2 [233]. Expression of HBx alone has been shown to induce DNA re-replication and polyploidy through increased expression of Cdc6 and Cdt1 and down-regulation of geminin [234]. DNA re-replication resulted in increased DNA damage and the activation of ATR leading to phosphorylation of Rad17 and H2AX but not CHK1. It was also demonstrated that HBx-expressing cells are able to progress to mitosis despite the presence of DNA damage [235]. Activation of Polo-like kinase 1 (Plk1) in the G2 phase of the cell cycle by

HBx reduced levels of Claspin, leading to CHK1 inactivation. This led to attenuation of the G2/M cell cycle checkpoint and subsequently suppressed DNA repair and p53-mediated apoptosis. Treatment of HBV infected cells with theophylline, a compound that inhibits ATR and ATM signalling, significantly reduces HBV replication suggesting a role for DDR signalling in the HBV lifecycle [236].

10.4. Summary

It is clear that HBV infection can increase oxidative stress leading to elevated levels of DNA damage in infected hepatocytes. HBV also appears to interfere with several DNA repair pathways, primarily through the actions of HBx, potentially exacerbating the increase in DNA damage. In addition, HBx can activate the ATR pathway, interfere with checkpoint activation and promote cell cycle progression in the presence of DNA damage that could ultimately result in genetic aberrations.

Despite BER being the primary pathway for repair of oxidative DNA damage, the majority of reports concerning HBV and DNA repair have focused on NER. Although NER can play a part in repair of oxidative damage, it is still unclear whether modulation of this pathway has a substantial role in tumour development following viral infection. As with HPV, DNA damage and abrogated repair can increase the likelihood of HBV integration, which has been linked to deleterious genetic alterations and altered expression of cellular genes. The fact that 80%–90% of HBV-related HCCs contain integrated HBV sequences highlights the link between viral integration and tumourigenesis [237].

11. Hepatitis C virus (HCV)

Belonging to the *Flaviviridae* family, the Hepatitis C virus (HCV) chronically infects over 170 million people worldwide and is responsible for around a third of cases of HCC [238]. While primarily a hepatotrophic virus, HCV can also replicate in lymphocytes and has been linked to several lymphoproliferative disorders including B-cell non-Hodgkin's lymphoma (NHL) [239].

HCV has a positive-sense single-stranded RNA genome of 9.6 kb that contains 5´and 3´untranslated regions (UTRs) that border a single ORF. An inteRNAl ribosome entry site (IRES) in the 5' UTR initiates translation of the HCV genome. The HCV ORF encodes a viral polyprotein of approximately 3010 amino acids that is subsequently cleaved by host proteases to produce a core protein, the E1 and E2 glycoproteins and the p7 ion channel protein. Additional cleavage by viral proteases produces six non-structural proteins NS2, NS3, NS4A, NS4B, NS5A, and NS5B.

Like all positive-strand RNA viruses, HCV reorganises intracellular membranes, such as those associated with mitochondria or endoplasmic reticulum, to form replication structures in the cytoplasm known as "membranous webs" [240,241]. Remodelling of endoplasmic reticulum has been observed following expression of NS4B suggesting that this protein is primarily responsible for the formation of HCV replication complexes [240].

11.1. Introduction of Oxidative DNA Damage by HCV

As with HBV, infection with HCV can lead to elevated levels of oxidative stress that subsequently increase the occurrence of DNA damage. Expression of HCV core and NS3 proteins have been shown to stimulate the inducible NO synthase (iNOS) gene leading to increased production of nitric oxide

(NO) and formation of DSBs in cellular DNA [242]. Expression of E1 during the study also caused a moderate increase in DSB formation but by a mechanism independent of NO production. It was subsequently demonstrated that HCV infection leads to a reduction in mitochondrial membrane potential and an increase in ROS levels [243]. Individual expression of core, E1, and NS3 confirmed that each protein is able to induce ROS that subsequently leads to an increase in DSB formation.

HCV infection can also lead to overexpression of 3β-hydroxysterol Δ24-reductase (DHCR24) which has been linked to attenuation of the p53-mediated response to oxidative stress [244]. Activation of Akt by NS5A can increase c-Myc transcription through stabilisation of the transcription factor β-catenin [245]. This increased expression of c-Myc enhances ROS production and results in increased DNA damage and cell cycle arrest.

11.2. Interference with DNA Repair by HCV

Several studies have demonstrated that interference with DNA repair pathways by HCV could contribute to the development of HCC. Reduced expression of several genes involved in the MMR pathway including MSH2, MLH1, GTBP and PMS2, has been observed in HCV-positive tissues from patients with HCC [246]. Another study demonstrated that ROS levels were elevated by 30–60 fold in HCV HCC cells compared to uninfected controls and that expression of the DNA glycosylase NEIL1, involved in the initial steps of BER, was suppressed [247]. Treatment with the antioxidant NAC or antiviral interferon (IFN) led to a partial restoration in NEIL1 expression indicating that virally-induced ROS could potentially impair BER. Down-regulation of Gadd45β, that plays a role in NER, was observed in HCV-infected cell lines and tissues, as well as transgenic mice expressing the entire HCV ORF [248]. Hypermethylation of the Gadd45β promoter in the presence of HCV was found to be responsible for the defect and led to impaired cell cycle arrest and reduced DNA excision repair. It has also been shown that expression of the HCV core protein in hepatocellular carcinoma cells leads to an impaired ability to repair UV-induced DNA damage [249].

As well as attenuating excision repair pathways, HCV can also interfere with DSB repair. Infection of lymphocytes with HCV was found to cause chromosomal aberrations, which are at least partially attributed to elevated NO and ROS levels [250]. In the same study, expression of Core and NS3 HCV proteins sensitised cells to DNA damaging agents by inhibiting NHEJ. In addition, HCV core protein was shown to interact with NBS1 and prevent formation of the MRN complex, which impairs ATM-mediated repair of DSBs.

11.3. Interaction between HCV Proteins and the ATM Pathway

In addition to inducing DNA damage, HCV can also modulate the DDR through interaction with the ATM-CHK2 pathway. NS3/4A can interact directly with ATM while NS5B interacts with both ATM and CHK2 [251]. In the same study, knockdown of ATM and CHK2 reduced replication of HCV RNA suggesting a functional ATM pathway is required for efficient viral replication. The interaction between NS3/4A and ATM was confirmed in a separate study and shown to sensitise cells to IR via retention of ATM in the cytoplasm that subsequently impairs phosphorylation of H2AX following DNA damage [252]. In addition, expression of the HCV non-structural transmembrane protein NS2 can enhance cellular proliferation and activate the ATM-CHK2 pathway [253]. Following DDR activation, p53 was retained in the cytoplasm in NS2-expressing cells resulting in impaired downstream signalling through p21 activation.

11.4. Summary

As with HBV, infection with HCV can lead to elevated intracellular oxidative stress that increases the occurrence of DNA damage. HCV proteins can also interact with several DDR factors resulting in a reduced capacity to repair DNA lesions. Expression of HCV proteins activates the ATM pathway although the virus appears to deregulate downstream signalling while using key components for viral replication. There is also evidence that HCV exploits the DDR to modulate cell cycle progression [254,255]. NS5B was shown to interact with cyclin-dependent kinase 2-interacting protein (CINP), involvedinthe ATR-CHK1 pathway, preventing its localisation to the nucleus and ultimately causing a delay in S-phase progression [255].

Despite having an RNA genome and replicating in the cytoplasm, HCV can still impact significantly on host DDR pathways. While the HCV lifecycle does not include a nuclear stage, truncated or mutated versions of several HCV proteins have been observed in the nucleus where they can interact with cellular proteins including those associated with the DDR [250,256,257]. There is some doubt, however, about the nuclear localisation of these proteins during realistic models of infection [258]. To this end, the development of superior murine models of HCV pathogenesis will be invaluable in assessing the relative contribution of DDR deregulation and other factors to the progression of HCC.

12. Conclusions

It is clear from the literature summarised here that the interaction between human tumour viruses and the DDR can contribute to an increase in genomic instability during viral infection. As is apparent in high-risk HPV types, the accumulation of deleterious mutations in the presence of viral oncoproteins that promote cellular survival and proliferation will inevitably increase the likelihood of cellular transformation. While the DDR can represent an antiviral defence and barrier to tumourigenesis, chronic activation also creates selection pressure for the deactivation of key components. In all the viruses covered here, DDR activation is an inevitable consequence of viral infection and can be the direct result of the recognition of foreign DNA or expression of viral proteins, or can occur more indirectly through elevated oxidative stress or aberrant cellular proliferation. Since cell cycle arrest and apoptosis are consequences of DDR activation, viruses typically inhibit downstream signalling that would have negative consequences for viral propagation. It is also notable that, in HBV and HPV, DNA damage inflicted during infection can increase the chances of viral integration. This, in turn, can contribute to malignant transformation through host genomic alterations and elevated expression of viral oncogenes [259].

While there have been many excellent studies in this field, in certain cases, experimental limitations have led to some contradictory findings that have impeded progress. The use of different cell culture models and non-specific kinase inhibitors has resulted in inconsistent conclusions regarding the role of DDR activation during replication of viruses such as EBV. A more detailed mechanistic understanding of the precise roles of DDR proteins during synthesis of viral genomes will help confirm their importance during the viral lifecycle. While the ectopic expression of viral genes is a typical way of assessing their contribution to DDR deregulation, it may be misleading in cell types that are not naturalviraltargets *in vivo*. In the case of EBV, for example, the BZLF1 lytic protein has contrasting effects on cell cycle progression when expressed in different cell lines [260]. It is also apparent that viral proteins may have dual effects on the DDR depending on levels of expression; an example mentioned above is the effect of HTLV-1 Tax on p53-dependent NER [195]. In these cases, results must be considered in the context of gene expression levels during natural viral infection. Furthermore, possible contributory effects of other viral proteins should be borne in mind.

Reports demonstrating the involvement of DDR factors in viral replication have led to suggestions that these proteins could be targeted as a novel therapeutic strategy [251]. This is particularly appealing in the case of viruses with RNA genomes where higher rates of mutation have limited efforts to target the virus directly [261]. In addition, it has also been proposed that inactivation of key DNA repair pathways by viruses could open the door for the use of synthetic lethality to specifically target tumours containing viral genomes [262]. While these are attractive possibilities, the DDR is a rapidly evolving area of research with new components and novel regulatory mechanisms being identified frequently. Virologists must keep abreast of the most recent findings to gain a more complete understanding of how viruses modulate these pathways. While it remains to be seen whether the study of viruses and the DDR will yield effective therapeutic interventions, at the very least it has shed new light on how these pathogens modulate host cell functions and uncovered new facets of DDR regulation.

Acknowledgments

We are most grateful to Anoushka Thomas for the illustrations used here and to Cancer Research UK for funding.

References

1. Weitzman, M.D.; Lilley, C.E.; Chaurushiya, M.S. Genomes in conflict: Maintaining genome integrity during virus infection. *Annu. Rev. Microbiol.* **2010**, *64*, 61–81. [CrossRef] [PubMed]
2. Turnell, A.S.; Grand, R.J. DNA viruses and the cellular DNA-damage response. *J. Gen. Virol.* **2012**, *93*, 2076–2097. [CrossRef] [PubMed]
3. Meerbrey, K.L.; Hu, G.; Kessler, J.D.; Roarty, K.; Li, M.Z.; Fang, J.E.; Herschkowitz, J.I.; Burrows, A.E.; Ciccia, A.; Sun, T.; *et al.* The pinducer lentiviral toolkit for inducible RNA interference in vitro and in vivo. *Proc. Natl. Acad. Sci. USA* **2011**, *108*, 3665–3670. [CrossRef] [PubMed]
4. Higgs, M.R.; Chouteau, P.; Lerat, H. 'Liver let die': Oxidative DNA damage and hepatotropic viruses. *J. Gen. Virol.* **2014**, *95*, 991–1004. [CrossRef] [PubMed]
5. Marriott, S.J.; Semmes, O.J. Impact of HTLV-I tax on cell cycle progression and the cellular DNA damage repair response. *Oncogene* **2005**, *24*, 5986–5995. [CrossRef] [PubMed]
6. Arias, C.; Weisburd, B.; Stern-Ginossar, N.; Mercier, A.; Madrid, A.S.; Bellare, P.; Holdorf, M.; Weissman, J.S.; Ganem, D. KSHV 2.0: A comprehensive annotation of the kaposi's sarcoma-associated herpesvirus genome using next-generation sequencing reveals novel genomic

and functional features. *PLoS Pathog.* **2014**, *10*, e1003847. [CrossRef] [PubMed]

7. Nichols, W.W.; Levan, A.; Aula, P.; Norrby, E. Chromosome damage associated with the measles virus *in vitro*. *Hereditas* **1965**, *54*, 101–118. [CrossRef] [PubMed]
8. Fortunato, E.A.; Spector, D.H. Viral induction of site-specific chromosome damage. *Rev. Med. Virol.* **2003**, *13*, 21–37. [CrossRef] [PubMed]
9. Ashley, A.K.; Shrivastav, M.; Nie, J.; Amerin, C.; Troksa, K.; Glanzer, J.G.; Liu, S.; Opiyo, S.O.; Dimitrova, D.D.; Le, P.; *et al.* DNA-pk phosphorylation of rpa32 ser4/ser8 regulates replication stress checkpoint activation, fork restart, homologous recombination and mitotic catastrophe. *DNA Repair* **2014**, *21*, 131–139. [CrossRef] [PubMed]
10. Weitzman, M.D.; Lilley, C.E.; Chaurushiya, M.S. Changing the ubiquitin landscape during viral manipulation of the DNA damage response. *FEBS Lett.* **2011**, *585*, 2897–2906. [CrossRef] [PubMed]
11. Lilley, C.E.; Chaurushiya, M.S.; Weitzman, M.D. Chromatin at the intersection of viral infection and DNA damage. *Biochim. Biophys. Acta* **2010**, *1799*, 319–327. [CrossRef] [PubMed]
12. Liu, S.; Bekker-Jensen, S.; Mailand, N.; Lukas, C.; Bartek, J.; Lukas, J. Claspin operates downstream of topbp1 to direct atr signaling towards chk1 activation. *Mol. Cell. Biol.* **2006**, *26*, 6056–6064. [CrossRef] [PubMed]
13. Jackson, S.P.; Bartek, J. The DNA-damage response in human biology and disease. *Nature* **2009**, *461*, 1071–1078. [CrossRef] [PubMed]
14. Reynolds, J.J.; Stewart, G.S. A single strand that links multiple neuropathologies in human disease. *Brain* **2013**, *136*, 14–27. [CrossRef] [PubMed]
15. Jeggo, P.A.; Lobrich, M. DNA double-strand breaks: Their cellular and clinical impact? *Oncogene* **2007**, *26*, 7717–7719. [CrossRef] [PubMed]
16. Davis, A.J.; Chen, B.P.; Chen, D.J. DNA-pk: A dynamic enzyme in a versatile dsb repair pathway. *DNA Repair* **2014**, *17*, 21–29. [CrossRef] [PubMed]
17. Cimprich, K.A.; Cortez, D. Atr: An essential regulator of genome integrity. *Nat. Rev. Mol. Cell. Biol.* **2008**, *9*, 616–627. [CrossRef] [PubMed]
18. Falck, J.; Coates, J.; Jackson, S.P. Conserved modes of recruitment of atm, atr and DNA-pkcs to sites of DNA damage. *Nature* **2005**, *434*, 605–611. [CrossRef] [PubMed]
19. Petrini, J.H.; Stracker, T.H. The cellular response to DNA double-strand breaks: Defining the sensors and mediators. *Trends Cell Biol.* **2003**, *13*, 458–462. [CrossRef] [PubMed]
20. Bekker-Jensen, S.; Lukas, C.; Kitagawa, R.; Melander, F.; Kastan, M.B.; Bartek, J.; Lukas, J. Spatial organization of the mammalian genome surveillance machinery in response to DNA strand breaks. *J. Cell Biol.* **2006**, *173*, 195–206. [CrossRef] [PubMed]
21. Bakkenist, C.J.; Kastan, M.B. DNA damage activates atm through intermolecular autophosphorylation and dimer dissociation. *Nature* **2003**, *421*, 499–506. [CrossRef] [PubMed]
22. Sun, Y.; Jiang, X.; Chen, S.; FeRNAndes, N.; Price, B.D. A role for the tip60 histone acetyltransferase in the acetylation and activation of atm. *Proc. Natl. Acad. Sci. USA* **2005**, *102*, 13182–13187. [CrossRef] [PubMed]
23. Lou, Z.; Minter-Dykhouse, K.; Franco, S.; Gostissa, M.; Rivera, M.A.; Celeste, A.; Manis, J.P.; van Deursen, J.; Nussenzweig, A.; Paull, T.T.; *et al.* Mdc1 maintains genomic stability by

participating in the amplification of atm-dependent DNA damage signals. *Mol. Cell* **2006**, *21*, 187–200. [CrossRef] [PubMed]

24. Ciccia, A.; Elledge, S.J. The DNA damage response: Making it safe to play with knives. *Mol. Cell* **2010**, *40*, 179–204. [CrossRef] [PubMed]
25. Stewart, G.S.; Panier, S.; Townsend, K.; Al-Hakim, A.K.; Kolas, N.K.; Miller, E.S.; Nakada, S.; Ylanko, J.; Olivarius, S.; Mendez, M.; *et al.* The riddle syndrome protein mediates a ubiquitin-dependent signaling cascade at sites of DNA damage. *Cell* **2009**, *136*, 420–434. [CrossRef] [PubMed]
26. Bekker-Jensen, S.; Rendtlew Danielsen, J.; Fugger, K.; Gromova, I.; Nerstedt, A.; Lukas, C.; Bartek, J.; Lukas, J.; Mailand, N. Herc2 coordinates ubiquitin-dependent assembly of DNA repair factors on damaged chromosomes. *Nat. Cell Biol.* **2010**, *12*, 80–86. [CrossRef] [PubMed]
27. Ellison, V.; Stillman, B. Biochemical characterization of DNA damage checkpoint complexes: Clamp loader and clamp complexes with specificity for 5' recessed DNA. *PLoS Biol.* **2003**, *1*, e33. [CrossRef] [PubMed]
28. Kumagai, A.; Kim, S.M.; Dunphy, W.G. Claspin and the activated form of atr-atrip collaborate in the activation of chk1. *J. Biol. Chem.* **2004**, *279*, 49599–49608. [CrossRef] [PubMed]
29. Kemp, M.G.; Akan, Z.; Yilmaz, S.; Grillo, M.; Smith-Roe, S.L.; Kang, T.H.; Cordeiro-Stone, M.; Kaufmann, W.K.; Abraham, R.T.; Sancar, A.; *et al.* Tipin-replication protein a interaction mediates chk1 phosphorylation by atr in response to genotoxic stress. *J. Biol. Chem.* **2010**, *285*, 16562–16571. [CrossRef] [PubMed]
30. Nam, E.A.; Cortez, D. Atr signalling: More than meeting at the fork. *Biochem. J.* **2011**, *436*, 527–536. [CrossRef] [PubMed]
31. Lukas, J.; Lukas, C.; Bartek, J. Mammalian cell cycle checkpoints: Signalling pathways and their organization in space and time. *DNA Repair* **2004**, *3*, 997–1007. [CrossRef] [PubMed]
32. DeCaprio, J.A. How the rb tumor suppressor structure and function was revealed by the study of adenovirus and sv40. *Virology* **2009**, *384*, 274–284. [CrossRef] [PubMed]
33. Jazayeri, A.; Falck, J.; Lukas, C.; Bartek, J.; Smith, G.C.; Lukas, J.; Jackson, S.P. Atm- and cell cycle-dependent regulation of atr in response to DNA double-strand breaks. *Nat. Cell Biol.* **2006**, *8*, 37–45. [CrossRef] [PubMed]
34. Sancar, A.; Lindsey-Boltz, L.A.; Unsal-Kacmaz, K.; Linn, S. Molecular mechanisms of mammalian DNA repair and the DNA damage checkpoints. *Annu. Rev. Biochem.* **2004**, *73*, 39–85. [CrossRef] [PubMed]
35. Fridman, J.S.; Lowe, S.W. Control of apoptosis by p53. *Oncogene* **2003**, *22*, 9030–9040. [CrossRef] [PubMed]
36. Fuentes-Gonzalez, A.M.; Contreras-Paredes, A.; Manzo-Merino, J.; Lizano, M. The modulation of apoptosis by oncogenic viruses. *Virol. J.* **2013**, *10*, e182. [CrossRef]
37. Cheng, E.H.; Nicholas, J.; Bellows, D.S.; Hayward, G.S.; Guo, H.G.; Reitz, M.S.; Hardwick, J.M. A bcl-2 homolog encoded by kaposi sarcoma-associated virus, human herpesvirus 8, inhibits apoptosis but does not heterodimerize with bax or bak. *Proc. Natl. Acad. Sci. USA* **1997**, *94*, 690–694. [CrossRef] [PubMed]
38. Henderson, S.; Rowe, M.; Gregory, C.; Croom-Carter, D.; Wang, F.; Longnecker, R.; Kieff, E.;

Rickinson, A. Induction of bcl-2 expression by epstein-barr virus latent membrane protein 1 protects infected b cells from programmed cell death. *Cell* **1991**, *65*, 1107–1115. [CrossRef] [PubMed]

39. Gross-Mesilaty, S.; Reinstein, E.; Bercovich, B.; Tobias, K.E.; Schwartz, A.L.; Kahana, C.; Ciechanover, A. Basal and human papillomavirus e6 oncoprotein-induced degradation of myc proteins by the ubiquitin pathway. *Proc. Natl. Acad. Sci. USA* **1998**, *95*, 8058–8063. [CrossRef] [PubMed]
40. Howley, P.M. Warts, cancer and ubiquitylation: Lessons from the papillomaviruses. *Trans. Am. Clin. Climatol. Assoc.* **2006**, *117*, 113–126, discussion 126–117. [PubMed]
41. Krueger, A.; Fas, S.C.; Giaisi, M.; Bleumink, M.; Merling, A.; Stumpf, C.; Baumann, S.; Holtkotte, D.; Bosch, V.; Krammer, P.H.; *et al.* HTLV-1 tax protects against cd95-mediated apoptosis by induction of the cellular flice-inhibitory protein (c-flip). *Blood* **2006**, *107*, 3933–3939. [CrossRef] [PubMed]
42. Hewitt, G.; Jurk, D.; Marques, F.D.; Correia-Melo, C.; Hardy, T.; Gackowska, A.; Anderson, R.; Taschuk, M.; Mann, J.; Passos, J.F. Telomeres are favoured targets of a persistent DNA damage response in ageing and stress-induced senescence. *Nat. Commun.* **2012**, *3*, 708. [CrossRef] [PubMed]
43. Chen, X.; Kamranvar, S.A.; Masucci, M.G. Tumor viruses and replicative immortality—avoiding the telomere hurdle. *Semin. Cancer Biol.* **2014**, *26*, 43–51. [CrossRef] [PubMed]
44. Zhang, A.; Wang, J.; Zheng, B.; Fang, X.; Angstrom, T.; Liu, C.; Li, X.; Erlandsson, F.; Bjorkholm, M.; Nordenskjord, M.; *et al.* Telomere attrition predominantly occurs in precursor lesions during in vivo carcinogenic process of the uterine cervix. *Oncogene* **2004**, *23*, 7441–7447. [CrossRef] [PubMed]
45. Miura, N.; Horikawa, I.; Nishimoto, A.; Ohmura, H.; Ito, H.; Hirohashi, S.; Shay, J.W.; Oshimura, M. Progressive telomere shortening and telomerase reactivation during hepatocellular carcinogenesis. *Cancer Genet. Cytogenet.* **1997**, *93*, 56–62. [CrossRef] [PubMed]
46. Oh, S.T.; Kyo, S.; Laimins, L.A. Telomerase activation by human papillomavirus type 16 e6 protein: Induction of human telomerase reverse transcriptase expression through myc and gc-rich sp1 binding sites. *J. Virol.* **2001**, *75*, 5559–5566. [CrossRef] [PubMed]
47. Zhang, X.; Dong, N.; Zhang, H.; You, J.; Wang, H.; Ye, L. Effects of Hepatitis B virus x protein on human telomerase reverse transcriptase expression and activity in hepatoma cells. *J. Lab. Clin. Med.* **2005**, *145*, 98–104. [CrossRef] [PubMed]
48. Bais, C.; van Geelen, A.; Eroles, P.; Mutlu, A.; Chiozzini, C.; Dias, S.; Silverstein, R.L.; Rafii, S.; Mesri, E.A. Kaposi's sarcoma associated herpesvirus g protein-coupled receptor immortalizes human endothelial cells by activation of the vegf receptor-2/ kdr. *Cancer Cell* **2003**, *3*, 131–143. [CrossRef] [PubMed]
49. Yamamoto, A.; Kumakura, S.; Uchida, M.; Barrett, J.C.; Tsutsui, T. Immortalization of normal human embryonic fibroblasts by introduction of either the human papillomavirus type 16 e6 or e7 gene alone. *Int. J. Cancer* **2003**, *106*, 301–309. [CrossRef] [PubMed]
50. Srivenugopal, K.S.; Ali-Osman, F. The DNA repair protein, o(6)-methylguanine-DNA

methyltransferase is a proteolytic target for the e6 human papillomavirus oncoprotein. *Oncogene* **2002**, *21*, 5940–5945. [CrossRef] [PubMed]

51. Iftner, T.; Elbel, M.; Schopp, B.; Hiller, T.; Loizou, J.I.; Caldecott, K.W.; Stubenrauch, F. Interference of papillomavirus e6 protein with single-strand break repair by interaction with xrcc1. *EMBO J.* **2002**, *21*, 4741–4748. [CrossRef] [PubMed]
52. Jeang, K.T.; Widen, S.G.; Semmes, O.J.t.; Wilson, S.H. HTLV-I trans-activator protein, tax, is a trans-repressor of the human beta-polymerase gene. *Science* **1990**, *247*, 1082–1084. [CrossRef] [PubMed]
53. Demetriou, S.K.; Ona-Vu, K.; Sullivan, E.M.; Dong, T.K.; Hsu, S.W.; Oh, D.H. Defective DNA repair and cell cycle arrest in cells expressing merkel cell polyomavirus T antigen. *Int. J. Cancer* **2012**, *131*, 1818–1827. [CrossRef] [PubMed]
54. Kao, S.Y.; Marriott, S.J. Disruption of nucleotide excision repair by the human T-cell leukemia virus type 1 tax protein. *J. Virol.* **1999**, *73*, 4299–4304. [PubMed]
55. Whitehurst, C.B.; Vaziri, C.; Shackelford, J.; Pagano, J.S. Epstein-barr virus bplf1 deubiquitinates pcna and attenuates polymerase eta recruitment to DNA damage sites. *J. Virol.* **2012**, *86*, 8097–8106. [CrossRef] [PubMed]
56. Lee, T.H.; Elledge, S.J.; Butel, J.S. Hepatitis B virus x protein interacts with a probable cellular DNA repair protein. *J. Virol.* **1995**, *69*, 1107–1114. [PubMed]
57. Sitterlin, D.; Lee, T.H.; Prigent, S.; Tiollais, P.; Butel, J.S.; Transy, C. Interaction of the UV-damaged DNA-binding protein with Hepatitis B virus x protein is conserved among mammalian hepadnaviruses and restricted to transactivation-proficient x-insertion mutants. *J. Virol.* **1997**, *71*, 6194–6199. [PubMed]
58. Qadri, I.; Conaway, J.W.; Conaway, R.C.; Schaack, J.; Siddiqui, A. Hepatitis B virus transactivator protein, hbx, associates with the components of tfiih and stimulates the DNA helicase activity of tfiih. *Proc. Natl. Acad. Sci. USA* **1996**, *93*, 10578–10583. [CrossRef] [PubMed]
59. Qadri, I.; Fatima, K.; Abde, L.H.H. Hepatitis B virus x protein impedes the DNA repair via its association with transcription factor, tfiih. *BMC Microbiol.* **2011**, *11*, e48. [CrossRef]
60. Wang, Y.; Li, H.; Tang, Q.; Maul, G.G.; Yuan, Y. Kaposi's sarcoma-associated herpesvirus ori-lyt-dependent DNA replication: Involvement of host cellular factors. *J. Virol.* **2008**, *82*, 2867–2882. [CrossRef] [PubMed]
61. Morimoto, H.; Tsukada, J.; Kominato, Y.; Tanaka, Y. Reduced expression of human mismatch repair genes in adult T-cell leukemia. *Am. J. Hematol.* **2005**, *78*, 100–107. [CrossRef] [PubMed]
62. Daikoku, T.; Kudoh, A.; Sugaya, Y.; Iwahori, S.; Shirata, N.; Isomura, H.; Tsurumi, T. Postreplicative mismatch repair factors are recruited to epstein-barr virus replication compartments. *J. Biol. Chem.* **2006**, *281*, 11422–11430. [CrossRef] [PubMed]
63. Park, J.W.; Nickel, K.P.; Torres, A.D.; Lee, D.; Lambert, P.F.; Kimple, R.J. Human papillomavirus type 16 e7 oncoprotein causes a delay in repair of DNA damage. *Radiother Oncol.* **2014**, *113*, 337–344. [CrossRef] [PubMed]
64. Kudoh, A.; Iwahori, S.; Sato, Y.; Nakayama, S.; Isomura, H.; Murata, T.; Tsurumi, T. Homologous recombinational repair factors are recruited and loaded onto the viral DNA genome in epstein-barr virus replication compartments. *J. Virol.* **2009**, *83*, 6641–6651. [CrossRef] [PubMed]

65. Gillespie, K.A.; Mehta, K.P.; Laimins, L.A.; Moody, C.A. Human papillomaviruses recruit cellular DNA repair and homologous recombination factors to viral replication centers. *J. Virol.* **2012**, *86*, 9520–9526. [CrossRef] [PubMed]
66. Belgnaoui, S.M.; Fryrear, K.A.; Nyalwidhe, J.O.; Guo, X.; Semmes, O.J. The viral oncoprotein tax sequesters DNA damage response factors by tethering mdc1 to chromatin. *J. Biol. Chem.* **2010**, *285*, 32897–32905. [CrossRef] [PubMed]
67. Xiao, Y.; Chen, J.; Liao, Q.; Wu, Y.; Peng, C.; Chen, X. Lytic infection of kaposi's sarcoma-associated herpesvirus induces DNA double-strand breaks and impairs non-homologous end joining. *J. Gen. Virol.* **2013**, *94*, 1870–1875. [CrossRef] [PubMed]
68. Gottlieb, T.M.; Jackson, S.P. The DNA-dependent protein kinase: Requirement for DNA ends and association with ku antigen. *Cell* **1993**, *72*, 131–142. [CrossRef] [PubMed]
69. Nick McElhinny, S.A.; Snowden, C.M.; McCarville, J.; Ramsden, D.A. Ku recruits the xrcc4-ligase iv complex to DNA ends. *Mol. Cell. Biol.* **2000**, *20*, 2996–3003. [CrossRef] [PubMed]
70. Hartlerode, A.J.; Scully, R. Mechanisms of double-strand break repair in somatic mammalian cells. *Biochem. J.* **2009**, *423*, 157–168. [CrossRef] [PubMed]
71. Grawunder, U.; Wilm, M.; Wu, X.; Kulesza, P.; Wilson, T.E.; Mann, M.; Lieber, M.R. Activity of DNA ligase iv stimulated by complex formation with xrcc4 protein in mammalian cells. *Nature* **1997**, *388*, 492–495. [CrossRef] [PubMed]
72. Ahnesorg, P.; Smith, P.; Jackson, S.P. Xlf interacts with the xrcc4-DNA ligase iv complex to promote DNA nonhomologous end-joining. *Cell* **2006**, *124*, 301–313. [CrossRef] [PubMed]
73. Sartori, A.A.; Lukas, C.; Coates, J.; Mistrik, M.; Fu, S.; Bartek, J.; Baer, R.; Lukas, J.; Jackson, S.P. Human CtIP promotes DNA end resection. *Nature* **2007**, *450*, 509–514. [CrossRef] [PubMed]
74. Symington, L.S.; Gautier, J. Double-strand break end resection and repair pathway choice. *Annu. Rev. Genet.* **2011**, *45*, 247–271. [CrossRef] [PubMed]
75. Nimonkar, A.V.; Sica, R.A.; Kowalczykowski, S.C. Rad52 promotes second-end DNA capture in double-stranded break repair to form complement-stabilized joint molecules. *Proc. Natl. Acad. Sci. USA* **2009**, *106*, 3077–3082. [CrossRef] [PubMed]
76. Nimonkar, A.V.; Genschel, J.; Kinoshita, E.; Polaczek, P.; Campbell, J.L.; Wyman, C.; Modrich, P.; Kowalczykowski, S.C. Blm-dna2-rpa-mrn and exo1-blm-rpa-mrn constitute two DNA end resection machineries for human DNA break repair. *Genes Dev.* **2011**, *25*, 350–362. [CrossRef] [PubMed]
77. McIlwraith, M.J.; West, S.C. DNA repair synthesis facilitates rad52-mediated second-end capture during dsb repair. *Mol. Cell* **2008**, *29*, 510–516. [CrossRef] [PubMed]
78. Nimonkar, A.V.; Kowalczykowski, S.C. Second-end DNA capture in double-strand break repair: How to catch a DNA by its tail. *Cell Cycle* **2009**, *8*, 1816–1817. [CrossRef] [PubMed]
79. Caldecott, K.W. DNA single-strand break repair. *Exp. Cell Res.* **2014**, *329*, 2–8. [CrossRef] [PubMed]
80. D'Amours, D.; Desnoyers, S.; D'Silva, I.; Poirier, G.G. Poly(adp-ribosyl)ation reactions in the regulation of nuclear functions. *Biochem. J.* **1999**, *342*, 249–268. [CrossRef] [PubMed]

81. Caldecott, K.W. Single-strand break repair and genetic disease. *Nat. Rev. Genet.* **2008**, *9*, 619–631. [PubMed]
82. Caldecott, K.W.; Aoufouchi, S.; Johnson, P.; Shall, S. Xrcc1 polypeptide interacts with DNA polymerase beta and possibly poly(adp-ribose) polymerase, and DNA ligase iii is a novel molecular 'nick-sensor' in vitro. *Nucl. Acids Res.* **1996**, *24*, 4387–4394. [CrossRef] [PubMed]
83. Whitehouse, C.J.; Taylor, R.M.; Thistlethwaite, A.; Zhang, H.; Karimi-Busheri, F.; Lasko, D.D.; Weinfeld, M.; Caldecott, K.W. Xrcc1 stimulates human polynucleotide kinase activity at damaged DNA termini and accelerates DNA single-strand break repair. *Cell* **2001**, *104*, 107–117. [CrossRef] [PubMed]
84. Caldecott, K.W. Mammalian single-strand break repair: Mechanisms and links with chromatin. *DNA Repair* **2007**, *6*, 443–453. [CrossRef] [PubMed]
85. Sedgwick, B. Repairing DNA-methylation damage. *Nat Rev Mol. Cell. Biol.* **2004**, *5*, 148–157. [CrossRef] [PubMed]
86. Sedgwick, B.; Bates, P.A.; Paik, J.; Jacobs, S.C.; Lindahl, T. Repair of alkylated DNA: Recent advances. *DNA Repair* **2007**, *6*, 429–442. [CrossRef] [PubMed]
87. Parsons, J.L.; Dianov, G.L. Co-ordination of base excision repair and genome stability. *DNA Repair* **2013**, *12*, 326–333. [CrossRef] [PubMed]
88. Dutta, A.; Yang, C.; Sengupta, S.; Mitra, S.; Hegde, M.L. New paradigms in the repair of oxidative damage in human genome: Mechanisms ensuring repair of mutagenic base lesions during replication and involvement of accessory proteins. *Cell. Mol. Life Sci.* **2015**, *72*, 1679–1698. [CrossRef] [PubMed]
89. Wallace, S.S. Base excision repair: A critical player in many games. *DNA Repair* **2014**, *19*, 14–26. [CrossRef] [PubMed]
90. Alekseev, S.; Coin, F. Orchestral maneuvers at the damaged sites in nucleotide excision repair. *Cell. Mol. Life Sci.* **2015**, *72*, 2177–2186. [CrossRef] [PubMed]
91. Vermeulen, W.; Fousteri, M. Mammalian transcription-coupled excision repair. *Cold Spring Harb. Perspect. Biol.* **2013**, *5*. [CrossRef]
92. de Laat, W.L.; Jaspers, N.G.; Hoeijmakers, J.H. Molecular mechanism of nucleotide excision repair. *Genes Dev.* **1999**, *13*, 768–785. [CrossRef] [PubMed]
93. Marteijn, J.A.; Lans, H.; Vermeulen, W.; Hoeijmakers, J.H. Understanding nucleotide excision repair and its roles in cancer and ageing. *Nat. Rev. Mol. Cell. Biol.* **2014**, *15*, 465–481. [CrossRef] [PubMed]
94. Li, G.M. New insights and challenges in mismatch repair: Getting over the chromatin hurdle. *DNA Repair* **2014**, *19*, 48–54. [CrossRef] [PubMed]
95. Kunkel, T.A.; Erie, D.A. DNA mismatch repair. *Annu. Rev. Biochem.* **2005**, *74*, 681–710. [CrossRef] [PubMed]
96. Jiricny, J. The multifaceted mismatch-repair system. *Nat Rev Mol. Cell. Biol.* **2006**, *7*, 335–346. [CrossRef] [PubMed]
97. Genschel, J.; Modrich, P. Mechanism of 5'-directed excision in human mismatch repair. *Mol. Cell* **2003**, *12*, 1077–1086. [CrossRef] [PubMed]
98. Williams, J.S.; Kunkel, T.A. Ribonucleotides in DNA: Origins, repair and consequences. *DNA Repair* **2014**, *19*, 27–37. [CrossRef] [PubMed]

99. Walden, H.; Deans, A.J. The fanconi anemia DNA repair pathway: Structural and functional insights into a complex disorder. *Annu. Rev. Biophys.* **2014**, *43*, 257–278. [CrossRef] [PubMed]
100. Kim, H.; D'Andrea, A.D. Regulation of DNA cross-link repair by the fanconi anemia/brca pathway. *Genes Dev.* **2012**, *26*, 1393–1408. [CrossRef] [PubMed]
101. Branzei, D.; Foiani, M. Regulation of DNA repair throughout the cell cycle. *Nat. Rev. Mol. Cell. Biol.* **2008**, *9*, 297–308. [CrossRef] [PubMed]
102. You, Z.; Bailis, J.M. DNA damage and decisions: CtIP coordinates DNA repair and cell cycle checkpoints. *Trends Cell Biol.* **2010**, *20*, 402–409. [CrossRef] [PubMed]
103. Germani, A.; Prabel, A.; Mourah, S.; Podgorniak, M.P.; Di Carlo, A.; Ehrlich, R.; Gisselbrecht, S.; Varin-Blank, N.; Calvo, F.; Bruzzoni-Giovanelli, H. Siah-1 interacts with CtIP and promotes its degradation by the proteasome pathway. *Oncogene* **2003**, *22*, 8845–8851. [CrossRef] [PubMed]
104. Schroering, A.G.; Edelbrock, M.A.; Richards, T.J.; Williams, K.J. The cell cycle and DNA mismatch repair. *Exp. Cell Res.* **2007**, *313*, 292–304. [CrossRef] [PubMed]
105. Chaudhry, M.A. Base excision repair of ionizing radiation-induced DNA damage in g1 and g2 cell cycle phases. *Cancer Cell Int.* **2007**, *7*, e15. [CrossRef]
106. Ghosal, G.; Chen, J. DNA damage tolerance: A double-edged sword guarding the genome. *Transl. Cancer Res.* **2013**, *2*, 107–129. [PubMed]
107. Walboomers, J.M.; Jacobs, M.V.; Manos, M.M.; Bosch, F.X.; Kummer, J.A.; Shah, K.V.; Snijders, P.J.; Peto, J.; Meijer, C.J.; Munoz, N. Human papillomavirus is a necessary cause of invasive cervical cancer worldwide. *J. Pathol.* **1999**, *189*, 12–19. [CrossRef] [PubMed]
108. Clifford, G.M.; Rana, R.K.; Franceschi, S.; Smith, J.S.; Gough, G.; Pimenta, J.M. Human papillomavirus genotype distribution in low-grade cervical lesions: Comparison by geographic region and with cervical cancer. *Cancer Epidemiol. Biomarkers Prev.* **2005**, *14*, 1157–1164. [CrossRef] [PubMed]
109. Cooper, K.; Herrington, C.S.; Stickland, J.E.; Evans, M.F.; McGee, J.O. Episomal and integrated human papillomavirus in cervical neoplasia shown by non-isotopic in situ hybridisation. *J. Clin. Pathol.* **1991**, *44*, 990–996. [CrossRef] [PubMed]
110. Zheng, Z.M.; Baker, C.C. Papillomavirus genome structure, expression, and post-transcriptional regulation. *Front. Biosci.* **2006**, *11*, 2286–2302. [CrossRef] [PubMed]
111. Crook, T.; Tidy, J.A.; Vousden, K.H. Degradation of p53 can be targeted by HPV e6 sequences distinct from those required for p53 binding and trans-activation. *Cell* **1991**, *67*, 547–556. [CrossRef] [PubMed]
112. Jones, D.L.; Munger, K. Interactions of the human papillomavirus e7 protein with cell cycle regulators. *Semin. Cancer Biol.* **1996**, *7*, 327–337. [CrossRef] [PubMed]
113. Moody, C.A.; Laimins, L.A. Human papillomaviruses activate the atm DNA damage pathway for viral genome amplification upon differentiation. *PLoS Pathog.* **2009**, *5*, e1000605. [CrossRef] [PubMed]
114. Fradet-Turcotte, A.; Bergeron-Labrecque, F.; Moody, C.A.; Lehoux, M.; Laimins, L.A.; Archambault, J. Nuclear accumulation of the papillomavirus e1 helicase blocks s-phase progression and triggers an atm-dependent DNA damage response. *J. Virol.* **2011**, *85*, 8996–9012. [CrossRef] [PubMed]

115. Sakakibara, N.; Mitra, R.; McBride, A.A. The papillomavirus e1 helicase activates a cellular DNA damage response in viral replication foci. *J. Virol.* **2011**, *85*, 8981–8995. [CrossRef] [PubMed]
116. Reinson, T.; Toots, M.; Kadaja, M.; Pipitch, R.; Allik, M.; Ustav, E.; Ustav, M. Engagement of the atr-dependent DNA damage response at the human papillomavirus 18 replication centers during the initial amplification. *J. Virol.* **2013**, *87*, 951–964. [CrossRef] [PubMed]
117. Kadaja, M.; Isok-Paas, H.; Laos, T.; Ustav, E.; Ustav, M. Mechanism of genomic instability in cells infected with the high-risk human papillomaviruses. *PLoS Pathog.* **2009**, *5*, e1000397. [CrossRef] [PubMed]
118. Kadaja, M.; Sumerina, A.; Verst, T.; Ojarand, M.; Ustav, E.; Ustav, M. Genomic instability of the host cell induced by the human papillomavirus replication machinery. *EMBO J.* **2007**, *26*, 2180–2191. [CrossRef] [PubMed]
119. Sun, R.; Lin, S.F.; Gradoville, L.; Yuan, Y.; Zhu, F.; Miller, G. A viral gene that activates lytic cycle expression of kaposi's sarcoma-associated herpesvirus. *Proc. Natl. Acad. Sci. USA* **1998**, *95*, 10866–10871. [CrossRef] [PubMed]
120. Spardy, N.; Duensing, A.; Charles, D.; Haines, N.; Nakahara, T.; Lambert, P.F.; Duensing, S. The human papillomavirus type 16 e7 oncoprotein activates the fanconi anemia (fa) pathway and causes accelerated chromosomal instability in fa cells. *J. Virol.* **2007**, *81*, 13265–13270. [CrossRef] [PubMed]
121. Park, J.W.; Pitot, H.C.; Strati, K.; Spardy, N.; Duensing, S.; Grompe, M.; Lambert, P.F. Deficiencies in the fanconi anemia DNA damage response pathway increase sensitivity to HPV-associated head and neck cancer. *Cancer Res.* **2010**, *70*, 9959–9968. [CrossRef] [PubMed]
122. Donaldson, M.M.; Mackintosh, L.J.; Bodily, J.M.; DoRNAn, E.S.; Laimins, L.A.; Morgan, I.M. An interaction between human papillomavirus 16 e2 and topbp1 is required for optimum viral DNA replication and episomal genome establishment. *J. Virol.* **2012**, *86*, 12806–12815. [CrossRef] [PubMed]
123. Chen, B.; Simpson, D.A.; Zhou, Y.; Mitra, A.; Mitchell, D.L.; Cordeiro-Stone, M.; Kaufmann, W.K. Human papilloma virus type16 e6 deregulates chk1 and sensitizes human fibroblasts to environmental carcinogens independently of its effect on p53. *Cell Cycle* **2009**, *8*, 1775–1787. [CrossRef] [PubMed]
124. Wallace, N.A.; Robinson, K.; Howie, H.L.; Galloway, D.A. HPV 5 and 8 e6 abrogate atr activity resulting in increased persistence of uvb induced DNA damage. *PLoS Pathog.* **2012**, *8*, e1002807. [CrossRef] [PubMed]
125. Winder, D.M.; Pett, M.R.; Foster, N.; Shivji, M.K.; Herdman, M.T.; Stanley, M.A.; Venkitaraman, A.R.; Coleman, N. An increase in DNA double-strand breaks, induced by ku70 depletion, is associated with human papillomavirus 16 episome loss and de novo viral integration events. *J. Pathol.* **2007**, *213*, 27–34. [CrossRef] [PubMed]
126. Williams, V.M.; Filippova, M.; Filippov, V.; Payne, K.J.; Duerksen-Hughes, P. Human papillomavirus type 16 e6* induces oxidative stress and DNA damage. *J. Virol.* **2014**, *88*, 6751–6761. [CrossRef] [PubMed]
127. Feng, H.; Shuda, M.; Chang, Y.; Moore, P.S. Clonal integration of a polyomavirus in human merkel cell carcinoma. *Science* **2008**, *319*, 1096–1100. [CrossRef] [PubMed]

128. Sastre-Garau, X.; Peter, M.; Avril, M.F.; Laude, H.; Couturier, J.; Rozenberg, F.; Almeida, A.; Boitier, F.; Carlotti, A.; Couturaud, B.; *et al.* Merkel cell carcinoma of the skin: Pathological and molecular evidence for a causative role of mcv in oncogenesis. *J. Pathol.* **2009**, *218*, 48–56. [CrossRef] [PubMed]
129. Shuda, M.; Kwun, H.J.; Feng, H.; Chang, Y.; Moore, P.S. Human merkel cell polyomavirus small T antigen is an oncoprotein targeting the 4e-bp1 translation regulator. *J. Clin. Invest.* **2011**, *121*, 3623–3634. [CrossRef] [PubMed]
130. Griffiths, D.A.; Abdul-Sada, H.; Knight, L.M.; Jackson, B.R.; Richards, K.; Prescott, E.L.; Peach, A.H.; Blair, G.E.; Macdonald, A.; Whitehouse, A. Merkel cell polyomavirus small T antigen targets the nemo adaptor protein to disrupt inflammatory signaling. *J. Virol.* **2013**, *87*, 13853–13867. [CrossRef] [PubMed]
131. Shuda, M.; Feng, H.; Kwun, H.J.; Rosen, S.T.; Gjoerup, O.; Moore, P.S.; Chang, Y. T antigen mutations are a human tumor-specific signature for merkel cell polyomavirus. *Proc. Natl. Acad. Sci. USA* **2008**, *105*, 16272–16277. [CrossRef] [PubMed]
132. Kwun, H.J.; Guastafierro, A.; Shuda, M.; Meinke, G.; Bohm, A.; Moore, P.S.; Chang, Y. The minimum replication origin of merkel cell polyomavirus has a unique large T-antigen loading architecture and requires small T-antigen expression for optimal replication. *J. Virol.* **2009**, *83*, 12118–12128. [CrossRef] [PubMed]
133. Li, J.; Wang, X.; Diaz, J.; Tsang, S.H.; Buck, C.B.; You, J. Merkel cell polyomavirus large T antigen disrupts host genomic integrity and inhibits cellular proliferation. *J. Virol.* **2013**, *87*, 9173–9188. [CrossRef] [PubMed]
134. Tsang, S.H.; Wang, X.; Li, J.; Buck, C.B.; You, J. Host DNA damage response factors localize to merkel cell polyomavirus DNA replication sites to support efficient viral DNA replication. *J. Virol.* **2014**, *88*, 3285–3297. [CrossRef] [PubMed]
135. Martin, D.F.; Kuppermann, B.D.; Wolitz, R.A.; Palestine, A.G.; Li, H.; Robinson, C.A. Oral ganciclovir for patients with cytomegalovirus retinitis treated with a ganciclovir implant. Roche ganciclovir study group. *N. Engl. J. Med.* **1999**, *340*, 1063–1070. [CrossRef] [PubMed]
136. Li, J.; Diaz, J.; Wang, X.; Tsang, S.H.; You, J. Phosphorylation of merkel cell polyomavirus large tumor antigen at serine 816 by atm kinase induces apoptosis in host cells. *J. Biol. Chem.* **2015**, *290*, 1874–1884. [CrossRef] [PubMed]
137. Chang, C.M.; Yu, K.J.; Mbulaiteye, S.M.; Hildesheim, A.; Bhatia, K. The extent of genetic diversity of epstein-barr virus and its geographic and disease patterns: A need for reappraisal. *Virus Res.* **2009**, *143*, 209–221. [CrossRef] [PubMed]
138. Grundhoff, A.; Ganem, D. Inefficient establishment of KSHV latency suggests an additional role for continued lytic replication in kaposi sarcoma pathogenesis. *J. Clin. Invest.* **2004**, *113*, 124–136. [CrossRef] [PubMed]
139. Young, L.S.; Rickinson, A.B. Epstein-barr virus: 40 years on. *Nat. Rev. Cancer* **2004**, *4*, 757–768. [CrossRef] [PubMed]
140. Kamranvar, S.A.; Gruhne, B.; Szeles, A.; Masucci, M.G. Epstein-barr virus promotes genomic instability in burkitt's lymphoma. *Oncogene* **2007**, *26*, 5115–5123. [CrossRef] [PubMed]
141. Gruhne, B.; Kamranvar, S.A.; Masucci, M.G.; Sompallae, R. Ebv and genomic instability—a new

look at the role of the virus in the pathogenesis of burkitt's lymphoma. *Semin. Cancer Biol.* **2009**, *19*, 394–400. [CrossRef] [PubMed]

142. Kamranvar, S.A.; Masucci, M.G. The epstein-barr virus nuclear antigen-1 promotes telomere dysfunction via induction of oxidative stress. *Leukemia* **2011**, *25*, 1017–1025. [CrossRef] [PubMed]
143. Liu, M.T.; Chen, Y.R.; Chen, S.C.; Hu, C.Y.; Lin, C.S.; Chang, Y.T.; Wang, W.B.; Chen, J.Y. Epstein-barr virus latent membrane protein 1 induces micronucleus formation, represses DNA repair and enhances sensitivity to DNA-damaging agents in human epithelial cells. *Oncogene* **2004**, *23*, 2531–2539. [CrossRef] [PubMed]
144. Chen, Y.R.; Liu, M.T.; Chang, Y.T.; Wu, C.C.; Hu, C.Y.; Chen, J.Y. Epstein-barr virus latent membrane protein 1 represses DNA repair through the pi3k/akt/foxo3a pathway in human epithelial cells. *J. Virol.* **2008**, *82*, 8124–8137. [CrossRef] [PubMed]
145. Chiu, S.H.; Wu, C.C.; Fang, C.Y.; Yu, S.L.; Hsu, H.Y.; Chow, Y.H.; Chen, J.Y. Epstein-barr virus balf3 mediates genomic instability and progressive malignancy in nasopharyngeal carcinoma. *Oncotarget* **2014**, *5*, 8583–8601. [PubMed]
146. Chang, Y.H.; Lee, C.P.; Su, M.T.; Wang, J.T.; Chen, J.Y.; Lin, S.F.; Tsai, C.H.; Hsieh, M.J.; Takada, K.; Chen, M.R. Epstein-barr virus bglf4 kinase retards cellular s-phase progression and induces chromosomal abnormality. *PLoS ONE* **2012**, *7*, e39217. [CrossRef] [PubMed]
147. Wu, C.C.; Liu, M.T.; Chang, Y.T.; Fang, C.Y.; Chou, S.P.; Liao, H.W.; Kuo, K.L.; Hsu, S.L.; Chen, Y.R.; Wang, P.W.; *et al.* Epstein-barr virus dnase (bglf5) induces genomic instability in human epithelial cells. *Nucl. Acids Res.* **2010**, *38*, 1932–1949. [CrossRef] [PubMed]
148. Kudoh, A.; Fujita, M.; Zhang, L.; Shirata, N.; Daikoku, T.; Sugaya, Y.; Isomura, H.; Nishiyama, Y.; Tsurumi, T. Epstein-barr virus lytic replication elicits atm checkpoint signal transduction while providing an s-phase-like cellular environment. *J. Biol. Chem.* **2005**, *280*, 8156–8163. [CrossRef] [PubMed]
149. Bailey, S.G.; Verrall, E.; Schelcher, C.; Rhie, A.; Doherty, A.J.; Sinclair, A.J. Functional interaction between epstein-barr virus replication protein zta and host DNA damage response protein 53bp1. *J. Virol.* **2009**, *83*, 11116–11122. [CrossRef] [PubMed]
150. Li, R.; Zhu, J.; Xie, Z.; Liao, G.; Liu, J.; Chen, M.R.; Hu, S.; Woodard, C.; Lin, J.; TaveRNA, S.D.; *et al.* Conserved herpesvirus kinases target the DNA damage response pathway and tip60 histone acetyltransferase to promote virus replication. *Cell Host Microbe* **2011**, *10*, 390–400. [CrossRef] [PubMed]
151. Hagemeier, S.R.; Barlow, E.A.; Meng, Q.; Kenney, S.C. The cellular ataxia telangiectasia-mutated kinase promotes epstein-barr virus lytic reactivation in response to multiple different types of lytic reactivation-inducing stimuli. *J. Virol.* **2012**, *86*, 13360–13370. [CrossRef] [PubMed]
152. Hau, P.M.; Deng, W.; Jia, L.; Yang, J.; Tsurumi, T.; Chiang, A.K.; Huen, M.S.; Tsao, S.W. Role of atm in the formation of the replication compartment during lytic replication of epstein-barr virus in nasopharyngeal epithelial cells. *J. Virol.* **2015**, *89*, 652–668. [CrossRef] [PubMed]
153. Nikitin, P.A.; Yan, C.M.; Forte, E.; Bocedi, A.; Tourigny, J.P.; White, R.E.; Allday, M.J.; Patel, A.; Dave, S.S.; Kim, W.; *et al.* An atm/chk2-mediated DNA damage-responsive signaling pathway

suppresses epstein-barr virus transformation of primary human b cells. *Cell Host Microbe* **2010**, *8*, 510–522. [CrossRef] [PubMed]

154. Koganti, S.; Hui-Yuen, J.; McAllister, S.; Gardner, B.; Grasser, F.; Palendira, U.; Tangye, S.G.; Freeman, A.F.; Bhaduri-McIntosh, S. Stat3 interrupts atr-chk1 signaling to allow oncovirus-mediated cell proliferation. *Proc. Natl. Acad. Sci. USA* **2014**, *111*, 4946–4951. [CrossRef] [PubMed]
155. Choudhuri, T.; Verma, S.C.; Lan, K.; Murakami, M.; Robertson, E.S. The atm/atr signaling effector chk2 is targeted by epstein-barr virus nuclear antigen 3c to release the g2/m cell cycle block. *J. Virol.* **2007**, *81*, 6718–6730. [CrossRef] [PubMed]
156. Jha, H.C.; A, J.M.; Saha, A.; Banerjee, S.; Lu, J.; Robertson, E.S. Epstein-barr virus essential antigen ebna3c attenuates h2ax expression. *J. Virol.* **2014**, *88*, 3776–3788. [CrossRef] [PubMed]
157. Deng, W.; Pang, P.S.; Tsang, C.M.; Hau, P.M.; Yip, Y.L.; Cheung, A.L.; Tsao, S.W. Epstein-barr virus-encoded latent membrane protein 1 impairs g2 checkpoint in human nasopharyngeal epithelial cells through defective chk1 activation. *PLoS ONE* **2012**, *7*, e39095. [CrossRef] [PubMed]
158. Dheekollu, J.; Deng, Z.; Wiedmer, A.; Weitzman, M.D.; Lieberman, P.M. A role for mre11, nbs1, and recombination junctions in replication and stable maintenance of ebv episomes. *PLoS ONE* **2007**, *2*, e1257. [CrossRef] [PubMed]
159. Chang, Y.; Cesarman, E.; Pessin, M.S.; Lee, F.; Culpepper, J.; Knowles, D.M.; Moore, P.S. Identification of herpesvirus-like DNA sequences in aids-associated kaposi's sarcoma. *Science* **1994**, *266*, 1865–1869. [CrossRef] [PubMed]
160. Cesarman, E.; Chang, Y.; Moore, P.S.; Said, J.W.; Knowles, D.M. Kaposi's sarcoma-associated herpesvirus-like DNA sequences in aids-related body-cavity-based lymphomas. *N. Engl. J. Med.* **1995**, *332*, 1186–1191. [CrossRef] [PubMed]
161. Soulier, J.; Grollet, L.; Oksenhendler, E.; Cacoub, P.; Cazals-Hatem, D.; Babinet, P.; d'Agay, M.F.; Clauvel, J.P.; Raphael, M.; Degos, L.; *et al.* Kaposi's sarcoma-associated herpesvirus-like DNA sequences in multicentric castleman's disease. *Blood* **1995**, *86*, 1276–1280. [PubMed]
162. Dittmer, D.P. Transcription profile of kaposi's sarcoma-associated herpesvirus in primary kaposi's sarcoma lesions as determined by real-time pcr arrays. *Cancer Res.* **2003**, *63*, 2010–2015. [PubMed]
163. Guito, J.; Lukac, D.M. KSHV reactivation and novel implications of protein isomerization on lytic switch control. *Viruses* **2015**, *7*, 72–109. [CrossRef] [PubMed]
164. Uppal, T.; Banerjee, S.; Sun, Z.; Verma, S.C.; Robertson, E.S. KSHV lana—the master regulator of KSHV latency. *Viruses* **2014**, *6*, 4961–4998. [CrossRef] [PubMed]
165. Mesri, E.A.; Cesarman, E.; Boshoff, C. Kaposi's sarcoma and its associated herpesvirus. *Nat. Rev. Cancer* **2010**, *10*, 707–719. [CrossRef] [PubMed]
166. Jha, H.C.; Upadhyay, S.K.; M, A.J.P.; Lu, J.; Cai, Q.; Saha, A.; Robertson, E.S. H2ax phosphorylation is important for lana-mediated kaposi's sarcoma-associated herpesvirus episome persistence. *J. Virol.* **2013**, *87*, 5255–5269. [CrossRef] [PubMed]
167. Singh, V.V.; Dutta, D.; Ansari, M.A.; Dutta, S.; Chandran, B. Kaposi's sarcoma-associated

herpesvirus induces the atm and h2ax DNA damage response early during de novo infection of primary endothelial cells, which play roles in latency establishment. *J. Virol.* **2014**, *88*, 2821–2834. [CrossRef] [PubMed]

168. Koopal, S.; Furuhjelm, J.H.; Jarviluoma, A.; Jaamaa, S.; Pyakurel, P.; Pussinen, C.; Wirzenius, M.; Biberfeld, P.; Alitalo, K.; Laiho, M.; *et al.* Viral oncogene-induced DNA damage response is activated in kaposi sarcoma tumorigenesis. *PLoS Pathog.* **2007**, *3*, 1348–1360. [CrossRef] [PubMed]
169. Verschuren, E.W.; Klefstrom, J.; Evan, G.I.; Jones, N. The oncogenic potential of kaposi's sarcoma-associated herpesvirus cyclin is exposed by p53 loss in vitro and in vivo. *Cancer Cell* **2002**, *2*, 229–241. [CrossRef] [PubMed]
170. Pan, H.; Zhou, F.; Gao, S.J. Kaposi's sarcoma-associated herpesvirus induction of chromosome instability in primary human endothelial cells. *Cancer Res.* **2004**, *64*, 4064–4068. [CrossRef] [PubMed]
171. Kumar, A.; Sahu, S.K.; Mohanty, S.; Chakrabarti, S.; Maji, S.; Reddy, R.R.; Jha, A.K.; Goswami, C.; Kundu, C.N.; Rajasubramaniam, S.; *et al.* Kaposi sarcoma herpes virus latency associated nuclear antigen protein release the g2/m cell cycle blocks by modulating atm/atr mediated checkpoint pathway. *PLoS ONE* **2014**, *9*, e100228. [CrossRef] [PubMed]
172. Gwack, Y.; Nakamura, H.; Lee, S.H.; Souvlis, J.; Yustein, J.T.; Gygi, S.; Kung, H.J.; Jung, J.U. Poly(adp-ribose) polymerase 1 and ste20-like kinase hkfc act as transcriptional repressors for gamma-2 herpesvirus lytic replication. *Mol. Cell. Biol.* **2003**, *23*, 8282–8294. [CrossRef] [PubMed]
173. Jackson, B.R.; Noerenberg, M.; Whitehouse, A. A novel mechanism inducing genome instability in kaposi's sarcoma-associated herpesvirus infected cells. *PLoS Pathog.* **2014**, *10*, e1004098. [CrossRef] [PubMed]
174. Shin, Y.C.; Nakamura, H.; Liang, X.; Feng, P.; Chang, H.; Kowalik, T.F.; Jung, J.U. Inhibition of the atm/p53 signal transduction pathway by kaposi's sarcoma-associated herpesvirus interferon regulatory factor 1. *J. Virol.* **2006**, *80*, 2257–2266. [CrossRef] [PubMed]
175. Krishnan, H.H.; Naranatt, P.P.; Smith, M.S.; Zeng, L.; Bloomer, C.; Chandran, B. Concurrent expression of latent and a limited number of lytic genes with immune modulation and antiapoptotic function by kaposi's sarcoma-associated herpesvirus early during infection of primary endothelial and fibroblast cells and subsequent decline of lytic gene expression. *J. Virol.* **2004**, *78*, 3601–3620. [CrossRef] [PubMed]
176. Ma, S.D.; Hegde, S.; Young, K.H.; Sullivan, R.; Rajesh, D.; Zhou, Y.; Jankowska-Gan, E.; Burlingham, W.J.; Sun, X.; Gulley, M.L.; *et al.* A new model of epstein-barr virus infection reveals an important role for early lytic viral protein expression in the development of lymphomas. *J. Virol.* **2011**, *85*, 165–177. [CrossRef] [PubMed]
177. Franchini, G.; Nicot, C.; Johnson, J.M. Seizing of t cells by human T-cell leukemia/lymphoma virus type 1. *Adv. Cancer Res.* **2003**, *89*, 69–132. [PubMed]
178. Matsuoka, M.; Jeang, K.T. Human T-cell leukaemia virus type 1 (HTLV-1) infectivity and cellular transformation. *Nat. Rev. Cancer* **2007**, *7*, 270–280. [CrossRef] [PubMed]

179. Korber, B.; Okayama, A.; Donnelly, R.; Tachibana, N.; Essex, M. Polymerase chain reaction analysis of defective human T-cell leukemia virus type i proviral genomes in leukemic cells of patients with adult T-cell leukemia. *J. Virol.* **1991**, *65*, 5471–5476. [PubMed]

180. Grassmann, R.; Dengler, C.; Muller-Fleckenstein, I.; Fleckenstein, B.; McGuire, K.; Dokhelar, M.C.; Sodroski, J.G.; Haseltine, W.A. Transformation to continuous growth of primary human T lymphocytes by human T-cell leukemia virus type i x-region genes transduced by a herpesvirus saimiri vector. *Proc. Natl. Acad. Sci. USA* **1989**, *86*, 3351–3355. [CrossRef] [PubMed]

181. Grassmann, R.; Berchtold, S.; Radant, I.; Alt, M.; Fleckenstein, B.; Sodroski, J.G.; Haseltine, W.A.; Ramstedt, U. Role of human T-cell leukemia virus type 1 x region proteins in immortalization of primary human lymphocytes in culture. *J. Virol.* **1992**, *66*, 4570–4575. [PubMed]

182. Hara, T.; Matsumura-Arioka, Y.; Ohtani, K.; Nakamura, M. Role of human T-cell leukemia virus type i tax in expression of the human telomerase reverse transcriptase (htert) gene in human T-cells. *Cancer Sci* **2008**, *99*, 1155–1163. [CrossRef] [PubMed]

183. Pise-Masison, C.A.; Mahieux, R.; Jiang, H.; Ashcroft, M.; Radonovich, M.; Duvall, J.; Guillerm, C.; Brady, J.N. Inactivation of p53 by human T-cell lymphotropic virus type 1 tax requires activation of the nf-kappab pathway and is dependent on p53 phosphorylation. *Mol. Cell. Biol.* **2000**, *20*, 3377–3386. [CrossRef] [PubMed]

184. Kehn, K.; Fuente Cde, L.; Strouss, K.; Berro, R.; Jiang, H.; Brady, J.; Mahieux, R.; Pumfery, A.; Bottazzi, M.E.; Kashanchi, F. The HTLV-I tax oncoprotein targets the retinoblastoma protein for proteasomal degradation. *Oncogene* **2005**, *24*, 525–540. [CrossRef] [PubMed]

185. Semmes, O.J.; Jeang, K.T. Localization of human T-cell leukemia virus type 1 tax to subnuclear compartments that overlap with interchromatin speckles. *J. Virol.* **1996**, *70*, 6347–6357. [PubMed]

186. Bex, F.; McDowall, A.; Burny, A.; Gaynor, R. The human T-cell leukemia virus type 1 transactivator protein tax colocalizes in unique nuclear structures with nf-kappab proteins. *J. Virol.* **1997**, *71*, 3484–3497. [PubMed]

187. Majone, F.; Semmes, O.J.; Jeang, K.T. Induction of micronuclei by HTLV-I tax: A cellular assay for function. *Virology* **1993**, *193*, 456–459. [CrossRef] [PubMed]

188. Philpott, S.M.; Buehring, G.C. Defective DNA repair in cells with human T-cell leukemia/bovine leukemia viruses: Role of tax gene. *J. Natl. Cancer Inst.* **1999**, *91*, 933–942. [CrossRef] [PubMed]

189. Baydoun, H.H.; Bai, X.T.; Shelton, S.; Nicot, C. HTLV-I tax increases genetic instability by inducing DNA double strand breaks during DNA replication and switching repair to nhej. *PLoS ONE* **2012**, *7*, e42226. [CrossRef] [PubMed]

190. Mihaylova, V.T.; Green, A.M.; Khurgel, M.; Semmes, O.J.; Kupfer, G.M. Human T-cell leukemia virus i tax protein sensitizes p53-mutant cells to DNA damage. *Cancer Res.* **2008**, *68*, 4843–4852. [CrossRef] [PubMed]

191. Kinjo, T.; Ham-Terhune, J.; Peloponese, J.M., Jr.; Jeang, K.T. Induction of reactive oxygen species by human T-cell leukemia virus type 1 tax correlates with DNA damage and expression of cellular

senescence marker. *J. Virol.* **2010** *84*, 5431–5437. [CrossRef] [PubMed]

192. Chaib-Mezrag, H.; Lemacon, D.; Fontaine, H.; Bellon, M.; Bai, X.T.; Drac, M.; Coquelle, A.; Nicot, C. Tax impairs DNA replication forks and increases DNA breaks in specific oncogenic genome regions. *Mol. Cancer* **2014**, *13*, e205. [CrossRef]
193. Miyake, H.; Suzuki, T.; Hirai, H.; Yoshida, M. Trans-activator tax of human T-cell leukemia virus type 1 enhances mutation frequency of the cellular genome. *Virology* **1999**, *253*, 155–161. [CrossRef] [PubMed]
194. Cannon, J.S.; Hamzeh, F.; Moore, S.; Nicholas, J.; Ambinder, R.F. Human herpesvirus 8-encoded thymidine kinase and phosphotransferase homologues confer sensitivity to ganciclovir. *J. Virol.* **1999**, *73*, 4786–4793. [PubMed]
195. Schavinsky-Khrapunsky, Y.; Priel, E.; Aboud, M. Dose-dependent dual effect of HTLV-1 tax oncoprotein on p53-dependent nucleotide excision repair in human T-cells. *Int. J. Cancer* **2008**, *122*, 305–316. [CrossRef] [PubMed]
196. Chandhasin, C.; Ducu, R.I.; Berkovich, E.; Kastan, M.B.; Marriott, S.J. Human T-cell leukemia virus type 1 tax attenuates the atm-mediated cellular DNA damage response. *J. Virol.* **2008**, *82*, 6952–6961. [CrossRef] [PubMed]
197. Dayaram, T.; Lemoine, F.J.; Donehower, L.A.; Marriott, S.J. Activation of wip1 phosphatase by HTLV-1 tax mitigates the cellular response to DNA damage. *PLoS ONE* **2013**, *8*, e55989. [CrossRef] [PubMed]
198. Majone, F.; Luisetto, R.; Zamboni, D.; Iwanaga, Y.; Jeang, K.T. Ku protein as a potential human T-cell leukemia virus type 1 (HTLV-1) tax target in clastogenic chromosomal instability of mammalian cells. *Retrovirology* **2005**, *2*, e45. [CrossRef]
199. Ducu, R.I.; Dayaram, T.; Marriott, S.J. The HTLV-1 tax oncoprotein represses ku80 gene expression. *Virology* **2011**, *416*, 1–8. [CrossRef] [PubMed]
200. Baydoun, H.H.; Pancewicz, J.; Nicot, C. Human T-lymphotropic type 1 virus p30 inhibits homologous recombination and favors unfaithful DNA repair. *Blood* **2011**, *117*, 5897–5906. [CrossRef] [PubMed]
201. Haoudi, A.; Daniels, R.C.; Wong, E.; Kupfer, G.; Semmes, O.J. Human T-cell leukemia virus-i tax oncoprotein functionally targets a subnuclear complex involved in cellular DNA damage-response. *J. Biol. Chem.* **2003**, *278*, 37736–37744. [CrossRef] [PubMed]
202. Park, H.U.; Jeong, J.H.; Chung, J.H.; Brady, J.N. Human T-cell leukemia virus type 1 tax interacts with chk1 and attenuates DNA-damage induced g2 arrest mediated by chk1. *Oncogene* **2004**, *23*, 4966–4974. [CrossRef] [PubMed]
203. Gupta, S.K.; Guo, X.; Durkin, S.S.; Fryrear, K.F.; Ward, M.D.; Semmes, O.J. Human T-cell leukemia virus type 1 tax oncoprotein prevents DNA damage-induced chromatin egress of hyperphosphorylated chk2. *J. Biol. Chem.* **2007**, *282*, 29431–29440. [CrossRef] [PubMed]
204. Durkin, S.S.; Guo, X.; Fryrear, K.A.; Mihaylova, V.T.; Gupta, S.K.; Belgnaoui, S.M.; Haoudi, A.; Kupfer, G.M.; Semmes, O.J. HTLV-1 tax oncoprotein subverts the cellular DNA damage response via binding to DNA-dependent protein kinase. *J. Biol. Chem.* **2008**, *283*, 36311–36320. [CrossRef] [PubMed]

205. Chlichlia, K.; Khazaie, K. HTLV-1 tax: Linking transformation, DNA damage and apoptotic T-cell death. *Chem Biol Interact* **2010**, *188*, 359–365. [CrossRef] [PubMed]
206. Bellon, M.; Baydoun, H.H.; Yao, Y.; Nicot, C. HTLV-I tax-dependent and -independent events associated with immortalization of human primary t lymphocytes. *Blood* **2010**, *115*, 2441–2448. [CrossRef] [PubMed]
207. Kumar, P.; Wood, C. Kaposi's sarcoma-associated herpesvirus transactivator rta induces cell cycle arrest in g0/g1 phase by stabilizing and promoting nuclear localization of p27kip. *J. Virol.* **2013**, *87*, 13226–13238. [CrossRef] [PubMed]
208. Chini, C.C.; Chen, J. Human claspin is required for replication checkpoint control. *J. Biol. Chem.* **2003**, *278*, 30057–30062. [CrossRef] [PubMed]
209. Jarviluoma, A.; Koopal, S.; Rasanen, S.; Makela, T.P.; Ojala, P.M. KSHV viral cyclin binds to p27kip1 in primary effusion lymphomas. *Blood* **2004**, *104*, 3349–3354. [CrossRef] [PubMed]
210. Bouchard, M.J.; Schneider, R.J. The enigmatic x gene of hepatitis b virus. *J. Virol.* **2004**, *78*, 12725–12734. [CrossRef] [PubMed]
211. Feitelson, M.A.; Zhu, M.; Duan, L.X.; London, W.T. Hepatitis b x antigen and p53 are associated in vitro and in liver tissues from patients with primary hepatocellular carcinoma. *Oncogene* **1993**, *8*, 1109–1117. [PubMed]
212. Wang, X.W.; Forrester, K.; Yeh, H.; Feitelson, M.A.; Gu, J.R.; Harris, C.C. Hepatitis B virus x protein inhibits p53 sequence-specific DNA binding, transcriptional activity, and association with transcription factor ercc3. *Proc. Natl. Acad. Sci. USA* **1994**, *91*, 2230–2234. [CrossRef] [PubMed]
213. Lee, S.G.; Rho, H.M. Transcriptional repression of the human p53 gene by hepatitis B viral x protein. *Oncogene* **2000**, *19*, 468–471. [CrossRef] [PubMed]
214. Rothkamm, K.; Kruger, I.; Thompson, L.H.; Lobrich, M. Pathways of DNA double-strand break repair during the mammalian cell cycle. *Mol. Cell. Biol.* **2003**, *23*, 5706–5715. [CrossRef] [PubMed]
215. Lieber, M.R. The mechanism of double-strand DNA break repair by the nonhomologous DNA end-joining pathway. *Annu. Rev. Biochem.* **2010**, *79*, 181–211. [CrossRef] [PubMed]
216. Nakamura, H.; Lu, M.; Gwack, Y.; Souvlis, J.; Zeichner, S.L.; Jung, J.U. Global changes in kaposi's sarcoma-associated virus gene expression patterns following expression of a tetracycline-inducible rta transactivator. *J. Virol.* **2003**, *77*, 4205–4220. [CrossRef] [PubMed]
217. Hagen, T.M.; Huang, S.; Curnutte, J.; Fowler, P.; Martinez, V.; Wehr, C.M.; Ames, B.N.; Chisari, F.V. Extensive oxidative DNA damage in hepatocytes of transgenic mice with chronic active hepatitis destined to develop hepatocellular carcinoma. *Proc. Natl. Acad. Sci. USA* **1994**, *91*, 12808–12812. [CrossRef] [PubMed]
218. Hsieh, Y.H.; Su, I.J.; Wang, H.C.; Chang, W.W.; Lei, H.Y.; Lai, M.D.; Chang, W.T.; Huang, W. Pre-s mutant surface antigens in chronic Hepatitis B virus infection induce oxidative stress and DNA damage. *Carcinogenesis* **2004**, *25*, 2023–2032. [CrossRef] [PubMed]
219. Matthews, T.; Boehme, R. Antiviral activity and mechanism of action of ganciclovir. *Rev. Infect. Dis.* **1988**, *10* Suppl. 3, S490–S494. [CrossRef] [PubMed]
220. Ward, I.M.; Chen, J. Histone h2ax is phosphorylated in an atr-dependent manner in response to

replicational stress. *J. Biol. Chem.* **2001** *276*, 47759–47762. [CrossRef] [PubMed]

221. Dandri, M.; Burda, M.R.; Burkle, A.; Zuckerman, D.M.; Will, H.; Rogler, C.E.; Greten, H.; Petersen, J. Increase in de novo hbv DNA integrations in response to oxidative DNA damage or inhibition of poly(adp-ribosyl)ation. *Hepatology* **2002**, *35*, 217–223. [CrossRef] [PubMed]
222. Leupin, O.; Bontron, S.; Schaeffer, C.; Strubin, M. Hepatitis B virus x protein stimulates viral genome replication via a ddb1-dependent pathway distinct from that leading to cell death. *J. Virol.* **2005**, *79*, 4238–4245. [CrossRef] [PubMed]
223. Bresnahan, W.A.; Boldogh, I.; Thompson, E.A.; Albrecht, T. Human cytomegalovirus inhibits cellular DNA synthesis and arrests productively infected cells in late g1. *Virology* **1996**, *224*, 150–160. [CrossRef] [PubMed]
224. Bryan, B.A.; Dyson, O.F.; Akula, S.M. Identifying cellular genes crucial for the reactivation of kaposi's sarcoma-associated herpesvirus latency. *J. Gen. Virol.* **2006**, *87*, 519–529. [CrossRef] [PubMed]
225. Becker, S.A.; Lee, T.H.; Butel, J.S.; Slagle, B.L. Hepatitis B virus x protein interferes with cellular DNA repair. *J. Virol.* **1998**, *72*, 266–272. [PubMed]
226. Martin-Lluesma, S.; Schaeffer, C.; Robert, E.I.; van Breugel, P.C.; Leupin, O.; Hantz, O.; Strubin, M. Hepatitis B virus x protein affects s phase progression leading to chromosome segregation defects by binding to damaged DNA binding protein 1. *Hepatology* **2008**, *48*, 1467–1476. [CrossRef] [PubMed]
227. Jaitovich-Groisman, I.; Benlimame, N.; Slagle, B.L.; Perez, M.H.; Alpert, L.; Song, D.J.; Fotouhi-Ardakani, N.; Galipeau, J.; Alaoui-Jamali, M.A. Transcriptional regulation of the tfiih transcription repair components xpb and xpd by the Hepatitis B virus x protein in liver cells and transgenic liver tissue. *J. Biol. Chem.* **2001**, *276*, 14124–14132. [PubMed]
228. Prost, S.; Ford, J.M.; Taylor, C.; Doig, J.; Harrison, D.J. Hepatitis b x protein inhibits p53-dependent DNA repair in primary mouse hepatocytes. *J. Biol. Chem.* **1998**, *273*, 33327–33332. [CrossRef] [PubMed]
229. Lee, A.T.; Ren, J.; Wong, E.T.; Ban, K.H.; Lee, L.A.; Lee, C.G. The Hepatitis B virus x protein sensitizes hepg2 cells to uv light-induced DNA damage. *J. Biol. Chem.* **2005**, *280*, 33525–33535. [CrossRef] [PubMed]
230. Van de Klundert, M.A.; van Hemert, F.J.; Zaaijer, H.L.; Kootstra, N.A. The Hepatitis B virus x protein inhibits thymine DNA glycosylase initiated base excision repair. *PLoS ONE* **2012**, *7*, e48940. [CrossRef] [PubMed]
231. Chung, Y.L. Defective DNA damage response and repair in liver cells expressing Hepatitis B virus surface antigen. *FASEB J.* **2013**, *27*, 2316–2327. [CrossRef] [PubMed]
232. Wang, W.H.; Hullinger, R.L.; Andrisani, O.M. Hepatitis B virus x protein via the p38mapk pathway induces e2f1 release and atr kinase activation mediating p53 apoptosis. *J. Biol. Chem.* **2008**, *283*, 25455–25467. [CrossRef] [PubMed]
233. Zhao, F.; Hou, N.B.; Yang, X.L.; He, X.; Liu, Y.; Zhang, Y.H.; Wei, C.W.; Song, T.; Li, L.; Ma, Q.J.; *et al.* Ataxia telangiectasia-mutated-rad3-related DNA damage checkpoint signaling pathway triggered by Hepatitis B virus infection. *World J. Gastroenterol.* **2008**, *14*, 6163–6170. [CrossRef] [PubMed]

234. Rakotomalala, L.; Studach, L.; Wang, W.H.; Gregori, G.; Hullinger, R.L.; Andrisani, O. Hepatitis B virus x protein increases the cdt1-to-geminin ratio inducing DNA re-replication and polyploidy. *J. Biol. Chem.* **2008**, *283*, 28729–28740. [CrossRef] [PubMed]
235. Studach, L.; Wang, W.H.; Weber, G.; Tang, J.; Hullinger, R.L.; Malbrue, R.; Liu, X.; Andrisani, O. Polo-like kinase 1 activated by the Hepatitis B virus x protein attenuates both the DNA damage checkpoint and DNA repair resulting in partial polyploidy. *J. Biol. Chem.* **2010**, *285*, 30282–30293. [CrossRef] [PubMed]
236. Zheng, Z.; Li, J.; Sun, J.; Song, T.; Wei, C.; Zhang, Y.; Rao, G.; Chen, G.; Li, D.; Yang, G.; *et al.* Inhibition of hbv replication by theophylline. *Antiviral Res.* **2011**, *89*, 149–155. [CrossRef] [PubMed]
237. Izumiya, Y.; Lin, S.F.; Ellison, T.J.; Levy, A.M.; Mayeur, G.L.; Izumiya, C.; Kung, H.J. Cell cycle regulation by kaposi's sarcoma-associated herpesvirus k-bzip: Direct interaction with cyclin-cdk2 and induction of g1 growth arrest. *J. Virol.* **2003**, *77*, 9652–9661. [CrossRef] [PubMed]
238. Wu, F.Y.; Tang, Q.Q.; Chen, H.; ApRhys, C.; Farrell, C.; Chen, J.; Fujimuro, M.; Lane, M.D.; Hayward, G.S. Lytic replication-associated protein (rap) encoded by kaposi sarcoma-associated herpesvirus causes p21cip-1-mediated g1 cell cycle arrest through ccaat/enhancer-binding protein-alpha. *Proc. Natl. Acad. Sci. USA* **2002**, *99*, 10683–10688. [CrossRef] [PubMed]
239. Rodriguez, A.; Jung, E.J.; Flemington, E.K. Cell cycle analysis of epstein-barr virus-infected cells following treatment with lytic cycle-inducing agents. *J. Virol.* **2001**, *75*, 4482–4489. [CrossRef] [PubMed]
240. Lilley, C.E.; Chaurushiya, M.S.; Boutell, C.; Everett, R.D.; Weitzman, M.D. The intrinsic antiviral defense to incoming hsv-1 genomes includes specific DNA repair proteins and is counteracted by the viral protein icp0. *PLoS Pathog.* **2011**, *7*, e1002084. [CrossRef] [PubMed]
241. FeRNAndez-Capetillo, O.; Chen, H.T.; Celeste, A.; Ward, I.; Romanienko, P.J.; Morales, J.C.; Naka, K.; Xia, Z.; Camerini-Otero, R.D.; Motoyama, N.; *et al.* DNA damage-induced g2-m checkpoint activation by histone h2ax and 53bp1. *Nat. Cell Biol.* **2002**, *4*, 993–997. [CrossRef] [PubMed]
242. Machida, K.; Cheng, K.T.; Sung, V.M.; Lee, K.J.; Levine, A.M.; Lai, M.M. Hepatitis C virus infection activates the immunologic (type ii) isoform of nitric oxide synthase and thereby enhances DNA damage and mutations of cellular genes. *J. Virol.* **2004**, *78*, 8835–8843. [CrossRef] [PubMed]
243. Machida, K.; Cheng, K.T.; Lai, C.K.; Jeng, K.S.; Sung, V.M.; Lai, M.M. Hepatitis C virus triggers mitochondrial permeability transition with production of reactive oxygen species, leading to DNA damage and stat3 activation. *J. Virol.* **2006**, *80*, 7199–7207. [CrossRef] [PubMed]
244. Nishimura, T.; Kohara, M.; Izumi, K.; Kasama, Y.; Hirata, Y.; Huang, Y.; Shuda, M.; Mukaidani, C.; Takano, T.; Tokunaga, Y.; *et al.* Hepatitis C virus impairs p53 via persistent overexpression of 3beta-hydroxysterol delta24-reductase. *J. Biol. Chem.* **2009**, *284*, 36442–36452. [CrossRef] [PubMed]
245. Higgs, M.R.; Lerat, H.; Pawlotsky, J.M. Hepatitis C virus-induced activation of beta-catenin promotes c-myc expression and a cascade of pro-carcinogenetic events. *Oncogene* **2013**, *32*, 4683–4693. [CrossRef] [PubMed]

246. Zekri, A.R.; Sabry, G.M.; Bahnassy, A.A.; Shalaby, K.A.; Abdel-Wahabh, S.A.; Zakaria, S. Mismatch repair genes (hmlh1, hpms1, hpms2, gtbp/hmsh6, hmsh2) in the pathogenesis of hepatocellular carcinoma. *World J. Gastroenterol.* **2005**, *11*, 3020–3026. [CrossRef] [PubMed]

247. Pal, S.; Polyak, S.J.; Bano, N.; Qiu, W.C.; Carithers, R.L.; Shuhart, M.; Gretch, D.R.; Das, A. Hepatitis C virus induces oxidative stress, DNA damage and modulates the DNA repair enzyme neil1. *J Gastroenterol Hepatol* **2010**, *25*, 627–634. [CrossRef] [PubMed]

248. Higgs, M.R.; Lerat, H.; Pawlotsky, J.M. Downregulation of gadd45beta expression by Hepatitis C virus leads to defective cell cycle arrest. *Cancer Res.* **2010**, *70*, 4901–4911. [CrossRef] [PubMed]

249. van Pelt, J.F.; Severi, T.; Crabbe, T.; Eetveldt, A.V.; Verslype, C.; Roskams, T.; Fevery, J. Expression of Hepatitis C virus core protein impairs DNA repair in human hepatoma cells. *Cancer Lett* **2004**, *209*, 197–205. [CrossRef] [PubMed]

250. Machida, K.; McNamara, G.; Cheng, K.T.; Huang, J.; Wang, C.H.; Comai, L.; Ou, J.H.; Lai, M.M. Hepatitis C virus inhibits DNA damage repair through reactive oxygen and nitrogen species and by interfering with the atm-nbs1/mre11/rad50 DNA repair pathway in monocytes and hepatocytes. *J Immunol* **2010**, *185*, 6985–6998. [CrossRef] [PubMed]

251. Ariumi, Y.; Kuroki, M.; Dansako, H.; Abe, K.; Ikeda, M.; Wakita, T.; Kato, N. The DNA damage sensors ataxia-telangiectasia mutated kinase and checkpoint kinase 2 are required for Hepatitis C virus RNA replication. *J. Virol.* **2008**, *82*, 9639–9646. [CrossRef] [PubMed]

252. Lai, C.K.; Jeng, K.S.; Machida, K.; Cheng, Y.S.; Lai, M.M. Hepatitis C virus ns3/4a protein interacts with atm, impairs DNA repair and enhances sensitivity to ionizing radiation. *Virology* **2008**, *370*, 295–309. [CrossRef] [PubMed]

253. Bittar, C.; Shrivastava, S.; Bhanja Chowdhury, J.; Rahal, P.; Ray, R.B. Hepatitis C virus ns2 protein inhibits DNA damage pathway by sequestering p53 to the cytoplasm. *PLoS ONE* **2013**, *8*, e62581. [CrossRef] [PubMed]

254. Naka, K.; Dansako, H.; Kobayashi, N.; Ikeda, M.; Kato, N. Hepatitis C virus ns5b delays cell cycle progression by inducing interferon-beta via toll-like receptor 3 signaling pathway without replicating viral genomes. *Virology* **2006**, *346*, 348–362. [CrossRef] [PubMed]

255. Wang, Y.; Xu, Y.; Tong, W.; Pan, T.; Li, J.; Sun, S.; Shao, J.; Ding, H.; Toyoda, T.; Yuan, Z. Hepatitis C virus ns5b protein delays s phase progression in human hepatocyte-derived cells by relocalizing cyclin-dependent kinase 2-interacting protein (cinp). *J. Biol. Chem.* **2011**, *286*, 26603–26615. [CrossRef] [PubMed]

256. Qadri, I.; Iwahashi, M.; Simon, F. Hepatitis C virus ns5a protein binds tbp and p53, inhibiting their DNA binding and p53 interactions with tbp and ercc3. *Biochim. Biophys. Acta* **2002**, *1592*, 193–204. [CrossRef]

257. Luo, M.H.; Rosenke, K.; CzoRNAk, K.; Fortunato, E.A. Human cytomegalovirus disrupts both ataxia telangiectasia mutated protein (atm)- and atm-rad3-related kinase-mediated DNA damage responses during lytic infection. *J. Virol.* **2007**, *81*, 1934–1950. [CrossRef] [PubMed]

258. Levin, A.; Neufeldt, C.J.; Pang, D.; Wilson, K.; Loewen-Dobler, D.; Joyce, M.A.; Wozniak, R.W.; Tyrrell, D.L. Functional characterization of nuclear localization and export signals in Hepatitis C virus proteins and their role in the membranous web. *PLoS ONE* **2014**, *9*, e114629. [CrossRef] [PubMed]

259. Chen, Y.; Williams, V.; Filippova, M.; Filippov, V.; Duerksen-Hughes, P. Viral carcinogenesis: Factors inducing DNA damage and virus integration. *Cancers* **2014**, *6*, 2155–2186. [CrossRef] [PubMed]
260. Mauser, A.; Holley-Guthrie, E.; Zanation, A.; Yarborough, W.; Kaufmann, W.; Klingelhutz, A.; Seaman, W.T.; Kenney, S. The epstein-barr virus immediate-early protein bzlf1 induces expression of e2f-1 and other proteins involved in cell cycle progression in primary keratinocytes and gastric carcinoma cells. *J. Virol.* **2002**, *76*, 12543–12552. [CrossRef] [PubMed]
261. Mohni, K.N.; Dee, A.R.; Smith, S.; Schumacher, A.J.; Weller, S.K. Efficient herpes simplex virus 1 replication requires cellular atr pathway proteins. *J. Virol.* **2013**, *87*, 531–542. [CrossRef] [PubMed]
262. Carpentier, A.; Barez, P.Y.; Boxus, M.; Willems, L. Checkpoints modulation by the human T-lymphotropic virus type 1 tax protein. *Retrovirology* **2014**, *11*, e90. [CrossRef]

8

Human Viruses and Cancer

Abigail Morales-Sánchez [1,2] and Ezequiel M. Fuentes-Panana [1,*]

[1] Unidad de Investigación en Virología y Cáncer, Hospital Infantil de México Federico Gómez. Dr. Márquez 162, Col. Doctores, C.P. 06720. México D.F., Mexico; E-Mail: abimor2002@yahoo.com.mx

[2] Programa de Doctorado en Ciencias Biomédicas, Facultad de Medicina, Universidad Nacional Autónoma de Mexico. Av. Universidad 3000, Col. Universidad Nacional Autónoma de México, C.U., C.P. 04510 México D.F., México

* Author to whom correspondence should be addressed; E-Mail: empanana@yahoo.com;

External Editor: Joanna Parish

Abstract: The first human tumor virus was discovered in the middle of the last century by Anthony Epstein, Bert Achong and Yvonne Barr in African pediatric patients with Burkitt's lymphoma. To date, seven viruses -EBV, KSHV, high-risk HPV, MCPV, HBV, HCV and HTLV1- have been consistently linked to different types of human cancer, and infections are estimated to account for up to 20% of all cancer cases worldwide. Viral oncogenic mechanisms generally include: generation of genomic instability, increase in the rate of cell proliferation, resistance to apoptosis, alterations in DNA repair mechanisms and cell polarity changes, which often coexist with evasion mechanisms of the antiviral immune response. Viral agents also indirectly contribute to the development of cancer mainly through immunosuppression or chronic inflammation, but also through chronic antigenic stimulation. There is also evidence that viruses can modulate the malignant properties of an established tumor. In the present work, causation criteria for viruses and cancer will be described, as well as the viral agents that comply with these criteria in human tumors, their epidemiological and biological characteristics, the molecular mechanisms by which they induce cellular transformation and their associated cancers.

Keywords: infectious cancer; human oncogenic viruses; transforming mechanisms

---

1. Introduction: Historical and Epidemiological Aspects

The first observations about a possible infectious etiology of cancer arose at the beginning of the past century. Ellermann and Bang in 1908 and Rous in 1911 transmitted avian leukemias and sarcomas, respectively, through cell-free tumor extracts, suggesting a viral etiology [1–3]. About 50 years later, the first human tumor virus was discovered. Sir Anthony Epstein, Bert Achong and Yvonne Barr observed viral particles in cell cultures from equatorial African pediatric patients with Burkitt's lymphoma; this virus was named Epstein Barr virus (EBV) in honor of their discoverers [4]. In the following years, a set of experimental evidence demonstrated that EBV was the causative agent of endemic Burkitt's lymphoma and other neoplasias. Currently, there is clear evidence that several viruses are oncogenic to humans and the first century of tumor virology research has culminated with the Medicine Nobel Price granted to Harald zur Hausen for the discovery of HPV as the causative agent of cervical cancer [5,6]. To date, EBV, Kaposi's sarcoma-associated herpesvirus (KSHV), human high-risk papillomaviruses (HPV), Merkel cell polyomavirus (MCPV), hepatitis B virus (HBV), hepatitis C virus (HCV) and Human T-cell Lymphotropic virus type 1 (HTLV1) have been classified as type 1 carcinogenic agents (the most strongly associated with human cancers) by the International Agency for Research on Cancer (IARC) (reviewed in [7]). It is estimated that infections are responsible for up to 15% of cancer cases worldwide and about 20% in developing countries [8]. With advent of new technologies allowing genetic identification, it is very likely that this numbers will continue to increase.

Virus-mediated oncogenesis results from the cooperation of multiple events, including different mechanisms bound to the viral life cycle. The knowledge derived from the study of tumor viruses has allowed the construction of a conceptual biological framework to understand not only cancers of infectious origin but also of almost any type of cancer. However, to change the traditional scientific thinking to accept the participation of infectious agents in cancer was difficult, mostly because the biological processes involved do not adjust to the causation dogmatic principles postulated by Koch [9] (Table 1). Koch original observations about the transmission of acute infectious agents are difficult to apply to cancer because of the multi-factorial nature of cancer and because tumorigenic viruses are generally present in a large part of the population without causing disease. Sir Austin Bradford Hill's epidemiologic causation criteria, which were originally proposed to establish the causation between smoking and lung cancer, are more suitable as a base to infer a causative relationship between a viral infection and cancer (Table 1) [10].

It is also accepted that none of the Bradford Hill's criteria could by itself conclude causation, neither it is necessary to comply with all of them to accept the virus-cancer association. For example, the geographic distribution of endemic Burkitt's lymphoma (equatorial Africa) does not coincide with the world distribution of EBV. However, we know today that malaria, endemic to this region, is a critical co-factor to develop Burkitt's lymphoma (reviewed in [11]). The Bradford Hill criteria applied to virus and cancer associations consider that causation is established if the virus is present in the tumor cells and not in the surrounding healthy tissue and if there exists plausibility and coherence between infection and cancer. For example, EBV resides in B-lymphocytes that reactivate in the epithelium of the upper digestive tract and EBV has been associated to B-cell lymphomas and carcinomas in tongue, nasopharynx and stomach. Also, transgenic animals that express EBV latent proteins develop neoplasias [12]. These combined data grant a minimal context for biologic plausibility and coherence required by the Bradford Hill criteria.

Table 1. Koch and Bradford Hill's postulates for causative relations.

Henle Koch's Postulates [9]	Bradford Hill's Causative Principles [10]
1. The pathogen agent must be present in sick population and absent in healthy population. 2. The agent must not appear randomly in another disease. 3. The agent can be isolated and cultured from a diseased organism and should cause disease when introduced into a healthy organism. 4. The agent isolated from the new host should be identical to the original causative agent.	1. Strength of the association. The agent must be more common in cases than in healthy controls. 2. Consistency. Different researchers must corroborate the association. 3. Specificity. The disease must coexist with the agent in the same space, preferably over other associations of the same agent and another disease. 4. Temporality. Exposure to the agent must predict the appearance of the disease. 5. Gradient. A higher exposure must correlate with a higher probability to develop the disease. 6. Plausibility. The association must be founded on the known biological aspects of the causative agent. 7. Coherence. The association must be based on the known aspects of the disease. 8. Experimental. Controlled conditions must reproduced and coincide with the disease and the blockage of biological mechanisms involved must reduce or prevent its appearance. 9. Analogy. Agents with similar mechanisms must be associated to similar diseases.

Arguable, the most powerful tool to indicate direct association is the viral monoclonal analysis in the tumor; the presence of a specific viral variant or viral quasispecie in all tumor cells indicates that the event of infection preceded the malignant cell transformation. This strongly supports that the virus was part of the initial genetic lesion that allowed the appearance of the cancerous clone, satisfying the Bradford Hill criteria for temporality.

2. General Principles of Viral Oncogenic Mechanisms

Oncogenic viruses generally maintain chronic infections in which there is not or little production of viral particles, and that last for the whole life of the infected individual. These mechanisms of viral persistency and/or latency are biologically compatible with the carcinogenic process, because they avoid cell death most common in acute lytic infections, while maintaining the infectious agent hidden from the immune system. Viral persistence in the host is achieved by integrating the viral genome into the cell genome or by expressing viral proteins that equally segregate the viral genome into daughter cells during cell partitioning. Both mechanisms ensure that the virus is not lost during cellular replication. Viral persistence is usually characterized by expression of proteins that control cell death and proliferation; in this manner, oncogenic viruses nurture infection of a controlled number of cells establishing a balance between virus and host, preserving the integrity of both. Cell transformation is probably not an evolutionary viral strategy, but rather a biological accident that rarely occurs in the virus-host interaction. Cancer leads to the death of the host, and thus, it also represents the end of the virus. The existence of viral oncogenes is explained as part of the viral persistence mechanisms, which only under altered conditions may lead to cancer. All virus-associated tumors result from the cooperation of various events, involving more than persistent infection and viral transformation mechanisms. Additional oncogenic hits are necessary for full-blown transformation. The occurrence of mutations impairing expression and function of viral and/or cellular oncogenes is necessary in the carcinogenic process, in line with that, an increased mutation rate of infected over normal cells is frequently observed (reviewed in [13,14]). In this scenario, latently infected cells by oncogenic viruses might be more susceptible targets of additional oncogenic hits; e.g., due to smoking, a diet scarce in fruits and vegetables or/and increased exposure to environmental oncogenic agents. All these insults, plus the host genetic component driving inflammatory responses triggered by the infection itself result in cell transformation and cancer development.

2.1. Direct and Indirect Viral Carcinogenesis

Infectious agents can contribute to carcinogenesis by direct and/or indirect mechanisms (Figure 1). The direct-acting carcinogenic agents are generally found in a monoclonal form within the tumor cells. These agents help to keep the tumor phenotype through expression of either viral or cellular oncogenes (reviewed in [7]). Retroviruses, whose replication cycle requires the integration of the viral genome into the host genome, commonly transform because integration deregulates expression of cellular oncogenes or tumor suppressor genes (insertional mutagenesis, see Section 4.2). On the other hand, EBV is an example of a virus that does not need to integrate and transforms through expression of its own oncogenes.

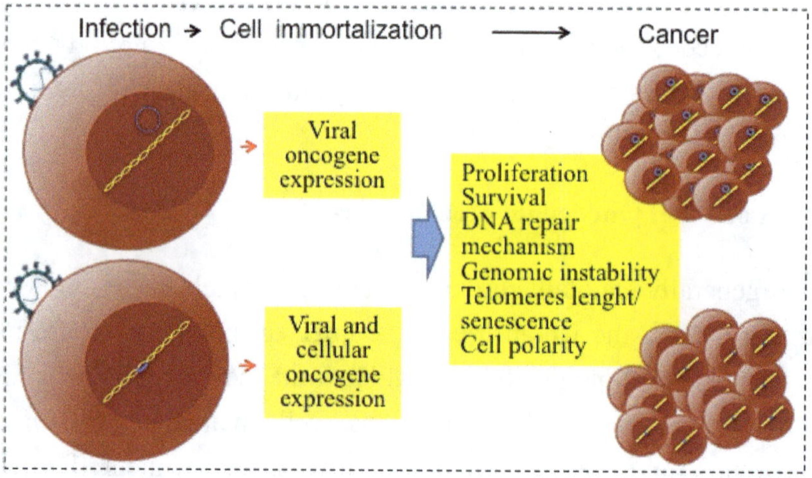

Figure 1. Direct mechanisms of viral carcinogenesis. After infecting target cells, tumor viruses are persistently maintained as genetic elements; viral genomes can form episomes (upper panel example, herpesviruses) or integrate into the host genomic DNA (lower panel example, retroviruses and HBV).

The indirect transforming viruses are not conditioned to exist within the cell that forms the tumor. These agents act through two main mechanisms: (i) triggering chronic inflammation and oxidative stress that persistently damage local tissues; and (ii) by producing immunosuppression that reduces or eliminates anti-tumor immune surveillance mechanisms (Figure 2). Among the most documented viral agents belonging to the first group are HBV and HCV; chronic inflammation produced by persistent infection associated with any of these viruses is a major risk to develop hepatocellular carcinoma (HCC) (reviewed in [15,16]). On the other hand, HIV belongs to the second group; patients with non-controlled infection and low T cell counts frequently develop lymphomas associated with EBV or KSV infection (reviewed in [17]).

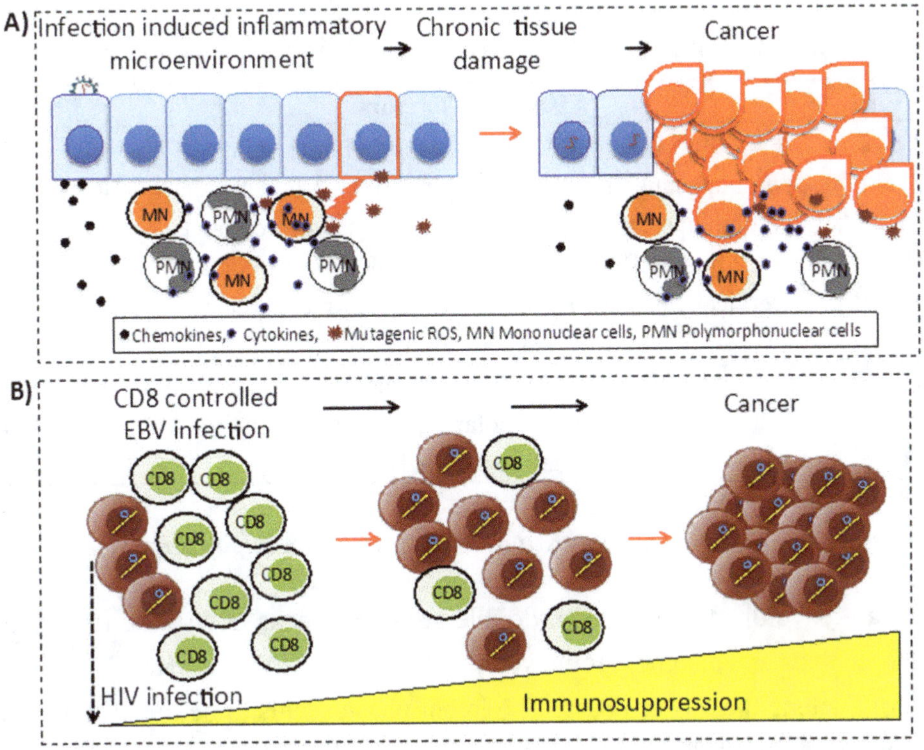

Figure 2. Indirect mechanisms of viral carcinogenesis. (**A**) Chronic inflammation. Infected cells produce chemokines attracting immune cells, which establish a chronic inflammatory microenvironment that persistently damage the local tissue. Cancer evolves within this cycle of infection, induced inflammation and tissue damage. (**B**) Immunosuppression. The prototype agent for immunosuppression is HIV. In immunocompetent individuals EBV infection is efficiently controlled by cytotoxic CD8 T cells; as HIV infection progresses and immune responses collapse, individuals become at increased risk of developing EBV associated lymphomas.

Tumorigenic viruses were previously considered either exclusively direct or indirect transforming agents. However, some agents may require both mechanisms to induce carcinogenesis; for instance HBV and HCV [15,16]. *Helicobacter pylori* is the prototype indirect carcinogen through chronic inflammation [18]. Nevertheless, the bacterium also encodes the CagA oncoprotein, which is translocated to epithelial cells though a type IV secretion system (reviewed in [19]). Therefore, direct and indirect mechanisms are not mutually exclusive and some tissues may be equally dependent in both mechanisms for oncogenic transformation, such as the liver and stomach.

3. Human Oncogenic Viruses and Associated Cancers

Many different viruses have direct transformation characteristics; however, they have not been convincingly associated to human neoplasias based in the Bradford Hill criteria, and the IARC does not include them in the group of human type 1 carcinogens. Thus, adenoviruses, polyomaviruses SV40, JCV and BKV and others, will not be discussed here. The human cancers associated with viral infection are summarized in Table 2.

Table 2. Human oncogenic viruses and their associated tumors.

Human Virus	Associated Tumors	Reference
EBV	Burkitt's lymphoma, Hodgkin's lymphoma, immunosuppression-related lymphoma, T and NK cell lymphomas; nasopharyngeal and stomach carcinomas.	Reviewed in [11]
KSHV	Primary effusion lymphoma and Kaposi sarcoma	[20]
High-risk HPVs	Cervical, head and neck and anogenital tract carcinomas	Reviewed in [21]
MCPV	Merkel cell carcinoma	[22]
HBV	Hepatocellular carcinoma	[23]
HCV	Hepatocellular carcinoma	[24]
HTLV1	Adult T-cell leukemia/lymphoma	[25]

3.1. Herpesviruses: Epstein Barr Virus and Kaposi Sarcoma-Associated Herpesvirus

Herpesviruses are enveloped viruses with double-stranded linear DNA that after infecting the host cell remain in the nucleus as episomes (reviewed in [26]). Both EBV and KSHV show a biphasic life cycle consisting of a latent and a lytic phase. The latent phase seems to be the primary choice in which most of viral gene expression is shut down. This phase allows these viruses to coexist with the host generally asymptomatically and only in unusual situations may cause disease, e.g., during pharmacological or HIV induced immunosuppression. The lytic phase occurs in healthy individuals only in poorly understood sporadic events of reactivation.

EBV, also known as HHV4 (Human *Herpesvirus Type 4*), is found in approximately 95% of the adult population worldwide [27]; its principal routes of transmission are oral and blood [28,29], while intrauterine transmission has been documented too [30,31]. Early acquisition of this agent does not cause disease but when primary infection occurs during adolescence or early adulthood it causes infectious mononucleosis (reviewed in [32]). Interestingly, this condition represents a risk factor for developing Hodgkin's lymphoma (reviewed in [33]).

B cells are the main target of EBV infection (reviewed in [34]); more rarely and less understood, EBV can also infect epithelial cells, mainly in the upper digestive tract, which is thought to occur in viral reactivation events [35]. EBV has mainly been associated with malignancies of B and epithelial cells of the upper digestive tract (Table 2), which provides biological plausibility and coherence to the role of EBV in these neoplasias.

EBV is found in a latent stage in both lymphomas and carcinomas, and within the latent genes, there are several with oncogenic properties. The viral protein best recognized as oncogenic is LMP1, a signaling protein that imitates a constitutively active TNF receptor. LMP1 activates MAP kinases and STAT and NFκB transcription factors in B cells, and also PI3K in epithelial cells [36]. LMP1 increases proliferation and survival of the infected cell. Of note, STAT and NFκB activation potentially stimulates expression of cytokines and chemokines important to establish the inflammatory microenvironment critical to create the niche from which infectious and non-infectious tumors emerge. LMP2A is another constitutively active viral protein with ITAM (*immunoreceptor tyrosine activated motif*) signaling domains [37]. LMP2A expression promotes the activation of PLCγ and PI3K pathways, which correlates with its capacity to transform epithelial cells and to confer a migratory phenotype to the transformed cell [38]. LMP1 and LMP2A provide antigen recognition-like signals to B cells, required for differentiation into long-lived memory cells in which the virus persists hidden from antagonistic immune responses. Although, both proteins can be expressed in EBV-induced carcinomas, their normal function in non-lymphoid tissue is not clear.

EBV-associated tumors are characterized by the expression of a different set of viral transcripts or latencies. In lymphomas arousing in immunosuppressed individuals (latency III) the family of EBNA proteins provides with additional oncogenic insults. For instance, EBNA-LP, -3A and -3C directly interfere with p53 and pRb functions, as well as with other proteins of the G0 to G1 phase transition. EBNA-1 is the common protein expressed in all EBV-associated neoplasias; it is expressed in latency III, latency II (Hodgkin's lymphoma and carcinomas) and it is the sole viral protein expressed in latency I (Burkitt's lymphoma). This absolute requirement for EBNA-1 is probably due to its capacity to equally segregate EBV episomes to both daughter cells during cell division [39].

The prevalence of KSHV infection varies among geographic regions, being 5% in Europe, Asia and some parts of North America and more than 50% in sub-Saharan Africa. KSHV is transmitted from casual contacts as well as through sexual contact, blood transfusion and organ transplant. In non-endemic regions, the main via of transmission is probably through sexual contact and the use of contaminated syringes [40]. KSHV is the etiological agent of both lymphomas and sarcomas [41] (Table 2). Neoplasias associated with KSVH were not frequent before the AIDS pandemic, but currently represent one of the most important signs of this disease [42,43].

Several KSVH genes have potential oncogenic properties, for example, modulation of transduction of signals by K1 and K5; regulation of cell cycle by v-Cyclin and LANA 1; apoptosis inhibition by K1, vFLIP and v-Bcl2 and immune modulation by v-IRF, K3 and K5 (reviewed in [41]). LANA1 cooperates with h-Ras to transform fibroblasts and immortalize endothelial cells [44]. v-FLIP induces the development of lymphomas in transgenic mice primarily through its anti-apoptosis activity, which has been related to the activation of NF*k*B [45,46]. K1 also contains an ITAM signaling domain similar to the one found in EBV LMP2A and activates PI3K. K1 expressed in mice as a transgene promotes the development of sarcomas and lymphomas [47]. These similarities in the transformation mechanisms of both herpesviruses satisfy the principle of analogy of Bradford Hill's causation criteria.

KSHV is often lytic in a small number of tumor cells [48], and some of its potentially oncogenic genes are products of the lytic cycle. Also similar to HCMV in gliomas, a few K1 lytic genes provide growth and angiogenic functions in a paracrine fashion, favoring tumor growth [49–52]. Of note, EBV defective viruses unable to switch to lytic cycle trigger less aggressive lymphomas in SCID mice than their wild type counterparts [53], and a small fraction of nasopharyngeal carcinomas (NPC) also harbors the virus in lytic phase [54]. Whether analogous mechanisms are in place for EBV, KSHV and HCMV in their paracrine requirement of lytic cycle proteins is not clear.

3.2. High-Risk Papillomaviruses

Human papilloma viruses belong to the *Papillomaviridae* family; they contain a double-strand DNA genome of approximately 8000 bp and are not enveloped viruses. More than 100 members of this family have been described and from them, more than a dozen (types 16, 18, 31, 33, 35, 45, 51, 52, 56, 58, 59, 62, 66 and 68) have been classified as high-risk due to their epidemiological association with cervical and other cancers (Table 2; reviewed in [21]). HPV subtypes 16 and 18 are the most frequently found in tumors; the first is mainly associated with invasive cervical cancer and the second is the most frequent in squamous cell carcinoma [55,56]. Low-risk HPVs generally cause benign lesions, such as warts (reviewed in [57]).

HPV is transmitted by skin contact, including genital contact during sexual intercourse; thus HPV infection in the genital area tents to be common in sexually active persons. Infection is generally controlled by the immune system and only in a low number of people, HPV persists, increasing the risk to develop epithelial lesions (reviewed in [58]). Viral persistence seems to be greatly helped by the inability of infected cells to present antigenic epitopes to adaptive immune cells, which is common in individuals with alterations in the HLA (Human Leucocyte Antigen) antigen presentation pathway (reviewed in [59]).

The neoplastic progression involves a series of histological changes that have been stratified in clinical stages, which correlate with differential expression of viral oncogenes and accumulation of mutations in the host genome. The main oncogenic proteins are E6 and E7, which are required since the first lesions and are necessary for the maintenance of the malignant phenotype. HPV is usually not integrated into the host genomic DNA, and E2 negatively regulates the expression of E6 and E7. An important event in the oncogenic process is the integration of the viral genome, a step usually resulting in loss of E2 and over-expression of E6 and E7 (reviewed in [60]). Increased expression of E6 and E7 correlates with progression to high grade lesions and eventually to carcinoma *in situ* (reviewed in [58]).

3.3. Merkel Cell Polyomavirus

Polyomaviruses are non-enveloped viruses with a circular, double-stranded DNA of approximately 5000 bp. The members of this family are present in all regions of the world infecting several species. Historically, it was considered that only JCV and BKV polyomaviruses infected humans, but next generation sequencing techniques have enabled the identification of at least nine other members in humans, among them MCPV. MCPV was identified in 2008 in an aggressive skin cancer denominated Merkel cell carcinoma (MCC) [22]. Virtually the whole adult population worldwide is infected by MCPV. Evidence supporting the participation of this agent in MCC carcinogenesis includes the presence of MCPV genomes in about 80% of the tumors but not in healthy tissue, and the clonal integration of the viral genome [22,61–63]. MCPV oncogenic transformation may result from loss of immune surveillance, as MCC mainly occurs in immunosuppressed individuals. MCC was a very rare cancer before the AIDS pandemia, and today, there are around 1700 new cases per year in the US [64,65].

The MCPV genome is inserted into the host genome during viral carcinogenesis. Integration is characterized by preserving the viral induced cell proliferation functions while abrogating viral replication; the latter probably due to deletion of some of the viral T antigen gene regions [66,67]. Viral integration also favors host resistance to cell death promoting viral persistence in a latent state [68]. This is a significant difference between the presence of the virus in MCC and in non-tumor tissue.

Due to the recent discovery of MCPV, we still do not understand the function of viral proteins. However, some viral proteins present homology in functional domains with tumorigenic polyomaviruses from non-human species. For example, like SV40 MCPV T antigens are generated by differential splicing to produce large T and small T antigens [69]. The large T antigen presents the structural motif that inactivates pRb (LXCXE) [70], and the T antigen is generally expressed in MCC, and even in its truncated form it maintains intact the pRb-inactivating domain [71]. Inactivation of the T antigen in MCC cell lines results in cell death, further supporting the causative role of MCPV in MCC [72]. Also, the small T antigen conserves the AKT/mTOR activating domain, which is responsible for loss of contact inhibition and promoting independent growth of substrate and serum [73].

3.4. Hepatitis B Virus

The *Hepadnaviridae* family groups a series of viruses that cause liver disease in animals, with Hepatitis B virus (HBV) infecting humans. HBV is an enveloped virus with an approximate 3.2 Kb genome of a partially double stranded DNA chain and a single stranded fragment. HBV replicates through an intermediary RNA via a viral reverse transcriptase. The main target of infection by HBV is the hepatocyte and infection can occur through vertical or horizontal transmission starting in the first years of life or during adulthood (reviewed in [74]).

Chronic infection by HBV is one of the main causes of hepatocellular carcinoma (HCC). The carcinogenesis process triggered by HBV is complex, involving direct and indirect mechanisms with the latter being driven by chronic inflammation (reviewed in [75]). Direct mechanisms such as expression of viral oncogenes and insertional mutagenesis have also been documented [76]. HBV X (HBx) is the main oncogenic viral protein. HBx is a viral replication protein that participates in transcription and DNA repair through which it regulates cell cycle, apoptosis and genomic instability [77]. Furthermore, HBx transgenic mice develop liver carcinomas [78].

3.5. Hepatitis C Virus

Hepatitis C virus (HCV) is a member of the *Flaviviridae* family; there are at least six genotypes that are regionally distributed and divided into subtypes [79]. The HCV genome consists of a single strand RNA of positive polarity of approximately 9600 nucleotides from which a polyprotein is translated from an unique open reading frame and later subdivided into different viral polypeptides by viral proteases (reviewed in [80]). HCV infects hepatocytes causing an acute infection that may turn chronic when the immune system cannot eliminate it. In those cases, the carrier may progress to hepatitis, cirrhosis and eventually to HCC (reviewed in [80]). It is estimated that more than 170 million persons worldwide are infected by HCV from which about 40% will develop some form of liver disease and 1%–4% HCC [81]. Transmission commonly occurs through blood and infected blood products.

Direct and indirect transforming mechanisms have also been described for HCV. The viral oncoprotein Core is the only viral product that in transgenic mice promotes the appearance of HCC [82]. Core is the main trigger of steatosis, an abnormal retention of lipids within the hepatocyte, and oxidative stress leading to chronic liver damage and HCC [83]. Different functions have been attributed to this protein, including altered cellular gene transcription, cell proliferation and cell death. For instance, Core expression correlates with changes in the activity of bona fide cellular tumor suppressors and oncogenes, and also of intermediaries of MAP kinases, NFκB and β-catenin signaling pathways [84]. Core protein regulates ROS production by inducing nitric oxide synthase (iNOS) which activates cyclooxygenase-2 (COX-2), importantly contributing with oxidative stress [85]. iNOS and COX-2 are also important components of the inflammatory pathway leading to cancer (reviewed in [86,87]). Core localizes in the mitochondria where it regulates levels of the mitochondrial chaperone prohibitin; it is proposed that altered binding of prohibitin and cytochrome c oxidase results in increased oxidative stress that favors DNA damage [88]. Taken together all these data has contributed to the formation of a model in which accelerated cell division by the inhibition of p53, pRb and other cell proteins in the presence of DNA damage by oxidative stress and the inflammatory response leads to the development of HCC.

3.6. Human T-Lymphotropic Virus Type 1

The *Retroviridae* family groups several viruses with two copies of a positive sense single stranded RNA genome that is retro-transcribed to DNA and integrated into the host cell genome. Retroviruses are classified as simple and complex. Simple retroviruses encode *gag*, *pol* and *env* genes from which structural proteins are expressed, plus other proteins involved in viral replication and integration. Complex viruses encode additional regulatory genes besides the mentioned above.

HTLV1 is a potent direct carcinogenic agent that has been associated with a spectrum of lymphoproliferative diseases collectively referred as adult T-cells leukemia/lymphoma (ATL) (reviewed in [89]). HTLV1 is endemic of Japan, the Western African coast, Central America and the Caribbean, with 15–25 million people infected worldwide [90]. There are three demonstrated ways of transmission for HTLV1: sexual contact, intravenous and breast feeding. The virus infects T- and B-lymphocytes and dendritic cells *in vivo*.

Although, the main retroviral mechanism of transformation is by insertional mutagenesis (see Section 4.2), HTLV1 is a complex retrovirus whose genome also encodes the Tax oncoprotein. Tax has the ability to immortalize cells *in vitro* and its enforced expression in transgenic mice results in development of leukemia/lymphoma [91–95]. Tax is a transcriptional activator/repressor capable of modulating expression of multiple cellular genes and it also directly interacts with a plethora of cellular proteins. Tax principal mechanism of transformation is related to reprogramming cell cycle and inhibition of DNA repair [96]. Tax induces NFκB activity, which stimulates the expression of cytokines and their receptors, including those of IL-13, IL-15, IL-2, IL-2Rα and co-stimulatory surface receptors (OX40/OX40L) [97–99]. Importantly, this activity mimics the chronic inflammatory process critical in the oncogenic progression of many types of cancers. These molecules trigger T cell proliferation, which may help to amplify the pool of HTLV1 infected cells. Thus, contrary to other cancers in which the inflammatory process is mediated by immune cells in response to the oncogenic insult, in HTLV1 infection this is directly induced by Tax. Besides NFkB promoters, Tax also regulates expression of cellular transcriptional promoters through interaction with cyclic-AMP response element binding protein (CREB) and serum response factor (SRF) (reviewed in [96]).

4. Common Mechanisms of Direct Carcinogenesis

4.1. Viral Oncogenes and Oncoproteins

4.1.1. p53 and pRb Inactivation and Other Targets of Increased Proliferation and Survival

Viral oncogenes often increase the rate of cell proliferation and resistance to apoptosis, which eventually leads to alterations in DNA repair mechanisms and genomic instability. Increased mutation rates then alter cell polarity, with substrate-independent growth, and acquisition of cell migration properties, among other malignancy-associated features. The mechanisms used by viruses to induce these cellular changes are similar and often converge on common signaling pathways and transcription factors. For instance, inactivation of p53 and pRb tumor suppressor genes is an event that occurs in most pathways of viral oncogenesis, both human and animal (reviewed in [100–102]). In conditions of DNA damage, p53 arrests cell cycle until the damage has been repaired. When this does not occur, p53 induces cell apoptosis or cell senescence (reviewed in [103,104]). pRb also arrests cell cycle progression after binding and inactivating members of the E2F family of transcription factors [102]. pRb specifically inhibits the G1-S transition in response to DNA damage. Thus, an accumulation of mutations and chromosomal abnormalities is favored in the absence of p53 and pRb function. Since tumorigenic viruses are not usually associated with the massive production of viral infectious particles that characterize acute-infecting viruses, they relay in triggering cell proliferation mechanisms to increase the pool of infected cells. Furthermore, the termini of the viral genomes could be sensed as nicked DNA by the p53 and pRb machinery, and this would trigger host cell apoptosis immediately after infection, if both proteins were not inactivated.

HPV E6 and E7 induce the degradation of tumor suppressor proteins, p53 and pRb, respectively. E6 catalyzes the degradation of p53 by binding to the E6 associated protein (E6AP), a cellular protein with ubiquitin-ligase activity. The E6/E6AP complex binds to the p53 central region, which is then ubiquitinated and subsequently degraded in the proteasome [105,106]. E6 also blocks the cell cycle inhibitor $p16^{INK4}$, which increases cell proliferation [107]. E7 directly induces release of E2F1-3 from pRb/E2F1-3 complexes, E2F1-3 in turn activates transcription of genes involved in cell cycle progression such as cyclins E and A [60,108]. HTLV1 Tax induces hyper-phosphorylation of pRb while promoting its degradation in the proteasome [109]. The mechanism by which Tax affects p53 function is less well understood and many mechanisms have been proposed, including hyper-phosphorylation, interfering with p53 function through competitive binding of cellular co-activators and through direct binding mediated by NFκB [110]. Tax also interferes with the activity and/or expression levels of cyclins and cyclin-dependent kinases [111–113]. Another HTLV1 protein, HBZ, induces over-expression of E2F1 target genes stimulating the proliferation of T lymphocytes [114]. KSHV LANA 1 inactivates p53 and it induces pRb phosphorylation and subsequent inactivation through its association with Cdk6 [115–117]. Most EBV latency III proteins target p53 and pRb for inactivation, along with other cell proliferation proteins: HA95, HAX1, cyclin A and D, p27kip1, p16INK4A and c-Myc [34].

Cell cycle progression and cell survival are conjointly regulated mechanisms. Still, tumor viruses often trigger additional survival mechanisms besides p53 and pRb inactivation. EBV LMP1 and LMP2A constitutively activate NFκB and PI3K/Akt signaling pathways, which results in increased activity of anti-apoptotic proteins Bcl-2, Bcl-xl, Mcl1 and A20 [118–120]. EBV also encodes BHRF1, a Bcl-2 homologue that in a subset of Burkitt's lymphoma seems to counteract c-Myc pro-apoptotic activity [121]. HTLV1 Tax is also an important activator of NFκB and PI3K/Akt signaling pathways, and HTLV p12 and p13 proteins regulate Bcl-2 and caspase 3 and 9 activity [122]. HPV E6 and E7 function has been associated with degradation of pro-apoptotic proteins pro-caspase 8, FADD and BAK, and upregulation of expression of anti-apoptotic proteins c-IAP2 and survivin [123–127]. E6 binds to the E6-associated protein ligase (E6AP), an ubiquitin ligase that targets E6-interacting pro-apoptotic proteins to the proteasome. HBV HBx interacts with Damaged DNA Binding Protein 1 (DDB1) inhibiting proteasome activity resulting in resistance to apoptosis [128]. Anti-apoptotic mechanisms have also been described for HCV core and NS5A proteins (reviewed in [129]). Because virally infected cells are at high risk of elimination by apoptosis, anti-apoptotic mechanisms are critical for viral persistence and carcinogenesis.

4.1.2. Genomic Instability

Another common carcinogenic route promoted by infectious agents is genomic instability, which leads to gene amplification and deletion, changes in the number of chromosomes (polyploidy and aneuploidy) and aberrant fusion of non-homologous chromosomes (translocations). For instance, HPV-16 E6 and E7 proteins promote gene amplification, structural chromosomal alterations and centrosome replication errors leading to aneuploidy and polyploidy. Thus, HPV immortalized cell lines are characterized by gain and loss of whole chromosomes [130–133]. In agreement, aneuploidy can be found as early as in HPV-associated noninvasive lesions (reviewed in [134]). HBV HBx also interferes with genomic instability. HBx forms complexes with HBx interacting protein (HBXIP) altering the formation of the mitotic spindle and the centrosome function [77]. EBV EBNA-1 may promote genomic instability through activation of the recombinase-activating genes RAG1 and RAG2 [7], which may be responsible for the Myc chromosomal translocation present in Burkitt's lymphoma [135]. Another enzyme associated with genomic instability is activation-induced cytidine deaminase (AID), whose expression is induced by EBV during the transit through germinal center reaction. Increased rate of mutations are observed in the variable regions of heavy and light chains after EBV infection [136]. Whether other host genomic regions are also targeted by AID is not know, but potentially this would facilitate EBV-induced transformation.

A mutator phenotype has also been attributed to Tax and both small and gross changes in DNA and chromosomes are often found in HTLV1 transformed cells [137,138]. On one hand, Tax multiple targets operating during the G2/M transition impair the DNA-damage-induced response, allowing cells to scape this transition with accumulated mutations [139]. On the other hand, Tax directly induces chromosomal instability by transcriptionally repressing various targets, including the DNA polymerase-β, an enzyme involved in base-excision repair [96]. Tax can also independently suppress the nucleotide excision repair mechanism, which is normally utilized by cells following UV irradiation [140]. Furthermore, ATL cells often contain an abnormal number of chromosomes (aneuploidy), and a role for Tax has been proposed, although the mechanism is not clear. Tax directly binds and inactivates MAD1, a mitotic spindle assembly checkpoint (SAC) kinetochore protein in charge of ensuring proper chromosomal segregation during mitosis [141]. Tax also promotes premature activation of the CDC20-associated anaphase promoting complex [142]. Overall these mechanisms would lead to faulty chromosomal segregation resulting in aneuploidy in HTLV1 infected cells.

4.1.3. Interfering with Telomere Shortening

Telomere shortening and cell senescence are the natural consequence of unlimited cell proliferation, and tumor viruses also display mechanisms of telomere maintenance. Telomere length maintenance is a fine regulated mechanism involving a complex set of proteins and the enzyme telomerase (reviewed in [143]). Expression of telomerase in physiological conditions is restricted to cells with stem properties, e.g., germinal cells or somatic stem/progenitor cells, but telomerase expression is turned off in differentiated cells. How tumor viruses regulate telomere length is not clear, but HPV E6, EBV LMP1, KSHV LANA, HTLV1 Tax and HBV HBx have all been shown to induce expression of telomerase [144–147]. Tumor viruses interference with DNA repair mechanisms and concomitant genomic instability may be in great measure a consequence of bypassing regulatory checkpoints of telomere length and p53- and pRb-dependent senescence (reviewed in [148]). In this scenario, tumor viruses have evolved with these mechanisms in order to achieve replicative immortality and thus persistency.

4.1.4. Interfering with Cell Polarity

Viral oncoproteins may also promote carcinogenesis by inactivating proteins related to cell polarity. Proteins containing PDZ (**p**ost synaptic density protein, drosophila **d**isc large tumor suppressor and **z**onula occludens-1 protein) domains function like scaffolds for both membrane and cytosolic supramolecular complexes, which have an important role in cell-cell contact and cell signaling. PDZ domains interact with target proteins through PBMs (PDZ domain-binding motif). A class I PBM was first described in the E4-ORF1 oncoprotein from adenovirus 9, and subsequently identified in other human virus oncoproteins, such as HPV E6 and HTLV1 Tax [149–152]. The E6 PBM is necessary for both *in vitro* and *in vivo* E6-mediated transformation [153,154]. On the other hand, mutational disruption of the Tax PBM reduces Tax-mediated cellular transformation and the capacity of HTLV1 to induce persistent infections [155,156]. Inactivation of cell polarity-associated proteins likely favors carcinogenesis by impairing morphogenesis, asymmetric division, migration and normal cell proliferation, survival and differentiation programs.

4.1.5. Viral miRNAs

MicroRNAs (miRNAs) have recently being shown to also participate in cell transformation. miRNAs are strongly conserved single stranded RNAs of approximately 22 nucleotide long that regulate expression of most genes. miRNAs inhibit mRNA translation mainly by translational repression based on base pair complementarity (reviewed in [157,158]). Almost all cancers present altered expression of cellular miRNAs (reviewed in [159,160]). However, a new and interesting topic in viral oncology concerns to viruses encoding miRNAs with oncogenic capabilities. The first five viral miRNAs were described in the EBV positive B95 cell line; to date, more than 40 miRNAs produced from the EBV BARTs and BHFR1 transcripts have been identified [161,162]. Those miRNAs are able to inhibit apoptosis, and some target cellular tumor suppressor genes, such as: PUMA, Bin, TOMM22 and WIF1 [163–166]. EBV infection of gastric carcinoma cells (AGS) induced anchorage independence in absence of viral protein synthesis, highlighting the importance of EBV miRNAs in the malignant process [167].

4.2. Insertional Mutagenesis

In the retrovirus life cycle, the integrated viral genome (the provirus) is replicated as a cellular genetic element during the host cell cycle. Expression of the provirus is controlled by viral regulatory elements, the long terminal repeats (LTRs), which are powerful transcriptional activators that often control the expression of cellular genes in the vicinity of the insertion area. When the provirus is close to a cell proto-oncogene, the LTR can upregulate its expression to oncogenic results. Although, all best characterized examples of cell transformation are due to upregulation of proto-oncogenes, retroviruses can potentially also interrupt tumor suppressor genes with similar effects (reviewed in [168]). During viral progeny formation, infective particles sometimes carry cellular oncogenes that were close to the insertion site and which are transduced to new hosts, now under the control of the LTRs. Among those genes frequently transduced by retroviruses are cell receptors such as ErbB and Fms, kinases such as Src and Abl and transcription factors such as Jun, Fos and Myc. These chimerical viruses become non-competent and unable to trigger lytic infections. Thus, these viruses have an augmented transforming capacity, as they are the only infectious agents capable of inducing tumors in just a few days. Due to this characteristic, such retroviruses are known as acute transformers. Preferential insertion sites are known as “hot spots”, for example, the murine mammary tumor virus (MMTV) responsible for breast cancer in several mouse species, frequently inserts in regions near to *Wnt* and *Notch* proto-oncogenes [169].

The mutagenesis mechanism by insertion or retro-transduction of cell proto-oncogenes has not been demonstrated in human retroviruses (HTLV1 mainly transforms by Tax expression. See Section 3.6) (reviewed in [170]). Next generation sequencing techniques have shown that HBV is preferably integrated in tumor cells in comparison to non-tumor infected hepatic tissue and its integration correlates with deregulated expression of *TERT*, *MLL4* and *CCNE* cellular oncogenes [76]. The similarity with animal retroviruses has granted analogy to this HBV mechanism of insertional mutagenesis. Although HPV and MCPV require integration to become oncogenic, in these cases the biological consequence is more similar to acute transforming retroviruses. Here, viral regulatory regions are lost and proviruses become defective and unable to produce infection competent progeny. Hence, integration correlates with the establishment of a latent stage, over-expression of viral oncogenes and host cell transformation (see Section 3.2 and 3.3).

5. Common Mechanisms of Indirect Carcinogenesis

The mechanisms of indirect oncogenesis are more difficult to demonstrate since they cannot be measured by *in vitro* assays, nor the expression of viral genes in transgenic animal models recapitulates the oncogenic process. These mechanisms have been proposed from epidemiologic evidence and coherence and plausibility principles are more difficult to fulfill. Besides chronic inflammation and immunosuppression (Figure 2), other proposed indirect mechanisms of transformation are described below (Figure 3).

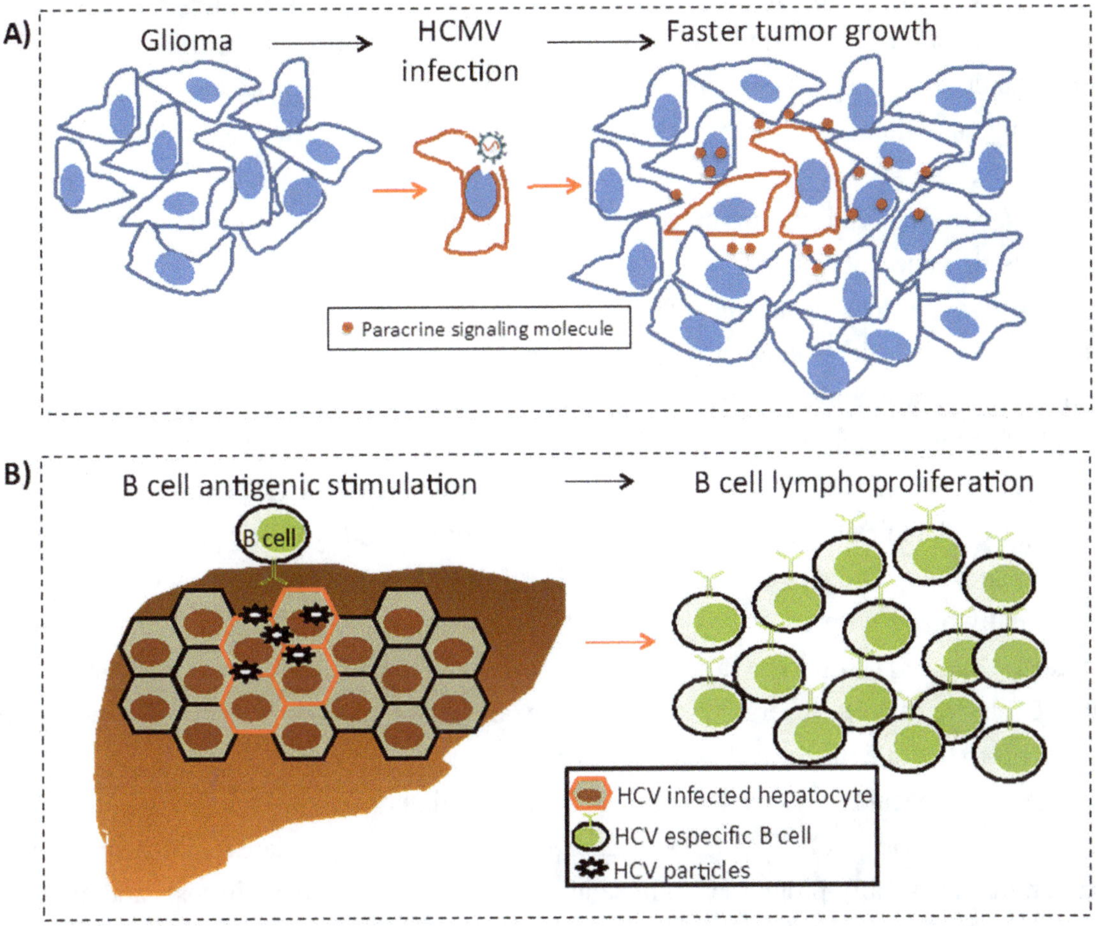

Figure 3. Other indirect mechanisms: Oncomodulation (**A**) and chronic antigen-driven lymphoproliferation (**B**). (**A**) In oncomodulation HCMV does not participate in the initial transformation of the glia; perhaps the virus has an increased tropism for tumor cells once the glioma has formed. Here, the virus only infects a fraction of the tumor cells activating signaling pathways that favor tumor growth; (**B**) B cells with antigen receptors specific for HCV antigens chronically respond to infected hepatocytes and free virus. This chronic stimulation increases the risk of unregulated lymphoproliferation and lymphoma.

5.1. Chronic Inflammation

Persistent infection is generally accompanied by local chronic inflammation, still in the presence of evasion mechanisms of the immune response. It has been proposed that this chronic inflammation induces a constant and progressive local damage, closely associated to regeneration events of the damaged tissue. The inflammatory response is characterized by local expression of pro-inflammatory cytokines, chemokines, adhesion molecules, growth factors and anti-apoptotic genes that regulate the sequential recruitment of leukocytes and stimulates fibroblasts and endothelial cells to divide and produce components of tissue remodeling and neovascularization (reviewed in [171]). A normal inflammatory response is self-limiting; chemoattraction of immune cells is gradually eliminated, pro-inflammatory cells already in the site of infection suffer apoptosis and are phagocytosed, while vascular changes are reversed. In contrast, in chronic inflammation associated with persistent infections, leukocytes remain in the lesion site and their apoptosis is suppressed. Additionally, to eliminate the infectious agent, immune cells produce oxygen and nitrogen free radicals, which are highly mutagenic. In this scenario, chronic inflammation favors the appearance of a cancerous clone, while tissue regeneration functions can also favor tumor growth, invasion and metastasis (for review, see [172], Figure 2A).

Helicobacter pylori is the prototype indirect carcinogen; it generates chronic gastric inflammation leading to gastric cancer through a series of progressive inflammatory lesions: non-atrophic gastritis, atrophic gastritis, intestinal metaplasia, dysplasia and gastric cancer [18]. *Helicobacter pylori* is also an IARC type I carcinogenic pathogen [173]. *Helicobacter pylori* stimulates the gastric epithelium to secrete IL-8 that attracts and activates neutrophils, favoring the establishment of a microenvironment populated by leukocytes and high concentrations of pro-inflammatory cytokines, such as TNF-α, IL-6, IL-1β and IL-12 [174]. Neutrophils release reactive oxygen species (superoxide anions, hydrogen peroxide, hydroxyl radicals and hydroperoxyl) and nitrogen oxides (nitric oxide, peroxynitrite and nitrogen dioxide) that induce mutations in cells of the gastric mucosa (reviewed in [175]). In agreement, individuals with IL-8, IL-1β and TNF-α polymorphisms present and increased risk to develop gastric cancer [176–179]. Of note, *Helicobacter pylori* pharmacological eradication in patients with pre-neoplastic lesions reverses tissue damage and halts the appearance of cancer, providing further support to the role of the bacterium in gastric cancer progression.

Although all oncogenic viruses maintain persistent infections, the role of inflammatory responses in oncogenesis is not clear. HCV and HBV triggered inflammation correlates with necrosis and tissue regeneration that eventually progresses to hepatic lesions such as steatosis, fibrosis and cirrhosis, from which liver cancer emerges. It has been observed that during steatosis and fibrosis, the liver is highly infiltrated by immune cells and there is a microenvironment of inflammatory cytokines and chemokines, among which TGF-β and IL-1β stand out (reviewed in [180]). We have also observed that increased EBV reactivation correlates with severe gastric inflammation and increased tissue damage leading to advanced gastric lesions, arguing for an important role for inflammation in the EBV-associated transformation of the gastric mucosa [181,182].

5.2. Immunosuppression

The role of the immune system in onco-surveillance has been clearly established since the AIDS pandemic. Although, HIV is not capable of inducing tumors in its host cell, 40% of patients with AIDS develop cancers associated to the disease. Thus, severe immunosuppression induced by HIV infection indirectly promotes the development of tumors (reviewed in [17,183]). Individuals with a low $CD8^+$ cytotoxic T lymphocyte count are more susceptible to infectious cancers [17], such as EBV- and

KSHV-associated lymphomas (exemplified in Figure 2B), KSHV sarcomas, HPV head and neck and cervical carcinomas, and MCPV Merkel cell carcinomas. Due to these features, HIV is classified as an indirect carcinogenic agent, while, direct transformation mechanisms mediated by EBV, KSHV, HPV and MCPV are still operating.

A similar phenomenon is observed in individuals with pharmacological immunosuppression due to solid organ or bone marrow transplants. The post-transplant lymphoproliferative disorders (PTLD) are often EBV-associated B-cell proliferations. PTLDs begin as polyclonal proliferations with a high risk to evolve into monoclonal aggressive lymphomas [184,185]. Although, most PTLD arise from host lymphocytes, a donor origin is possible too. The use of T-cell depleting agents is a risk factor for EBV-positive PTLD, highlighting the importance of T-cells in the antitumor immunosurveillance mechanisms (reviewed in [186]). Infusion of autologous T-cells specific to the immunodominant EBV EBNA3A/3B/3C proteins has proven a very successful therapy [187,188].

5.3. Oncomodulation

There is evidence that viruses also participate in tumor growth modulating the biological course of an already-established cancer (Figure 3A). The term "oncomodulation" was suggested by Martin Michaelis *et al.* to describe the role of human cytomegalovirus (HCMV) in tumor progression [189]. HCMV is a herpesvirus whose worldwide prevalence is between 50% and 100% in the adult population; infection is normally asymptomatic and only produces disease under immunosuppressive conditions.

Up to today, there is not enough evidence of HCMV being capable of participating in the transformation process. Nevertheless, HCMV may infect tumor cells and through the expression of viral genes affecting signaling pathways important for proliferation, survival, angiogenesis, invasiveness and immune modulation, could increase the aggressiveness of the tumor [190–194]. The best documented example is HCMV participation in high degree gliomas, a brain cancer with extremely bad prognosis. HCMV genome and proteins have been found more frequently in high degree gliomas than in other central nervous system tumors or non-tumorous brain samples (e.g., from epilepsy) [195–197]. However, even when HCMV resides in the tumor, it only infects a fraction of the tumor cells and does not exhibit viral monoclonality; therefore, the HCMV association with high grade gliomas does not fulfill the Bradford Hill's temporality criteria, arguing that infection happened after the event of transformation.

5.4. Chronic Antigen-Driven Lymphoproliferation

Cells of the immune system are expanded in response to infection; particularly, B cells exhibit extensive proliferation during the germinal center (GC) reaction in which they undergo antigen receptor isotype switch and increased target affinity (somatic hypermutation). The activation-induced cytidine deaminase (AID) is in charge of both processes in which the antigen receptor is modified. B cell lymphomas frequently emerge from the GC reaction due to the risky combination of increased proliferation and expression of mutagenic enzymes. EBV LMP1 and LMP2A provide decoy signals inducing infected B cells to go through the GC reaction and emerge as memory cells in which the virus can persist for the life-time of the host. EBV-associated lymphomas may partially result from this EBV-induced GC reaction [136]. Similarly, chronic antigenic stimulation resulting from other persistent infections can potentially increase the risk to develop lymphomas; among the most widely documented are, infection by bacteria *Helicobacter pylori*, *Borrelia burgdorferi*, *Campylobacter jejuni* and *Chlamydia psittaci* and by HCV. Concerning the latter, clonal B cell expansions have been observed in HCV infected patients correlating with longer chronic infections and with receptor specificity against HCV proteins [198–200]. Still, the most reliable evidence for a causal association comes from HCV pharmacological eradication, which is frequently associated with lymphoma remission [201]. Similarly, anti- *Helicobacter pylori* treatment results in regression of associated gastric MALT lymphomas [202].

6. Conclusions

The last 100 years have seen the birth and evolution of tumor virology with seven viral agents already been convincingly associated with the pathogenesis of cancer in humans. Tumor virology has importantly contributed to the understanding of the molecular mechanisms operating during carcinogenesis. However, causation is especially difficult to demonstrate because in most cases the tumor viruses are wide spread in the population without causing disease. It is essential to consider that infection by tumor viruses is never sufficient but always required for development of associated tumors. Cancer cannot be the aim of the virus since it compromises both host and virus survival. However, viral mechanisms of persistence in which cellular processes are impaired such as proliferation, survival, DNA repair, among others, provide a suitable substrate from which cancer can emerge after additional environmental aggressions and permissive host genetics. Today, Sir Austin Bradford Hill's causation criteria are considered the experimental, epidemiological and clinical conceptual base from which to infer a virus-cancer causative relationship.

Two different modes of cellular transformation have been documented based in whether the virus is acting from within (directly) or outside (indirectly) the cell that will form the tumor. Direct mechanisms infer expression of viral oncogenes together with deregulation of cellular oncogenes and/or tumor suppressor genes. Among the most important indirect mechanisms are (i) the establishment of an inflammatory milieu in which chronic production of mutagenic molecules is persistently damaging the surrounding tissue, and (ii) immunosuppression with loss of the cancer immunosurveillance mechanisms. However, all tumor viruses probably present direct and indirect mechanisms and this separation mostly alludes to the main mechanism of cell transformation. The tumor microenvironment is always inflammatory whether infectious or aseptic, and inflammatory molecules importantly contribute with tumor initiation and progression. *Helicobacter pylori* is considered the prototype infectious agent transforming through chronic inflammation, still a bacterial oncogene able to induce gastric tumors in transgenic mice has recently been described. Similarly, EBV importantly cooperates with gastric inflammation and progression though a series of inflammatory lesions of increased severity [181,182] and HBV- and HCV-mediated liver cancer also progresses from a series of precursor inflammatory lesions besides their known capacity to express viral and cellular oncogenes. It is also possible that the contribution of direct and indirect mechanisms is mandated by the transforming tissue, with liver and gastric tissue equally depending on both modes of transformation.

Infection-associated tumors are responsible for 15%–20% of all cancer cases worldwide, representing an important challenge in public health programs. With the advent of new technologies it is highly probably that this frequency will increase. Wide genome sequencing technologies have recently allowed the discovery of MCPV and have helped to establish its causal association with Merkel cell carcinoma. Together with new tumor agents, it is probably that new mechanisms of infection-induced transformation will emerge while others could be better understood. The hit-and-run transforming mechanism proposes that a viral agent takes part in the carcinogenesis but it is later lost as the tumor cell acquires additional oncogenic hits [203]. This "non classical" oncogenic pathway is not compatible with current causality criteria. However, it is very likely that current causation criteria will be modified and extended in the future. For instance, Birdwell *et al.* used a model of transient infection in EBV-infected keratinocytes to analyze the pattern of methylation in CpG islands. They found that the epigenetic changes caused by infection correlated with a tumorigenic phenotype, which was maintained even after of loss of the virus [204]. Although, there is not evidence of transient infection by EBV does not happen naturally, the Birdwell's work highlights the potential role of infections that are not maintained throughout cancer development. Also, facilitated by massive sequencing of tumor samples, a widespread APOBEC3B fingerprint was found among many types of cancers [205]. Because the APOBEC family of cytidine deaminases is part of an innate antiviral response, it is possible that this fingerprint reflects a history of past infections in which the antiviral response also collaterally triggered cellular somatic mutations leading to cancer.

The discovery of cancers with an infectious origin is critical to develop vaccines and preventive and therapeutic pharmacological therapies. This knowledge has already leaded to vaccines against HBV and high risk-HPV and targeted therapies against HIV and HCV.

Acknowledgments

This work constitutes a partial fulfillment of the Graduate Program of Doctor Degree in Biomedical Sciences, Medicine Faculty, National Autonomous University of Mexico, Mexico City, Mexico. A Morales-Sánchez acknowledges to the National Autonomous University of Mexico and the scholarship and financial support provided by the National Council of Science and Technology (CONACyT) and National Autonomous University of Mexico. This study was supported by grant HIM-2013-051 (to E.M. Fuentes Pananá) from Fondo de Apoyo a la Investigación Hospital Infantil de México Federico Gómez.

References and Notes

1. Rous, P. A transmissible avian neoplasm. (sarcoma of the common fowl.). *J. Exp. Med.* **1910**, *12*, 696–705.
2. Rous, P. A sarcoma of the fowl transmissible by an agent separable from the tumor cells. *J. Exp. Med.* **1911**, *13*, 397–411.
3. Ellerman, V.; Bang, O. Experimentelle leukämie bei hühnern. *Zent. Bakteriol. Parasitenkd. Infectionskr. Hyg. Abt. Orig.* **1908**, *46*, 595–609.
4. Epstein, M.A.; Achong, B.G.; Barr, Y.M. Virus particles in cultured lymphoblasts from burkitt's

lymphoma. *Lancet* **1964**, *1*, 702–703.

5. Durst, M.; Gissmann, L.; Ikenberg, H.; zur Hausen, H. A papillomavirus DNA from a cervical carcinoma and its prevalence in cancer biopsy samples from different geographic regions. *Proc. Natl. Acad. Sci. USA* **1983**, *80*, 3812–3815.
6. Boshart, M.; Gissmann, L.; Ikenberg, H.; Kleinheinz, A.; Scheurlen, W.; zur Hausen, H. A new type of papillomavirus DNA, its presence in genital cancer biopsies and in cell lines derived from cervical cancer. *EMBO J.* **1984**, *3*, 1151–1157.
7. Moore, P.S.; Chang, Y. Why do viruses cause cancer? Highlights of the first century of human tumour virology. *Nat. Rev. Cancer* **2010**, *10*, 878–889.
8. Parkin, D.M. The global health burden of infection-associated cancers in the year 2002. *Int. J. Cancer* **2006**, *118*, 3030–3044.
9. Koch, R. Untersuchungen über bakterien: V. Die ätiologie der milzbrand-krankheit, begründet auf die entwicklungsgeschichte des bacillus anthracis [investigations into bacteria: V. The etiology of anthrax, based on the ontogenesis of bacillus anthracis]. *Cohns Beitr. Biol. Pflanz.* **1876**, *2*, 277–310.
10. Hill, A.B. The environment and disease: Association or causation? *Proc. Royal Soc.Med.* **1965**, *58*, 295–300.
11. Thompson, M.P.; Kurzrock, R. Epstein-barr virus and cancer. *Clin. Cancer Res.* **2004**, *10*, 803–821.
12. Kulwichit, W.; Edwards, R.H.; Davenport, E.M.; Baskar, J.F.; Godfrey, V.; Raab-Traub, N. Expression of the epstein-barr virus latent membrane protein 1 induces b cell lymphoma in transgenic mice. *Proc. Natl. Acad. Sci. USA* **1998**, *95*, 11963–11968.
13. Loeb, L.A.; Springgate, C.F.; Battula, N. Errors in DNA replication as a basis of malignant changes. *Cancer Res.* **1974**, *34*, 2311–2321.
14. Prindle, M.J.; Fox, E.J.; Loeb, L.A. The mutator phenotype in cancer: Molecular mechanisms and targeting strategies. *Curr. Drug Targets* **2010**, *11*, 1296–1303.
15. Coleman, W.B. Mechanisms of human hepatocarcinogenesis. *Curr. Mol. Med.* **2003**, *3*, 573–588.
16. Zucman-Rossi, J.; Laurent-Puig, P. Genetic diversity of hepatocellular carcinomas and its potential impact on targeted therapies. *Pharmacogenomics* **2007**, *8*, 997–1003.
17. Chadburn, A.; Abdul-Nabi, A.M.; Teruya, B.S.; Lo, A.A. Lymphoid proliferations associated with human immunodeficiency virus infection. *Arch. Pathol. Lab. Med.* **2013**, *137*, 360–370.
18. Correa, P.; Piazuelo, M.B. The gastric precancerous cascade. *J. Dig. Dis.* **2012**, *13*, 2–9.
19. Hatakeyama, M.; Higashi, H. *Helicobacter pylori* caga: A new paradigm for bacterial carcinogenesis. *Cancer Sci.* **2005**, *96*, 835–843.
20. Chang, Y.; Cesarman, E.; Pessin, M.S.; Lee, F.; Culpepper, J.; Knowles, D.M.; Moore, P.S. Identification of herpesvirus-like DNA sequences in aids-associated kaposi's sarcoma. *Science* **1994**, *266*, 1865–1869.
21. Zur Hausen, H. Papillomaviruses and cancer: From basic studies to clinical application. *Nat. Rev. Cancer* **2002**, *2*, 342–350.
22. Feng, H.; Shuda, M.; Chang, Y.; Moore, P.S. Clonal integration of a polyomavirus in human merkel cell carcinoma. *Science* **2008**, *319*, 1096–1100.
23. Beasley, R.P.; Hwang, L.Y.; Lin, C.C.; Chien, C.S. Hepatocellular carcinoma and hepatitis b

virus. A prospective study of 22,707 men in taiwan. *Lancet* **1981**, *2*, 1129–1133.

24. Choo, Q.L.; Kuo, G.; Weiner, A.J.; Overby, L.R.; Bradley, D.W.; Houghton, M. Isolation of a cDNA clone derived from a blood-borne non-a, non-b viral hepatitis genome. *Science* **1989**, *244*, 359–362.
25. Poiesz, B.J.; Ruscetti, F.W.; Gazdar, A.F.; Bunn, P.A.; Minna, J.D.; Gallo, R.C. Detection and isolation of type c retrovirus particles from fresh and cultured lymphocytes of a patient with cutaneous t-cell lymphoma. *Proc. Natl. Acad. Sci. USA* **1980**, *77*, 7415–7419.
26. Rickinson, A.B.; Kieff, E. Epstein-barr virus. In *Fields Virology*, Lippincott-Raven Publishers: Philadelphia, PA, USA, 1996; Volume 2, pp. 2397–2446.
27. Henle, G.; Henle, W.; Clifford, P.; Diehl, V.; Kafuko, G.W.; Kirya, B.G.; Klein, G.; Morrow, R.H.; Munube, G.M.; Pike, P.; *et al.* Antibodies to epstein-barr virus in burkitt's lymphoma and control groups. *J. Natl. Cancer Inst.* **1969**, *43*, 1147–1157.
28. Gerber, P.; Walsh, J.H.; Rosenblum, E.N.; Purcell, R.H. Association of eb-virus infection with the post-perfusion syndrome. *Lancet* **1969**, *1*, 593–595.
29. Hoagland, R.J. The transmission of infectious mononucleosis. *Am. J. Med. Sci.* **1955**, *229*, 262–272.
30. Goldberg, G.N.; Fulginiti, V.A.; Ray, C.G.; Ferry, P.; Jones, J.F.; Cross, H.; Minnich, L. In utero epstein-barr virus (infectious mononucleosis) infection. *JAMA: J. Am. Med. Assoc.* **1981**, *246*, 1579–1581.
31. Meyohas, M.C.; Marechal, V.; Desire, N.; Bouillie, J.; Frottier, J.; Nicolas, J.C. Study of mother-to-child epstein-barr virus transmission by means of nested pcrs. *J. Virol.* **1996**, *70*, 6816–6819.
32. Stock, I. Infectious mononucleosis—A "childhood disease" of great medical concern. *Med. Mon. Pharma.* **2013**, *36*, 364–368.
33. Hjalgrim, H. On the aetiology of hodgkin lymphoma. *Dan. Med. J.* **2012**, *59*, B4485.
34. Klein, G.; Klein, E.; Kashuba, E. Interaction of epstein-barr virus (ebv) with human b-lymphocytes. *Biochem. Biophys. Res. Commun.* **2010**, *396*, 67–73.
35. Morgan, D.G.; Niederman, J.C.; Miller, G.; Smith, H.W.; Dowaliby, J.M. Site of epstein-barr virus replication in the oropharynx. *Lancet* **1979**, *2*, 1154–1157.
36. Shair, K.H.; Schnegg, C.I.; Raab-Traub, N. Ebv latent membrane protein 1 effects on plakoglobin, cell growth, and migration. *Cancer Res.* **2008**, *68*, 6997–7005.
37. Caldwell, R.G.; Wilson, J.B.; Anderson, S.J.; Longnecker, R. Epstein-barr virus lmp2a drives b cell development and survival in the absence of normal b cell receptor signals. *Immunity* **1998**, *9*, 405–411.
38. Scholle, F.; Bendt, K.M.; Raab-Traub, N. Epstein-barr virus lmp2a transforms epithelial cells, inhibits cell differentiation, and activates akt. *J. Virol.* **2000**, *74*, 10681–10689.
39. Yates, J.L.; Warren, N.; Sugden, B. Stable replication of plasmids derived from epstein-barr virus in various mammalian cells. *Nature* **1985**, *313*, 812–815.
40. Dukers, N.H.; Rezza, G. Human herpesvirus 8 epidemiology: What we do and do not know. *Aids* **2003**, *17*, 1717–1730.
41. Cai, Q.; Verma, S.C.; Lu, J.; Robertson, E.S. Molecular biology of kaposi's sarcoma-associated

herpesvirus and related oncogenesis. *Adv. Virus Res.* **2010**, *78*, 87–142.

42. Viejo-Borbolla, A.; Ottinger, M.; Schulz, T.F. Human herpesvirus 8: Biology and role in the pathogenesis of kaposi's sarcoma and other aids-related malignancies. *Curr. HIV/AIDS Rep.* **2004**, *1*, 5–11.
43. Beral, V.; Peterman, T.A.; Berkelman, R.L.; Jaffe, H.W. Kaposi's sarcoma among persons with aids: A sexually transmitted infection? *Lancet* **1990**, *335*, 123–128.
44. Radkov, S.A.; Kellam, P.; Boshoff, C. The latent nuclear antigen of kaposi sarcoma-associated herpesvirus targets the retinoblastoma-e2f pathway and with the oncogene hras transforms primary rat cells. *Nat. Med.* **2000**, *6*, 1121–1127.
45. Chugh, P.; Matta, H.; Schamus, S.; Zachariah, S.; Kumar, A.; Richardson, J.A.; Smith, A.L.; Chaudhary, P.M. Constitutive nf-kappab activation, normal fas-induced apoptosis, and increased incidence of lymphoma in human herpes virus 8 k13 transgenic mice. *Proc. Natl. Acad. Sci. USA* **2005**, *102*, 12885–12890.
46. Sun, Q.; Zachariah, S.; Chaudhary, P.M. The human herpes virus 8-encoded viral flice-inhibitory protein induces cellular transformation via nf-kappab activation. *J. Biol. Chem.* **2003**, *278*, 52437–52445.
47. Wang, L.; Dittmer, D.P.; Tomlinson, C.C.; Fakhari, F.D.; Damania, B. Immortalization of primary endothelial cells by the k1 protein of kaposi's sarcoma-associated herpesvirus. *Cancer Res.* **2006**, *66*, 3658–3666.
48. Staskus, K.A.; Zhong, W.; Gebhard, K.; Herndier, B.; Wang, H.; Renne, R.; Beneke, J.; Pudney, J.; Anderson, D.J.; Ganem, D.; *et al.* Kaposi's sarcoma-associated herpesvirus gene expression in endothelial (spindle) tumor cells. *J. Virol.* **1997**, *71*, 715–719.
49. Xie, J.; Pan, H.; Yoo, S.; Gao, S.J. Kaposi's sarcoma-associated herpesvirus induction of ap-1 and interleukin 6 during primary infection mediated by multiple mitogen-activated protein kinase pathways. *J. Virol.* **2005**, *79*, 15027–15037.
50. Naranatt, P.P.; Krishnan, H.H.; Svojanovsky, S.R.; Bloomer, C.; Mathur, S.; Chandran, B. Host gene induction and transcriptional reprogramming in kaposi's sarcoma-associated herpesvirus (kshv/hhv-8)-infected endothelial, fibroblast, and b cells: Insights into modulation events early during infection. *Cancer Res.* **2004**, *64*, 72–84.
51. Masood, R.; Cesarman, E.; Smith, D.L.; Gill, P.S.; Flore, O. Human herpesvirus-8-transformed endothelial cells have functionally activated vascular endothelial growth factor/vascular endothelial growth factor receptor. *Am. J. Pathol.* **2002**, *160*, 23–29.
52. Cerimele, F.; Curreli, F.; Ely, S.; Friedman-Kien, A.E.; Cesarman, E.; Flore, O. Kaposi's sarcoma-associated herpesvirus can productively infect primary human keratinocytes and alter their growth properties. *J. Virol.* **2001**, *75*, 2435–2443.
53. Hong, G.K.; Gulley, M.L.; Feng, W.H.; Delecluse, H.J.; Holley-Guthrie, E.; Kenney, S.C. Epstein-barr virus lytic infection contributes to lymphoproliferative disease in a scid mouse model. *J. Virol.* **2005**, *79*, 13993–14003.
54. Martel-Renoir, D.; Grunewald, V.; Touitou, R.; Schwaab, G.; Joab, I. Qualitative analysis of the expression of epstein-barr virus lytic genes in nasopharyngeal carcinoma biopsies. *J. Gen. Virol.* **1995**, *76*, 1401–1408.
55. Munoz, N.; Bosch, F.X.; de Sanjose, S.; Herrero, R.; Castellsague, X.; Shah, K.V.; Snijders, P.J.;

Meijer, C.J. International Agency for Research on Cancer Multicenter Cervical Cancer Study, G. Epidemiologic classification of human papillomavirus types associated with cervical cancer. *N. Engl. J. Med.* **2003**, *348*, 518–527.

56. Clifford, G.M.; Smith, J.S.; Plummer, M.; Munoz, N.; Franceschi, S. Human papillomavirus types in invasive cervical cancer worldwide: A meta-analysis. *Br. J. Cancer* **2003**, *88*, 63–73.
57. Chow, L.T.; Broker, T.R. Human papillomavirus infections: Warts or cancer? *Cold Spring Harbor Perspect. Biol.* **2013**, *5*, 10.1101/cshperspect.a012997.
58. Woodman, C.B.; Collins, S.I.; Young, L.S. The natural history of cervical hpv infection: Unresolved issues. *Nat. Rev. Cancer* **2007**, *7*, 11–22.
59. Zur Hausen, H. Papillomaviruses—To vaccination and beyond. *Biochem. Biokhimiia* **2008**, *73*, 498–503.
60. Ghittoni, R.; Accardi, R.; Hasan, U.; Gheit, T.; Sylla, B.; Tommasino, M. The biological properties of e6 and e7 oncoproteins from human papillomaviruses. *Virus Genes* **2010**, *40*, 1–13.
61. Becker, J.C.; Houben, R.; Ugurel, S.; Trefzer, U.; Pfohler, C.; Schrama, D. Mc polyomavirus is frequently present in merkel cell carcinoma of european patients. *J. Investig. Dermatol.* **2009**, *129*, 248–250.
62. Carter, J.J.; Paulson, K.G.; Wipf, G.C.; Miranda, D.; Madeleine, M.M.; Johnson, L.G.; Lemos, B.D.; Lee, S.; Warcola, A.H.; Iyer, J.G.; *et al.* Association of merkel cell polyomavirus-specific antibodies with merkel cell carcinoma. *J. Natl. Cancer Inst.* **2009**, *101*, 1510–1522.
63. Duncavage, E.J.; Zehnbauer, B.A.; Pfeifer, J.D. Prevalence of merkel cell polyomavirus in merkel cell carcinoma. *Mod. Pathol.* **2009**, *22*, 516–521.
64. Agelli, M.; Clegg, L.X. Epidemiology of primary merkel cell carcinoma in the United States. *J. Am. Acad. Dermatol.* **2003**, *49*, 832–841.
65. Hodgson, N.C. Merkel cell carcinoma: Changing incidence trends. *J. Surg. Oncol.* **2005**, *89*, 1–4.
66. Kassem, A.; Schopflin, A.; Diaz, C.; Weyers, W.; Stickeler, E.; Werner, M.; Zur Hausen, A. Frequent detection of merkel cell polyomavirus in human merkel cell carcinomas and identification of a unique deletion in the vp1 gene. *Cancer Res.* **2008**, *68*, 5009–5013.
67. Kwun, H.J.; Guastafierro, A.; Shuda, M.; Meinke, G.; Bohm, A.; Moore, P.S.; Chang, Y. The minimum replication origin of merkel cell polyomavirus has a unique large t-antigen loading architecture and requires small t-antigen expression for optimal replication. *J. Virol.* **2009**, *83*, 12118–12128.
68. Moens, U.; van Ghelue, M.; Johannessen, M. Oncogenic potentials of the human polyomavirus regulatory proteins. *Cell. Mol. Life Sci.* **2007**, *64*, 1656–1678.
69. Shuda, M.; Arora, R.; Kwun, H.J.; Feng, H.; Sarid, R.; Fernandez-Figueras, M.T.; Tolstov, Y.; Gjoerup, O.; Mansukhani, M.M.; Swerdlow, S.H.; *et al.* Human merkel cell polyomavirus infection i. Mcv t antigen expression in merkel cell carcinoma, lymphoid tissues and lymphoid tumors. *Int. J. Cancer* **2009**, *125*, 1243–1249.
70. Shuda, M.; Feng, H.; Kwun, H.J.; Rosen, S.T.; Gjoerup, O.; Moore, P.S.; Chang, Y. T antigen mutations are a human tumor-specific signature for merkel cell polyomavirus. *Proc. Natl. Acad. Sci. USA* **2008**, *105*, 16272–16277.
71. Houben, R.; Adam, C.; Baeurle, A.; Hesbacher, S.; Grimm, J.; Angermeyer, S.; Henzel, K.; Hauser,

S.; Elling, R.; Brocker, E.B.; *et al.* An intact retinoblastoma protein-binding site in merkel cell polyomavirus large t antigen is required for promoting growth of merkel cell carcinoma cells. *Int. J. Cancer* **2012**, *130*, 847–856.

72. Houben, R.; Shuda, M.; Weinkam, R.; Schrama, D.; Feng, H.; Chang, Y.; Moore, P.S.; Becker, J.C. Merkel cell polyomavirus-infected merkel cell carcinoma cells require expression of viral t antigens. *J. Virol.* **2010**, *84*, 7064–7072.
73. Shuda, M.; Kwun, H.J.; Feng, H.; Chang, Y.; Moore, P.S. Human merkel cell polyomavirus small t antigen is an oncoprotein targeting the 4e-bp1 translation regulator. *J. Clin. Investig.* **2011**, *121*, 3623–3634.
74. Kew, M.C. Epidemiology of chronic hepatitis b virus infection, hepatocellular carcinoma, and hepatitis b virus-induced hepatocellular carcinoma. *Pathol.-Biol.* **2010**, *58*, 273–277.
75. Tarocchi, M.; Polvani, S.; Marroncini, G.; Galli, A. Molecular mechanism of hepatitis b virus-induced hepatocarcinogenesis. *World J. Gastroenterol.* **2014**, *20*, 11630–11640.
76. Sung, W.K.; Zheng, H.; Li, S.; Chen, R.; Liu, X.; Li, Y.; Lee, N.P.; Lee, W.H.; Ariyaratne, P.N.; Tennakoon, C.; *et al.* Genome-wide survey of recurrent hbv integration in hepatocellular carcinoma. *Nat. Genet.* **2012**, *44*, 765–769.
77. Wen, Y.; Golubkov, V.S.; Strongin, A.Y.; Jiang, W.; Reed, J.C. Interaction of hepatitis b viral oncoprotein with cellular target hbxip dysregulates centrosome dynamics and mitotic spindle formation. *J. Biol. Chem.* **2008**, *283*, 2793–2803.
78. Kim, C.M.; Koike, K.; Saito, I.; Miyamura, T.; Jay, G. Hbx gene of hepatitis b virus induces liver cancer in transgenic mice. *Nature* **1991**, *351*, 317–320.
79. Simmonds, P.; Bukh, J.; Combet, C.; Deleage, G.; Enomoto, N.; Feinstone, S.; Halfon, P.; Inchauspe, G.; Kuiken, C.; Maertens, G.; *et al.* Consensus proposals for a unified system of nomenclature of hepatitis c virus genotypes. *Hepatology* **2005**, *42*, 962–973.
80. Tang, H.; Grise, H. Cellular and molecular biology of hcv infection and hepatitis. *Clin. Sci.* **2009**, *117*, 49–65.
81. Morgan, R.L.; Baack, B.; Smith, B.D.; Yartel, A.; Pitasi, M.; Falck-Ytter, Y. Eradication of hepatitis c virus infection and the development of hepatocellular carcinoma: A meta-analysis of observational studies. *Ann. Intern. Med.* **2013**, *158*, 329–337.
82. Moriya, K.; Fujie, H.; Shintani, Y.; Yotsuyanagi, H.; Tsutsumi, T.; Ishibashi, K.; Matsuura, Y.; Kimura, S.; Miyamura, T.; Koike, K. The core protein of hepatitis c virus induces hepatocellular carcinoma in transgenic mice. *Nat. Med.* **1998**, *4*, 1065–1067.
83. Moriya, K.; Yotsuyanagi, H.; Shintani, Y.; Fujie, H.; Ishibashi, K.; Matsuura, Y.; Miyamura, T.; Koike, K. Hepatitis c virus core protein induces hepatic steatosis in transgenic mice. *J. Gen. Virol.* **1997**, *78 (Pt 7)*, 1527–1531.
84. Pei, Y.; Zhang, T.; Renault, V.; Zhang, X. An overview of hepatocellular carcinoma study by omics-based methods. *Acta Biochim. Biophys. Sin.* **2009**, *41*, 1–15.
85. Nunez, O.; Fernandez-Martinez, A.; Majano, P.L.; Apolinario, A.; Gomez-Gonzalo, M.; Benedicto, I.; Lopez-Cabrera, M.; Bosca, L.; Clemente, G.; Garcia-Monzon, C.; *et al.* Increased intrahepatic cyclooxygenase 2, matrix metalloproteinase 2, and matrix metalloproteinase 9 expression is associated with progressive liver disease in chronic hepatitis c virus infection: Role of viral core and ns5a proteins. *Gut* **2004**, *53*, 1665–1672.

86. Murakami, A.; Ohigashi, H. Targeting nox, inos and cox-2 in inflammatory cells: Chemoprevention using food phytochemicals. *Int. J. Cancer* **2007**, *121*, 2357–2363.
87. Ohshima, H.; Tazawa, H.; Sylla, B.S.; Sawa, T. Prevention of human cancer by modulation of chronic inflammatory processes. *Mutat. Res.* **2005**, *591*, 110–122.
88. Fujinaga, H.; Tsutsumi, T.; Yotsuyanagi, H.; Moriya, K.; Koike, K. Hepatocarcinogenesis in hepatitis c: Hcv shrewdly exacerbates oxidative stress by modulating both production and scavenging of reactive oxygen species. *Oncology* **2011**, *81* (Suppl. S1), 11–17.
89. Kannian, P.; Green, P.L. Human t lymphotropic virus type 1 (htlv-1): Molecular biology and oncogenesis. *Viruses* **2010**, *2*, 2037–2077.
90. Proietti, F.A.; Carneiro-Proietti, A.B.; Catalan-Soares, B.C.; Murphy, E.L. Global epidemiology of htlv-i infection and associated diseases. *Oncogene* **2005**, *24*, 6058–6068.
91. Grassmann, R.; Dengler, C.; Muller-Fleckenstein, I.; Fleckenstein, B.; McGuire, K.; Dokhelar, M.C.; Sodroski, J.G.; Haseltine, W.A. Transformation to continuous growth of primary human t lymphocytes by human t-cell leukemia virus type i x-region genes transduced by a herpesvirus saimiri vector. *Proc. Natl. Acad. Sci. USA* **1989**, *86*, 3351–3355.
92. Grassmann, R.; Berchtold, S.; Radant, I.; Alt, M.; Fleckenstein, B.; Sodroski, J.G.; Haseltine, W.A.; Ramstedt, U. Role of human t-cell leukemia virus type 1 x region proteins in immortalization of primary human lymphocytes in culture. *J. Virol.* **1992**, *66*, 4570–4575.
93. Akagi, T.; Shimotohno, K. Proliferative response of tax1-transduced primary human t cells to anti-cd3 antibody stimulation by an interleukin-2-independent pathway. *J. Virol.* **1993**, *67*, 1211–1217.
94. Hasegawa, H.; Sawa, H.; Lewis, M.J.; Orba, Y.; Sheehy, N.; Yamamoto, Y.; Ichinohe, T.; Tsunetsugu-Yokota, Y.; Katano, H.; Takahashi, H.; *et al.* Thymus-derived leukemia-lymphoma in mice transgenic for the tax gene of human t-lymphotropic virus type i. *Nat. Med.* **2006**, *12*, 466–472.
95. Benvenisty, N.; Ornitz, D.M.; Bennett, G.L.; Sahagan, B.G.; Kuo, A.; Cardiff, R.D.; Leder, P. Brain tumours and lymphomas in transgenic mice that carry htlv-i ltr/c-myc and ig/tax genes. *Oncogene* **1992**, *7*, 2399–2405.
96. Azran, I.; Schavinsky-Khrapunsky, Y.; Aboud, M. Role of tax protein in human t-cell leukemia virus type-i leukemogenicity. *Retrovirology* **2004**, *1*, 20.
97. Li, X.H.; Gaynor, R.B. Mechanisms of nf-kappab activation by the htlv type 1 tax protein. *AIDS Res. Hum. Retrovir.* **2000**, *16*, 1583–1590.
98. Harhaj, E.W.; Harhaj, N.S.; Grant, C.; Mostoller, K.; Alefantis, T.; Sun, S.C.; Wigdahl, B. Human t cell leukemia virus type i tax activates cd40 gene expression via the nf-kappa b pathway. *Virology* **2005**, *333*, 145–158.
99. Mori, N.; Fujii, M.; Cheng, G.; Ikeda, S.; Yamasaki, Y.; Yamada, Y.; Tomonaga, M.; Yamamoto, N. Human t-cell leukemia virus type i tax protein induces the expression of anti-apoptotic gene bcl-xl in human t-cells through nuclear factor-kappab and c-amp responsive element binding protein pathways. *Virus Genes* **2001**, *22*, 279–287.
100. Hollstein, M.; Sidransky, D.; Vogelstein, B.; Harris, C.C. P53 mutations in human cancers. *Science* **1991**, *253*, 49–53.
101. Levine, A.J.; Momand, J.; Finlay, C.A. The p53 tumour suppressor gene. *Nature* **1991**, *351*, 453–456.

102. Khidr, L.; Chen, P.L. Rb, the conductor that orchestrates life, death and differentiation. *Oncogene* **2006**, *25*, 5210–5219.

103. Lee, J.M.; Bernstein, A. Apoptosis, cancer and the p53 tumour suppressor gene. *Cancer Metastasis Rev.* **1995**, *14*, 149–161.

104. Amundson, S.A.; Myers, T.G.; Fornace, A.J., Jr. Roles for p53 in growth arrest and apoptosis: Putting on the brakes after genotoxic stress. *Oncogene* **1998**, *17*, 3287–3299.

105. Scheffner, M.; Werness, B.A.; Huibregtse, J.M.; Levine, A.J.; Howley, P.M. The e6 oncoprotein encoded by human papillomavirus types 16 and 18 promotes the degradation of p53. *Cell* **1990**, *63*, 1129–1136.

106. Scheffner, M.; Huibregtse, J.M.; Vierstra, R.D.; Howley, P.M. The hpv-16 e6 and e6-ap complex functions as a ubiquitin-protein ligase in the ubiquitination of p53. *Cell* **1993**, *75*, 495–505.

107. Reznikoff, C.A.; Yeager, T.R.; Belair, C.D.; Savelieva, E.; Puthenveettil, J.A.; Stadler, W.M. Elevated p16 at senescence and loss of p16 at immortalization in human papillomavirus 16 e6, but not e7, transformed human uroepithelial cells. *Cancer Res.* **1996**, *56*, 2886–2890.

108. Dyson, N.; Howley, P.M.; Munger, K.; Harlow, E. The human papilloma virus-16 e7 oncoprotein is able to bind to the retinoblastoma gene product. *Science* **1989**, *243*, 934–937.

109. Giam, C.Z.; Jeang, K.T. Htlv-1 tax and adult t-cell leukemia. *Front. Biosci.: J. Virtual Libr.* **2007**, *12*, 1496–1507.

110. Pise-Masison, C.A.; Brady, J.N. Setting the stage for transformation: Htlv-1 tax inhibition of p53 function. *Front. Biosci.* **2005**, *10*, 919–930.

111. Haller, K.; Wu, Y.; Derow, E.; Schmitt, I.; Jeang, K.T.; Grassmann, R. Physical interaction of human t-cell leukemia virus type 1 tax with cyclin-dependent kinase 4 stimulates the phosphorylation of retinoblastoma protein. *Mol. Cell. Biol.* **2002**, *22*, 3327–3338.

112. Suzuki, T.; Narita, T.; Uchida-Toita, M.; Yoshida, M. Down-regulation of the ink4 family of cyclin-dependent kinase inhibitors by tax protein of htlv-1 through two distinct mechanisms. *Virology* **1999**, *259*, 384–391.

113. Suzuki, T.; Kitao, S.; Matsushime, H.; Yoshida, M. Htlv-1 tax protein interacts with cyclin-dependent kinase inhibitor p16ink4a and counteracts its inhibitory activity towards cdk4. *EMBO J.* **1996**, *15*, 1607–1614.

114. Satou, Y.; Yasunaga, J.; Yoshida, M.; Matsuoka, M. Htlv-i basic leucine zipper factor gene mrna supports proliferation of adult t cell leukemia cells. *Proc. Natl. Acad. Sci. USA* **2006**, *103*, 720–725.

115. Cai, Q.L.; Knight, J.S.; Verma, S.C.; Zald, P.; Robertson, E.S. Ec5s ubiquitin complex is recruited by kshv latent antigen lana for degradation of the vhl and p53 tumor suppressors. *PLoS Pathog.* **2006**, *2*, e116.

116. Friborg, J., Jr.; Kong, W.; Hottiger, M.O.; Nabel, G.J. P53 inhibition by the lana protein of kshv protects against cell death. *Nature* **1999**, *402*, 889–894.

117. Si, H.; Robertson, E.S. Kaposi's sarcoma-associated herpesvirus-encoded latency-associated nuclear antigen induces chromosomal instability through inhibition of p53 function. *J. Virol.* **2006**, *80*, 697–709.

118. Spender, L.C.; Cannell, E.J.; Hollyoake, M.; Wensing, B.; Gawn, J.M.; Brimmell, M.; Packham,

G.; Farrell, P.J. Control of cell cycle entry and apoptosis in b lymphocytes infected by epstein-barr virus. *J. Virol.* **1999**, *73*, 4678–4688.

119. Mei, Y.P.; Zhou, J.M.; Wang, Y.; Huang, H.; Deng, R.; Feng, G.K.; Zeng, Y.X.; Zhu, X.F. Silencing of lmp1 induces cell cycle arrest and enhances chemosensitivity through inhibition of akt signaling pathway in ebv-positive nasopharyngeal carcinoma cells. *Cell Cycle* **2007**, *6*, 1379–1385.
120. Portis, T.; Longnecker, R. Epstein-barr virus (ebv) lmp2a mediates b-lymphocyte survival through constitutive activation of the ras/pi3k/akt pathway. *Oncogene* **2004**, *23*, 8619–8628.
121. Desbien, A.L.; Kappler, J.W.; Marrack, P. The epstein-barr virus bcl-2 homolog, bhrf1, blocks apoptosis by binding to a limited amount of bim. *Proc. Natl. Acad. Sci. USA* **2009**, *106*, 5663–5668.
122. Saggioro, D.; Silic-Benussi, M.; Biasiotto, R.; D'Agostino, D.M.; Ciminale, V. Control of cell death pathways by htlv-1 proteins. *Front. Biosci.* **2009**, *14*, 3338–3351.
123. Underbrink, M.P.; Howie, H.L.; Bedard, K.M.; Koop, J.I.; Galloway, D.A. E6 proteins from multiple human betapapillomavirus types degrade bak and protect keratinocytes from apoptosis after uvb irradiation. *J. Virol.* **2008**, *82*, 10408–10417.
124. Garnett, T.O.; Filippova, M.; Duerksen-Hughes, P.J. Accelerated degradation of fadd and procaspase 8 in cells expressing human papilloma virus 16 e6 impairs trail-mediated apoptosis. *Cell Death Differ.* **2006**, *13*, 1915–1926.
125. Yuan, H.; Fu, F.; Zhuo, J.; Wang, W.; Nishitani, J.; An, D.S.; Chen, I.S.; Liu, X. Human papillomavirus type 16 e6 and e7 oncoproteins upregulate c-iap2 gene expression and confer resistance to apoptosis. *Oncogene* **2005**, *24*, 5069–5078.
126. Filippova, M.; Parkhurst, L.; Duerksen-Hughes, P.J. The human papillomavirus 16 e6 protein binds to fas-associated death domain and protects cells from fas-triggered apoptosis. *J. Biol. Chem.* **2004**, *279*, 25729–25744.
127. Du, J.; Chen, G.G.; Vlantis, A.C.; Chan, P.K.; Tsang, R.K.; van Hasselt, C.A. Resistance to apoptosis of hpv 16-infected laryngeal cancer cells is associated with decreased bak and increased bcl-2 expression. *Cancer Lett.* **2004**, *205*, 81–88.
128. Becker, S.A.; Lee, T.H.; Butel, J.S.; Slagle, B.L. Hepatitis b virus x protein interferes with cellular DNA repair. *J. Virol.* **1998**, *72*, 266–272.
129. Aweya, J.J.; Tan, Y.J. Modulation of programmed cell death pathways by the hepatitis c virus. *Front. Biosci.* **2011**, *16*, 608–618.
130. Plug-DeMaggio, A.W.; Sundsvold, T.; Wurscher, M.A.; Koop, J.I.; Klingelhutz, A.J.; McDougall, J.K. Telomere erosion and chromosomal instability in cells expressing the hpv oncogene 16e6. *Oncogene* **2004**, *23*, 3561–3571.
131. Duensing, S.; Munger, K. The human papillomavirus type 16 e6 and e7 oncoproteins independently induce numerical and structural chromosome instability. *Cancer Res.* **2002**, *62*, 7075–7082.
132. Duensing, S.; Duensing, A.; Crum, C.P.; Munger, K. Human papillomavirus type 16 e7 oncoprotein-induced abnormal centrosome synthesis is an early event in the evolving malignant phenotype. *Cancer Res.* **2001**, *61*, 2356–2360.

133. Duensing, S.; Lee, L.Y.; Duensing, A.; Basile, J.; Piboonniyom, S.; Gonzalez, S.; Crum, C.P.; Munger, K. The human papillomavirus type 16 e6 and e7 oncoproteins cooperate to induce mitotic defects and genomic instability by uncoupling centrosome duplication from the cell division cycle. *Proc. Natl. Acad. Sci. USA* **2000**, *97*, 10002–10007.
134. Chen, J.J. Genomic instability induced by human papillomavirus oncogenes. *North Am. J. Med. Sci.* **2010**, *3*, 43–47.
135. Bornkamm, G.W. Epstein-barr virus and its role in the pathogenesis of burkitt's lymphoma: An unresolved issue. *Semin. Cancer Biol.* **2009**, *19*, 351–365.
136. Heath, E.; Begue-Pastor, N.; Chaganti, S.; Croom-Carter, D.; Shannon-Lowe, C.; Kube, D.; Feederle, R.; Delecluse, H.J.; Rickinson, A.B.; Bell, A.I. Epstein-barr virus infection of naive b cells *in vitro* frequently selects clones with mutated immunoglobulin genotypes: Implications for virus biology. *PLoS Pathog.* **2012**, *8*, e1002697.
137. Marriott, S.J.; Lemoine, F.J.; Jeang, K.T. Damaged DNA and miscounted chromosomes: Human t cell leukemia virus type i tax oncoprotein and genetic lesions in transformed cells. *J. Biomed. Sci.* **2002**, *9*, 292–298.
138. Lemoine, F.J.; Marriott, S.J. Genomic instability driven by the human t-cell leukemia virus type i (htlv-i) oncoprotein, tax. *Oncogene* **2002**, *21*, 7230–7234.
139. Chandhasin, C.; Ducu, R.I.; Berkovich, E.; Kastan, M.B.; Marriott, S.J. Human t-cell leukemia virus type 1 tax attenuates the atm-mediated cellular DNA damage response. *J. Virol.* **2008**, *82*, 6952–6961.
140. Kao, S.Y.; Lemoine, F.J.; Marriott, S.J. P53-independent induction of apoptosis by the htlv-i tax protein following uv irradiation. *Virology* **2001**, *291*, 292–298.
141. Jin, D.Y.; Spencer, F.; Jeang, K.T. Human t cell leukemia virus type 1 oncoprotein tax targets the human mitotic checkpoint protein mad1. *Cell* **1998**, *93*, 81–91.
142. Liu, B.; Hong, S.; Tang, Z.; Yu, H.; Giam, C.Z. Htlv-i tax directly binds the cdc20-associated anaphase-promoting complex and activates it ahead of schedule. *Proc. Natl. Acad. Sci. USA* **2005**, *102*, 63–68.
143. Cohen, S.B.; Graham, M.E.; Lovrecz, G.O.; Bache, N.; Robinson, P.J.; Reddel, R.R. Protein composition of catalytically active human telomerase from immortal cells. *Science* **2007**, *315*, 1850–1853.
144. Terrin, L.; dal Col, J.; Rampazzo, E.; Zancai, P.; Pedrotti, M.; Ammirabile, G.; Bergamin, S.; Rizzo, S.; Dolcetti, R.; de Rossi, A. Latent membrane protein 1 of epstein-barr virus activates the htert promoter and enhances telomerase activity in b lymphocytes. *J. Virol.* **2008**, *82*, 10175–10187.
145. Zhang, X.; Dong, N.; Zhang, H.; You, J.; Wang, H.; Ye, L. Effects of hepatitis b virus x protein on human telomerase reverse transcriptase expression and activity in hepatoma cells. *J. Lab. Clin. Med.* **2005**, *145*, 98–104.
146. Verma, S.C.; Borah, S.; Robertson, E.S. Latency-associated nuclear antigen of kaposi's sarcoma-associated herpesvirus up-regulates transcription of human telomerase reverse transcriptase promoter through interaction with transcription factor sp1. *J. Virol.* **2004**, *78*, 10348–10359.

147. Gewin, L.; Myers, H.; Kiyono, T.; Galloway, D.A. Identification of a novel telomerase repressor that interacts with the human papillomavirus type-16 e6/e6-ap complex. *Genes Dev.* **2004**, *18*, 2269–2282.
148. Chen, X.; Kamranvar, S.A.; Masucci, M.G. Tumor viruses and replicative immortality—Avoiding the telomere hurdle. *Semin. Cancer Biol.* **2014**, *26*, 43–51.
149. Ohashi, M.; Sakurai, M.; Higuchi, M.; Mori, N.; Fukushi, M.; Oie, M.; Coffey, R.J.; Yoshiura, K.; Tanaka, Y.; Uchiyama, M.; *et al.* Human t-cell leukemia virus type 1 tax oncoprotein induces and interacts with a multi-pdz domain protein, magi-3. *Virology* **2004**, *320*, 52–62.
150. Glaunsinger, B.A.; Lee, S.S.; Thomas, M.; Banks, L.; Javier, R. Interactions of the pdz-protein magi-1 with adenovirus e4-orf1 and high-risk papillomavirus e6 oncoproteins. *Oncogene* **2000**, *19*, 5270–5280.
151. Rousset, R.; Fabre, S.; Desbois, C.; Bantignies, F.; Jalinot, P. The c-terminus of the htlv-1 tax oncoprotein mediates interaction with the pdz domain of cellular proteins. *Oncogene* **1998**, *16*, 643–654.
152. Lee, S.S.; Weiss, R.S.; Javier, R.T. Binding of human virus oncoproteins to hdlg/sap97, a mammalian homolog of the drosophila discs large tumor suppressor protein. *Proc. Natl. Acad. Sci. USA* **1997**, *94*, 6670–6675.
153. Spanos, W.C.; Hoover, A.; Harris, G.F.; Wu, S.; Strand, G.L.; Anderson, M.E.; Klingelhutz, A.J.; Hendriks, W.; Bossler, A.D.; Lee, J.H. The pdz binding motif of human papillomavirus type 16 e6 induces ptpn13 loss, which allows anchorage-independent growth and synergizes with ras for invasive growth. *J. Virol.* **2008**, *82*, 2493–2500.
154. Spanos, W.C.; Geiger, J.; Anderson, M.E.; Harris, G.F.; Bossler, A.D.; Smith, R.B.; Klingelhutz, A.J.; Lee, J.H. Deletion of the pdz motif of hpv16 e6 preventing immortalization and anchorage-independent growth in human tonsil epithelial cells. *Head Neck* **2008**, *30*, 139–147.
155. Xie, L.; Yamamoto, B.; Haoudi, A.; Semmes, O.J.; Green, P.L. Pdz binding motif of htlv-1 tax promotes virus-mediated t-cell proliferation *in vitro* and persistence *in vivo*. *Blood* **2006**, *107*, 1980–1988.
156. Hirata, A.; Higuchi, M.; Niinuma, A.; Ohashi, M.; Fukushi, M.; Oie, M.; Akiyama, T.; Tanaka, Y.; Gejyo, F.; Fujii, M. Pdz domain-binding motif of human t-cell leukemia virus type 1 tax oncoprotein augments the transforming activity in a rat fibroblast cell line. *Virology* **2004**, *318*, 327–336.
157. Bartel, D.P. Micrornas: Genomics, biogenesis, mechanism, and function. *Cell* **2004**, *116*, 281–297.
158. Lewis, B.P.; Burge, C.B.; Bartel, D.P. Conserved seed pairing, often flanked by adenosines, indicates that thousands of human genes are microrna targets. *Cell* **2005**, *120*, 15–20.
159. Calin, G.A.; Croce, C.M. Microrna signatures in human cancers. *Nat. Rev. Cancer* **2006**, *6*, 857–866.
160. Lu, J.; Getz, G.; Miska, E.A.; Alvarez-Saavedra, E.; Lamb, J.; Peck, D.; Sweet-Cordero, A.; Ebert, B.L.; Mak, R.H.; Ferrando, A.A.; *et al.* Microrna expression profiles classify human cancers. *Nature* **2005**, *435*, 834–838.
161. Cai, X.; Schafer, A.; Lu, S.; Bilello, J.P.; Desrosiers, R.C.; Edwards, R.; Raab-Traub, N.; Cullen, B.R. Epstein-barr virus micrornas are evolutionarily conserved and differentially expressed. *PLoS Pathog.* **2006** *2*, e23.

162. Pfeffer, S.; Zavolan, M.; Grasser, F.A.; Chien, M.; Russo, J.J.; Ju, J.; John, B.; Enright, A.J.; Marks, D.; Sander, C.; *et al.* Identification of virus-encoded micrornas. *Science* **2004**, *304*, 734–736.
163. Choy, E.Y.; Siu, K.L.; Kok, K.H.; Lung, R.W.; Tsang, C.M.; To, K.F.; Kwong, D.L.; Tsao, S.W.; Jin, D.Y. An epstein-barr virus-encoded microrna targets puma to promote host cell survival. *J. Exp. Med.* **2008**, *205*, 2551–2560.
164. Dolken, L.; Malterer, G.; Erhard, F.; Kothe, S.; Friedel, C.C.; Suffert, G.; Marcinowski, L.; Motsch, N.; Barth, S.; Beitzinger, M.; *et al.* Systematic analysis of viral and cellular microrna targets in cells latently infected with human gamma-herpesviruses by risc immunoprecipitation assay. *Cell Host Microbe* **2010**, *7*, 324–334.
165. Marquitz, A.R.; Mathur, A.; Nam, C.S.; Raab-Traub, N. The epstein-barr virus bart micrornas target the pro-apoptotic protein bim. *Virology* **2011**, *412*, 392–400.
166. Marquitz, A.R.; Raab-Traub, N. The role of mirnas and ebv barts in npc. *Semin. Cancer Biol.* **2012**, *22*, 166–172.
167. Marquitz, A.R.; Mathur, A.; Shair, K.H.; Raab-Traub, N. Infection of epstein-barr virus in a gastric carcinoma cell line induces anchorage independence and global changes in gene expression. *Proc. Natl. Acad. Sci. USA* **2012**, *109*, 9593–9598.
168. Blattner, W.A. Human retroviruses: Their role in cancer. *Proc. Assoc. Am. Phys.* **1999**, *111*, 563–572.
169. Kim, H.H.; van den Heuvel, A.P.; Schmidt, J.W.; Ross, S.R. Novel common integration sites targeted by mouse mammary tumor virus insertion in mammary tumors have oncogenic activity. *PLoS One* **2011**, *6*, e27425.
170. Sourvinos, G.; Tsatsanis, C.; Spandidos, D.A. Mechanisms of retrovirus-induced oncogenesis. *Folia Biol.* **2000**, *46*, 226–232.
171. Chimal-Ramirez, G.K.; Espinoza-Sanchez, N.A.; Fuentes-Panana, E.M. Protumor activities of the immune response: Insights in the mechanisms of immunological shift, oncotraining, and oncopromotion. *J. Oncol.* **2013**, *2013*, 835956.
172. Elinav, E.; Nowarski, R.; Thaiss, C.A.; Hu, B.; Jin, C.; Flavell, R.A. Inflammation-induced cancer: Crosstalk between tumours, immune cells and microorganisms. *Nat. Rev. Cancer* **2013**, *13*, 759–771.
173. Schistosomes, Liver Flukes and Helicobacter Pylori. Iarc working group on the evaluation of carcinogenic risks to humans. Lyon, 7–14 June 1994. *IARC Monogr. Eval. Carcinog. Risks Hum.* **1994**, *61*, 1–241.
174. Fuentes-Panana, E.; Camorlinga-Ponce, M.; Maldonado-Bernal, C. Infection, inflammation and gastric cancer. *Salud Publica Mex.* **2009**, *51*, 427–433.
175. Kusters, J.G.; van Vliet, A.H.; Kuipers, E.J. Pathogenesis of *Helicobacter pylori* infection. *Clin. Microbiol. Rev.* **2006**, *19*, 449–490.
176. Xu, J.; Yin, Z.; Cao, S.; Gao, W.; Liu, L.; Yin, Y.; Liu, P.; Shu, Y. Systematic review and meta-analysis on the association between il-1b polymorphisms and cancer risk. *PLoS One* **2013**, *8*, e63654.
177. Xue, H.; Lin, B.; Ni, P.; Xu, H.; Huang, G. Interleukin-1b and interleukin-1 rn polymorphisms and gastric carcinoma risk: A meta-analysis. *J. Gastroenterol. Hepatol.* **2010** *25*, 1604–1617.

178. Crusius, J.B.; Canzian, F.; Capella, G.; Pena, A.S.; Pera, G.; Sala, N.; Agudo, A.; Rico, F.; Del Giudice, G.; Palli, D.; *et al.* Cytokine gene polymorphisms and the risk of adenocarcinoma of the stomach in the european prospective investigation into cancer and nutrition (epic-eurgast). *Ann. Oncol.* **2008**, *19*, 1894–1902.

179. Cheng, D.; Hao, Y.; Zhou, W.; Ma, Y. Positive association between interleukin-8 -251a>t polymorphism and susceptibility to gastric carcinogenesis: A meta-analysis. *Cancer Cell Int.* **2013**, *13*, 100.

180. Poli, G. Pathogenesis of liver fibrosis: Role of oxidative stress. *Mol. Asp. Med.* **2000**, *21*, 49–98.

181. Cardenas-Mondragon, M.G.; Carreon-Talavera, R.; Camorlinga-Ponce, M.; Gomez-Delgado, A.; Torres, J.; Fuentes-Panana, E.M. Epstein barr virus and helicobacter pylori co-infection are positively associated with severe gastritis in pediatric patients. *PLoS One* **2013**, *8*, e62850.

182. Cárdenas-Mondragón, M.; Carreón-Talavera, R.; Flores-Luna, L.; Camorlinga-Ponce, M.; Gómez-Delgado, A.; Torres, J.; Fuentes-Pananá, E. Epstein barr virus reactivation is an important trigger of gastric inflammation and progression to intestinal type gastric cancer. In Proceedings of the Epstein Barr Virus 50th Anniversary Conference, Keble College, Oxford, UK, 23–25 March, 2014.

183. Bernstein, W.B.; Little, R.F.; Wilson, W.H.; Yarchoan, R. Acquired immunodeficiency syndrome-related malignancies in the era of highly active antiretroviral therapy. *Int. J. Hematol.* **2006**, *84*, 3–11.

184. Young, L.S.; Murray, P.G. Epstein-barr virus and oncogenesis: From latent genes to tumours. *Oncogene* **2003**, *22*, 5108–5121.

185. Young, L.; Alfieri, C.; Hennessy, K.; Evans, H.; O'Hara, C.; Anderson, K.C.; Ritz, J.; Shapiro, R.S.; Rickinson, A.; Kieff, E.; *et al.* Expression of epstein-barr virus transformation-associated genes in tissues of patients with ebv lymphoproliferative disease. *N. Engl. J. Med.* **1989**, *321*, 1080–1085.

186. Nourse, J.P.; Jones, K.; Gandhi, M.K. Epstein-barr virus-related post-transplant lymphoproliferative disorders: Pathogenetic insights for targeted therapy. *Am. J. Transplant.* **2011**, *11*, 888–895.

187. Gandhi, M.K.; Wilkie, G.M.; Dua, U.; Mollee, P.N.; Grimmett, K.; Williams, T.; Whitaker, N.; Gill, D.; Crawford, D.H. Immunity, homing and efficacy of allogeneic adoptive immunotherapy for posttransplant lymphoproliferative disorders. *Am. J. Transplant.* **2007**, *7*, 1293–1299.

188. Haque, T.; Wilkie, G.M.; Jones, M.M.; Higgins, C.D.; Urquhart, G.; Wingate, P.; Burns, D.; McAulay, K.; Turner, M.; Bellamy, C.; *et al.* Allogeneic cytotoxic t-cell therapy for ebv-positive posttransplantation lymphoproliferative disease: Results of a phase 2 multicenter clinical trial. *Blood* **2007**, *110*, 1123–1131.

189. Michaelis, M.; Doerr, H.W.; Cinatl, J. The story of human cytomegalovirus and cancer: Increasing evidence and open questions. *Neoplasia* **2009**, *11*, 1–9.

190. Boldogh, I.; Huang, E.S.; Rady, P.; Arany, I.; Tyring, S.; Albrecht, T. Alteration in the coding potential and expression of h-ras in human cytomegalovirus-transformed cells. *Intervirology* **1994**, *37*, 321–329.

191. Geder, K.M.; Lausch, R.; O'Neill, F.; Rapp, F. Oncogenic transformation of human embryo lung cells by human cytomegalovirus. *Science* **1976**, *192*, 1134–1137.

192. Geder, L.; Kreider, J.; Rapp, F. Human cells transformed *in vitro* by human cytomegalovirus: Tumorigenicity in athymic nude mice. *J. Natl. Cancer Inst.* **1977**, *58*, 1003–1009.

193. Geder, L.; Laychock, A.M.; Gorodecki, J.; Rapp, F. Alterations in biological properties of different lines of cytomegalorivus-transformed human embryo lung cells following *in vitro* cultivation. *IARC Sci. Publ.* **1978**, *24*, 591–601.

194. Cinatl, J.; Scholz, M.; Kotchetkov, R.; Vogel, J.U.; Doerr, H.W. Molecular mechanisms of the modulatory effects of hcmv infection in tumor cell biology. *Trends Mol. Med.* **2004**, *10*, 19–23.

195. Scheurer, M.E.; Bondy, M.L.; Aldape, K.D.; Albrecht, T.; El-Zein, R. Detection of human cytomegalovirus in different histological types of gliomas. *Acta Neuropathol.* **2008**, *116*, 79–86.

196. Cobbs, C.S.; Soroceanu, L.; Denham, S.; Zhang, W.; Kraus, M.H. Modulation of oncogenic phenotype in human glioma cells by cytomegalovirus ie1-mediated mitogenicity. *Cancer Res.* **2008**, *68*, 724–730.

197. Maussang, D.; Verzijl, D.; van Walsum, M.; Leurs, R.; Holl, J.; Pleskoff, O.; Michel, D.; van Dongen, G.A.; Smit, M.J. Human cytomegalovirus-encoded chemokine receptor us28 promotes tumorigenesis. *Proc. Natl. Acad. Sci. USA* **2006**, *103*, 13068–13073.

198. Vallat, L.; Benhamou, Y.; Gutierrez, M.; Ghillani, P.; Hercher, C.; Thibault, V.; Charlotte, F.; Piette, J.C.; Poynard, T.; Merle-Beral, H.; *et al.* Clonal b cell populations in the blood and liver of patients with chronic hepatitis c virus infection. *Arthritis Rheum.* **2004**, *50*, 3668–3678.

199. Quinn, E.R.; Chan, C.H.; Hadlock, K.G.; Foung, S.K.; Flint, M.; Levy, S. The b-cell receptor of a hepatitis c virus (hcv)-associated non-hodgkin lymphoma binds the viral e2 envelope protein, implicating hcv in lymphomagenesis. *Blood* **2001**, *98*, 3745–3749.

200. Chan, C.H.; Hadlock, K.G.; Foung, S.K.; Levy, S. V(h)1–69 gene is preferentially used by hepatitis c virus-associated b cell lymphomas and by normal b cells responding to the e2 viral antigen. *Blood* **2001**, *97*, 1023–1026.

201. Hermine, O.; Lefrere, F.; Bronowicki, J.P.; Mariette, X.; Jondeau, K.; Eclache-Saudreau, V.; Delmas, B.; Valensi, F.; Cacoub, P.; Brechot, C.; *et al.* Regression of splenic lymphoma with villous lymphocytes after treatment of hepatitis c virus infection. *N. Engl. J. Med.* **2002**, *347*, 89–94.

202. Zullo, A.; Hassan, C.; Cristofari, F.; Andriani, A.; de Francesco, V.; Ierardi, E.; Tomao, S.; Stolte, M.; Morini, S.; Vaira, D. Effects of helicobacter pylori eradication on early stage gastric mucosa-associated lymphoid tissue lymphoma. *Clin. Gastroenterol. Hepatol.* **2010**, *8*, 105–110.

203. Skinner, G.R. Transformation of primary hamster embryo fibroblasts by type 2 simplex virus: Evidence for a "hit and run" mechanism. *Br. J. Exp. Pathol.* **1976**, *57*, 361–376.

204. Birdwell, C.E.; Queen, K.J.; Kilgore, P.C.; Rollyson, P.; Trutschl, M.; Cvek, U.; Scott, R.S. Genome-wide DNA methylation as an epigenetic consequence of epstein-barr virus infection of immortalized keratinocytes. *J. Virol.* **2014**, *88*, 11442–11458.

205. Burns, M.B.; Temiz, N.A.; Harris, R.S. Evidence for apobec3b mutagenesis in multiple human cancers. *Nat. Genet.* **2013**, *45*, 977–983.

9

The Role of the DNA Damage Response throughout the Papillomavirus Life Cycle

Caleb C. McKinney †, Katherine L. Hussmann † and Alison A. McBride *

Laboratory of Viral Diseases, National Institute of Allergy and Infectious Diseases, National Institutes of Health, Bethesda, MD 20892, USA; E-Mails: caleb.mckinney@nih.gov (C.C.M.); katherine.hussmann@nih.gov (K.L.H.)

† These authors contributed equally to this work.

* Author to whom correspondence should be addressed; E-Mail: amcbride@nih.gov;

Academic Editor: Joanna Parish

Abstract: The DNA damage response (DDR) maintains genomic integrity through an elaborate network of signaling pathways that sense DNA damage and recruit effector factors to repair damaged DNA. DDR signaling pathways are usurped and manipulated by the replication programs of many viruses. Here, we review the papillomavirus (PV) life cycle, highlighting current knowledge of how PVs recruit and engage the DDR to facilitate productive infection.

Keywords: HPV; papillomavirus; replication; DNA damage response; homologous recombination; keratinocyte; replication foci; DNA repair; partitioning; episome

---

1. Introduction

Papillomaviruses (PVs) are an ancient group of small, double-stranded (ds) DNA viruses that infect the highly adapted niche of the stratified epithelium of the skin or mucosa in specific host species. Although HPV infection can be asymptomatic, HPVs are also the etiological agent of a wide range of benign papillomas or warts [1]. A subset of HPVs cause infections that can transition to cancer after long-term, persistent infection [2,3]. As the causative agent of over 99% of cervical cancers and an increasing number of anogenital and oropharyngeal cancers, HPVs remain a serious health threat [4].

There are several hundred different PVs that infect a multitude of individual host species, yet the basic genomic scheme and life cycle strategy of each virus are remarkably consistent. Each virus contains a small dsDNA circular genome of approximately 8 kb that encodes just six to eight genes [5] (Figure 1).

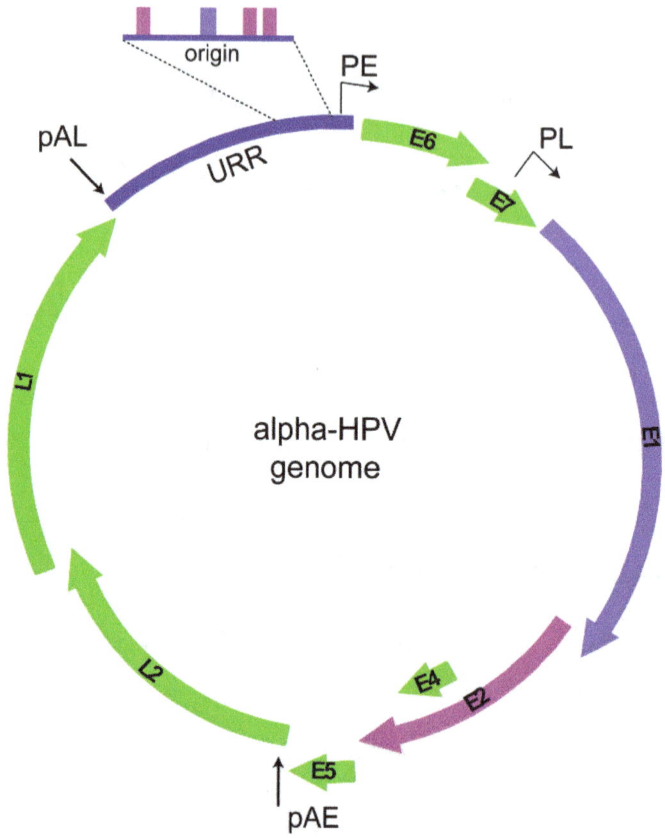

Figure 1. Viral genome. The circular dsDNA genome of an alpha-HPV genome is shown. Viral open reading frames are depicted as curved arrows. The URR (upstream regulatory region) is expanded to show the replication origin containing binding sites for the E2 protein (magenta boxes) and the E1 binding site (purple rectangle) are shown. The early promoter (PE), late promoter (PL) and early and late polyadenylation sites (pAE and pAL) are indicated.

Because of this limited coding capacity, PVs retain a strict dependence on host factors for viral replication [6]. Elucidation of the different replication mechanisms of HPV could identify novel targets that may prove effective in the development of therapies for preexisting HPV infections, where the multivalent vaccines are not readily useful. Recent studies have shown that the DNA damage response and repair (DDR) machinery is necessary for efficient HPV replication. Here, we review the mechanisms of genome replication in the HPV life cycle and summarize how the virus recruits and engages the DDR to facilitate viral DNA synthesis.

2. Replication Phases in the Papillomavirus Life Cycle

2.1. Overview of Phases of Replication in Papillomavirus Infection

Upon initial infection of cells in the basal epithelium, the HPV genome enters the nucleus and undergoes a limited number of rounds of DNA replication to establish a low copy number of genomes per infected cell. Subsequently, when the infected cells in the basal layer replicate and divide, the HPV genome replicates in synchrony as extrachromosomal elements tethered to the host genome. When these infected cells detach from the basement membrane and enter the suprabasal epithelial layer as part of the differentiation process, the HPV E6 and E7 proteins promote unscheduled cell cycle progression by manipulating cell cycle regulation and cellular differentiation programs (see Figure 2). As cells continue to advance through the epithelial layer, there is a switch in the mode of genome replication to productive viral DNA amplification concomitant with increased levels of the E1 and E2 replication proteins. In the terminally differentiated layers of the epithelium, L1 and L2, the viral capsid proteins, are synthesized, and viral particles are assembled.

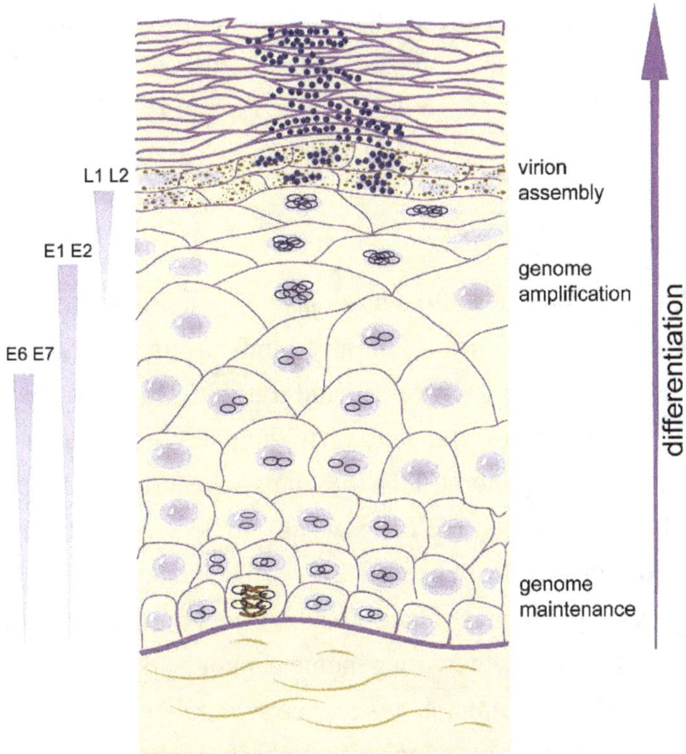

Figure 2. Model of a stratified epithelium. The layers of epithelium shown from bottom to top are stratum basale (with a mitotic cell), stratum spinosum, stratum granulosum (with brown keratohyalin granules), and stratum corneum. The dividing cells in the lowest layer of the epithelium maintain the viral genome as a plasmid (dark blue circles). As these cells progress upwards during the process of differentiation, viral genomes are amplified and packaged in viral particles (dark blue particles). The levels of viral proteins also increase with differentiation as shown on the left.

2.2. HPV Replication Proteins

The relatively small intrinsic coding capacity of HPV genomes warrants exquisite dependence on host factors, as well as viral factors, for replication. HPV encodes two proteins directly involved in replication: E1, a replicative helicase, and E2, a multifunctional protein that recruits E1 to the replication origin of the viral genome [7–9]. The replication origin, located in the Upstream Regulatory Region (URR) of the viral genome, contains binding sites for both E1 and E2 proteins [9]. In cooperation with E2, E1 binds specifically to the replication origin of HPV, but E2 is then displaced and E1 converts to a double hexamer that unwinds the DNA in an ATP-dependent manner [10]. The host DNA replication machinery is then recruited to synthesize the viral DNA. Both E1 and E2 are required for initial amplification and establishment of viral DNA and late vegetative replication [11]. However, in certain circumstances, E1 is dispensable for maintenance replication [11,12].

Additional HPV proteins are required to maintain an environment conducive to viral replication. The oncogenic HPV E6 and E7 proteins promote cellular proliferation, delay cellular differentiation, and promote immune evasion (reviewed in [2]). Both E6 and E7 are required for productive replication [13–15] and it was long thought that E6 and E7 were required to sustain differentiated cells in a pseudo-S phase to provide access to host DNA replication machinery. However, in a stratified epithelium, the differentiated cells that amplify viral genomes are in a G2 like phase that is also dependent on E7 expression [16,17]. As described below, E6 and E7 play essential roles in modulating the cellular DDR for viral replication.

2.3. Initial Amplification and Establishment

HPVs infect the dividing keratinocytes of the basal layer by entering the stratified epithelium through a microabrasion (reviewed in [18]). Virions initially bind through interactions with heparin sulfate proteoglycans [19], and the viral capsid is processed and trafficked through the endosomal pathway. The minor capsid protein, L2, is bound to the viral genome within the virion and, once the virion is processed through the endosome, delivers the genome into the nucleus where it localizes to ND10 bodies [20]. Nuclear access most likely occurs in mitotic cells, where nuclear envelope breakdown allows nuclear access, rather than entry through a nuclear pore [21,22].

Once in the nucleus, the viral genome replicates to a low level number of copies per cell. The genome copy number in the basal cells is low, as the viral genome cannot be detected by *in situ* techniques during this stage [23,24]. The infected cell maintains this low copy number as the viral DNA replicates during subsequent cell divisions in the maintenance replication phase (Figure 3).

A time course of HPV31 infection in HaCaT cells demonstrated that spliced messages which could encode E1 and E2 were present just four hours post-infection [25], consistent with the requirement of E1 and E2 for initial replication. Other viral transcripts appear at eight hours post-infection [25]. The E8^E2 transcript was also detected at four hours post-infection and this is very consistent with its role as a repressor of viral transcription and replication [26]. Expression of E8^E2 at this stage of infection could temper runaway replication and promote the switch to maintenance replication.

2.4. Maintenance Replication and Persistence

During the maintenance phase of replication, the viral genome is replicated in S-phase along with the host genome. Initial evidence using bovine papillomavirus type 1 (BPV1) suggested that viral genome replication is licensed during the maintenance phase [27,28], but later studies demonstrated that in S-phase cells, replication is by a random choice mechanism, whereby some genomes undergo multiple rounds of replication and others remain unreplicated [29,30]. A more recent study of cell lines maintaining HPV genomes revealed that, depending on the HPV type and cell line, both replication mechanisms could be detected in dividing cells [31]. High levels of E1 expression promoted random choice replication, which likely represents the unscheduled DNA synthesis characteristic of vegetative amplification [31].

The level of replication must be tightly controlled during the maintenance phase of the viral life cycle and this may occur via several mechanisms. The E1 protein is retained in the cytoplasm of cells that are not undergoing S-phase [32,33] and in certain circumstances the E1 protein might even be dispensable for maintenance replication [11,12]. The E8^E2 transcriptional repressor tightly regulates both transcription and replication and is required to regulate maintenance replication [26,34]. HPVs also regulate microRNA 145, which in turn binds to the E1 and E2 genes and down-regulates their expression [35]. In BPV1, E2 is a limiting factor in maintenance replication and phosphorylation of the E2 protein regulates its stability and modulates genome copy number in dividing cells [36].

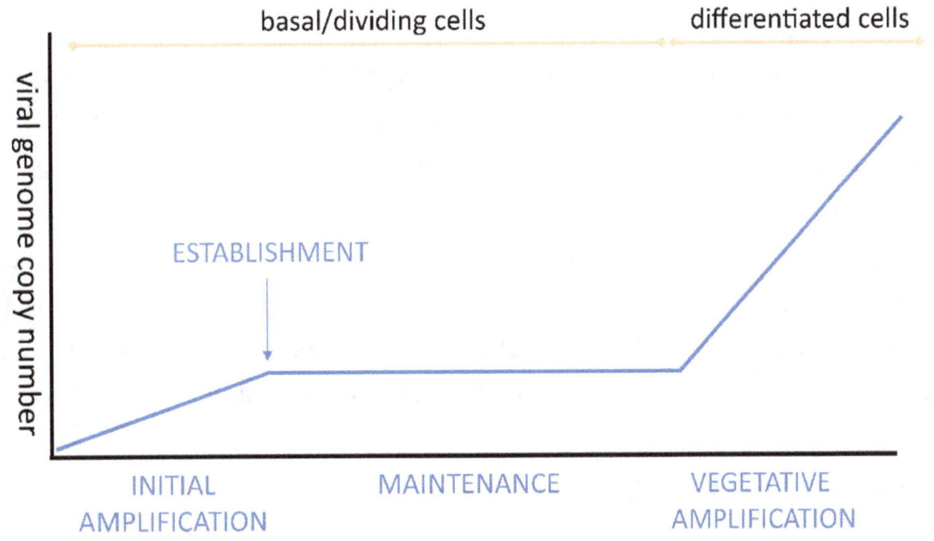

Figure 3. Viral Genome Copy Number during the Different Phases of Replication.

For HPV to persist in dividing cells, not only must the viral genomes be replicated in synchrony with host DNA, but nascent genomes must be efficiently partitioned to daughter cells. The partitioning model, best defined for BPV1, is that the E2 protein binds to multiple E2 binding motifs within the viral URR and tethers the viral genome to host chromatin, thus ensuring it is perpetuated within the basal layer of cells [37–39]. While this model likely applies to all PVs, it is probable that there are differences in the details [40]. For example, most HPVs do not have the large number of E2 binding sites found in BPV1 (and other delta PVs) and all PV E2 proteins do not bind tightly to host mitotic chromatin [41]. Nevertheless, the tethering strategy is likely to be universal for all PVs, as a similar mechanism is used by other persistent viruses that maintain their genomes as extrachromosomal plasmids.

Attachment of PV genomes to host chromatin is important for more than just partitioning of genomes to daughter cells because tethering to active, inactive or even genetically unstable regions of host chromatin could have important outcomes for the infection [42–44]. Extensive studies of the E2 protein have shown its interaction with several well characterized proteins involved in replication, transcription, and host cell cycle regulation [45] and reviewed in [46], and several proteins have been proposed to be the chromatin target responsible for partitioning the E2-PVgenome complex (reviewed in [46]). One of the best-studied (and most debated) targets is BRD4, a chromatin adaptor protein essential for transcriptional initiation and elongation, as well as mitotic bookmarking of host chromatin (reviewed in [47,48]). E2 binds to BRD4 and stabilizes its association with host chromatin [49–51], and BRD4 is a key regulator of PV transcription [52–56]. However, the role of BRD4 in the partitioning of the alpha-PV genomes seems to be more complex since these E2 proteins bind with lower affinity to BRD4 (and to host chromatin) [45,52]. Alpha-E2s and BRD4 are not observed on host mitotic chromosomes under conditions in which other E2 proteins are readily detected; however, the HPV16 E2-BRD4 complex has recently been discovered on chromosomes by bimolecular fluorescence complementation [57] or when E2 is expressed as a GFP-fusion protein [58]. However, HPV31 genomes that encode an E2 protein defective for BRD4 binding are maintained in stable cell lines [59,60], suggesting either that BRD4 is not essential for genome maintenance of all HPV strains, or that the interaction of BRD4 and E2 is more complex in the background of a viral infection. Accordingly, there is evidence that the latter situation is true, since BRD4 is associated with replication foci formed both by E1 and E2 overexpression and in HPV31 genome-containing differentiated cells [61–63]. In the latter situation BRD4 surrounds the replication foci in a satellite pattern [61], but its exact mechanistic role is not clear. BRD4 could facilitate viral transcription in replication factories, could directly function in replication, or might interface with components of the DDR. There are hints that BRD4 might function in the DDR; it interacts with the DDR associated RFC1 subunit, ATAD5 [53], a minor isoform of BRD4 protects adjacent chromatin from DNA damage signaling [64], and we find that BRD4 is associated with aphidicolin inducible fragile sites in C-33A cells [43,64]. Thus, BRD4, and possibly other host proteins required for maintenance replication, may play complex roles during the transition from maintenance replication to vegetative amplification.

2.5. Differentiation-Dependent Viral DNA Amplification

The third phase of HPV replication is tightly linked to the differentiation program of the stratified epithelium. HPVs must transition out of maintenance phase to induce high level viral DNA synthesis, late gene expression, and production and perpetuation of infectious particles. As proliferating cells that harbor HPV genomes transition through the differentiation process, the late promoter is activated, high levels of the E1 and E2 proteins are expressed and the mode of viral genome replication switches to support productive viral genome amplification (Figures 2 and 3 and [65]). Using laser microdissection to analyze viral genome copy number of OcPV1 (ROPV; rabbit oral papillomavirus) in the stratified layers of oral lesions, Maglennon *et al.* demonstrate a five log amplification of viral DNA in the superficial layers compared to the basal layers [66].

The exact mechanism of genome amplification has not been elucidated, but there has long been evidence that it might differ from the bidirectional theta mode characteristic of maintenance replication [67,68]. A breakthrough in the study of HPV replication was the observation that differentiation-dependent genome amplification required the cellular ATM DNA damage response and repair (DDR) pathway [69]. This finding opened up the possibility that genomes might be amplified in differentiated cells by a recombination-dependent replication mode supported by the DDR response.

The remainder of this review will focus on recent developments that uncover how HPV contests and hijacks the carefully crafted DDR network to recruit, engage, and manipulate the host DDR machinery for viral DNA replication at various stages of the life cycle.

3. Role of the DNA Damage Response (DDR) in HPV Replication

3.1. DNA Damage Response Overview

Cellular DNA constantly sustains endogenous and exogenous insults that result in mutations, crosslinks and single and double stranded breaks [70]. However, cells have evolved an elaborate pathway to correct these lesions known as the DNA damage and repair response (DDR) (Figure 4 and reviewed in [71]). The DDR consists of sensors, such as the MRE11-Rad50-Nbs1 complex (MRN) or replication protein A (RPA), that detect a wide range of DNA lesions and recruit the Ataxia telangiectasia mutated (ATM) and Ataxia telangiectasia and Rad3 related (ATR) transducer kinases to the site of damage. With the help of mediator proteins, these transducer kinases induce a signaling cascade through the effector kinases Chk1 and Chk2, activating cell cycle checkpoints to prevent cell cycle progression and ultimately recruiting the DNA repair machinery to the damaged DNA. Once the damage is repaired, the checkpoints are mitigated and cells return to their normal state. However, extensive DNA damage may warrant the initiation of cellular death pathways (Figure 4).

Some of the most severe types of damage are dsDNA breaks that result from ionizing radiation, replication stress, reactive metabolic intermediates, or exogenous chemicals and result in activation of the ATM pathway. dsDNA breaks are bound by the MRN complex that both bridges the gap and activates the ATM signaling cascade. This results in activation of a Chk2 dependent cell cycle checkpoint. dsDNA breaks can be repaired either through the low fidelity, non-homologous end joining (NHEJ) pathway or the high fidelity, homologous recombination (HR) pathway. In HR, a section of DNA adjacent to the 5′end of the break is resectioned by an exonuclease complex recruited by the MRN complex. This ssDNA becomes coated with Rad51 and invades the undamaged sister chromatid, which is used to provide a template for DNA synthesis to faithfully restore the sequence on the damaged strand. Since a homologous DNA sequence is required for proper repair, HR is restricted to S and G2 phases of the cell cycle, when a homologous sister chromatid is present to provide a template.

ATR is activated in response to the presence of persistent ssDNA that results from replication stress. RPA (replication protein A) binds this ssDNA and recruits ATRIP (ATR interacting partner) and ATR. The ring-shaped 9-1-1 complex (consisting of Rad9, Hus1, Rad1) is loaded onto collapsed replication forks and recruits TopBP1 (Topoisomerase II-binding protein 1), a multifaceted factor essential for maintaining genomic stability and facilitating DNA replication by recruiting replication factors to replication forks. 9-1-1 further enlists claspin, which recruits the kinase, Chk1. ATR-dependent phosphorylation of Chk1 activates a cell cycle checkpoint and facilitates stabilization of replication forks. The DDR pathway not only functions to accurately repair DNA, but must also regulate the cell cycle, pausing it to allow repair to be completed. The DDR activates specific downstream cell cycle checkpoints during each phase of the cell cycle to maintain DNA integrity. For example, a DDR mediated increase in stability of p53 can lead to increased expression of CDK inhibitor p21, which arrests cells in G1. Likewise, Chk1 and Chk2 phosphorylation inhibits Cdc25 family members, which are important for progression at several stages of the cell cycle (reviewed in [72]).

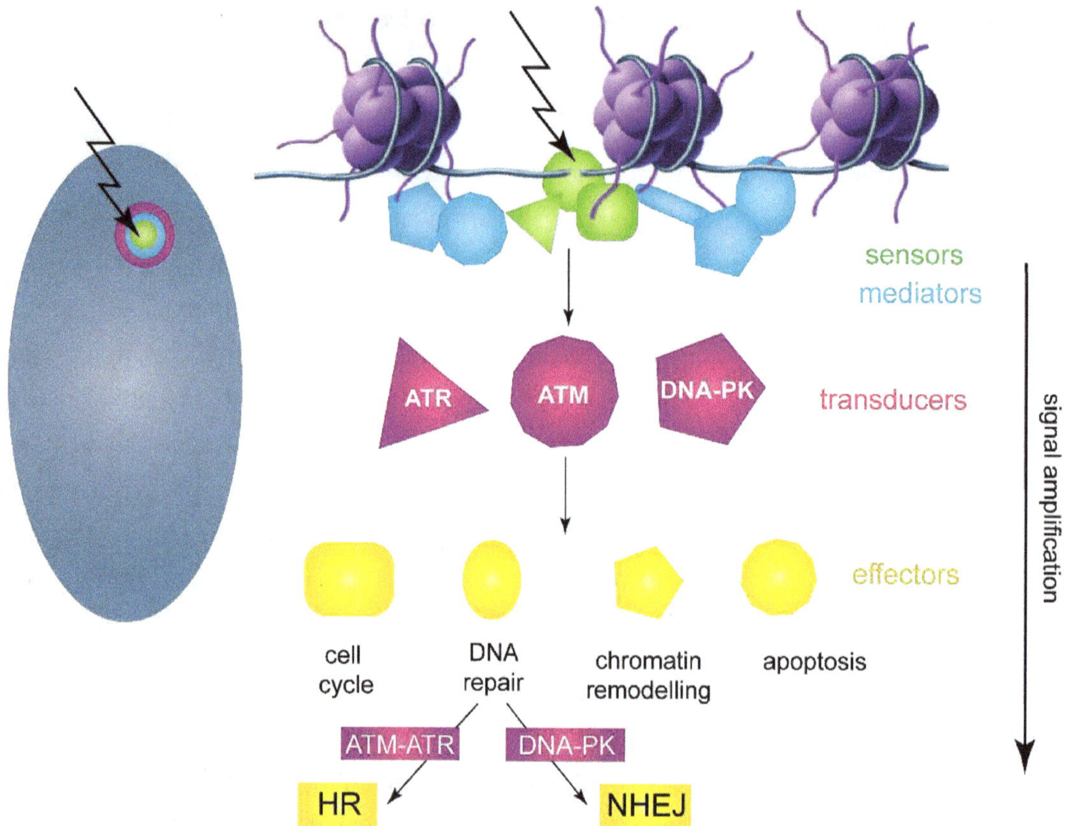

Figure 4. Diagram of the DNA Damage and Repair Response Pathway. DNA breaks or collapsed replication forks are detected by sensors that mark the site of damage. Three kinase signaling cascades (ATM, ATR, and DNA-PK) regulate and transduce the response to damage. With the help of mediator proteins, transducer and effector proteins transmit and greatly amplify the signal throughout the cell, resulting in a huge influx of factors to repair damage and remodel chromatin. Two major repair pathways, HR and NHEJ, are regulated by the ATM/ATR and DNA-PK pathways, respectively. The nucleus on the left contains an HPV replication focus that mimics a DDR focus. Adapted from [71].

The unusual structure of viral DNA (e.g., extrachromosomal linear or small circular molecules), unscheduled viral DNA synthesis, viral protein expression or aberrant cellular proliferation can induce a DDR in infected cells. While this can be detrimental to infection, many viruses disable certain components of the DDR and take advantage of others to synthesize and process viral DNA in productive infection [73,74]. Viral DNA synthesis can also result in additional unique structures that require processing. For example, studies in SV40 show that ATM and ATR are required for quality control of viral replication products and for maintenance of the replication foci; ATM signaling reduces unidirectional replication and ATR signaling prevents DNA breakage at the converging forks that result from bidirectional replication [75]. ATM also ensures that HR factors, and not NHEJ factors, are recruited to SV40 replication centers [76]. The use of repair pathways to synthesize viral DNA also enables replication in cells that are outwith S-phase. Not only does this reduce competition from host cell synthesis, but in the case of HPVs, the use of repair pathways to synthesize DNA allows replication in differentiated cells. A landmark study in the HPV field demonstrated that the ATM arm of the DDR response was required for amplification of HPV31 genomes in differentiated cells [69]. Subsequent studies have shown that several viral proteins, including E1 and E7, are involved in the recruitment of DSB repair factors to HPV replication factories [61,77–80]. HPV replication foci also recruit factors from both the ATM and ATR pathways, such as TopBP1, Rad51, pNBS1, MRN, RPA, BRCA1, and 53BP1 [61,63,69,77–81].

In the context of the life cycle, E6 and E7 play important roles in both promoting DDR pathways as well as inhibiting the downstream consequences. In general, E7 promotes the DDR to provide an environment conducive for viral replication while E6 mitigates the downstream effects of the DDR cascade to allow cells to tolerate chronic DDR activation, growth arrest and/or apoptosis. Thus, HPVs have usurped DNA damage sensing and repair strategies to promote viral DNA replication. The sections below will review current knowledge of the role of the DDR in the different phases of HPV DNA replication.

3.2. HPV Replication Foci Formation

High level amplification of viral DNA occurs as infected cells differentiate and progress toward the epithelial surface. Most viruses replicate their genomes in defined cellular regions that are designated replication foci, compartments, or factories. These regions serve to nucleate and concentrate the components required for viral DNA synthesis and other processes to specific regions of the cell, presumably to facilitate viral replication. Nuclear replication foci can be detected in differentiated cells that contain replicating HPV [61,69,82].

Studies from our lab as well as others have shown that HPV viral DNA replication occurs in nuclear foci and is dependent on the E1 and E2 proteins. Expression of the E1 and E2 replication proteins (along with an origin containing replicon) is sufficient for the formation of replication foci that recruit components of the DDR [77,78,80,83]. The E1 protein induces the DDR and this is concentrated into nuclear foci by the E2 protein [77,78]. Viral DNA is amplified to high levels in these foci and this does not require keratinocyte differentiation, most likely because E1 and E2 are provided from heterologous promoters. Remarkably, viral replication factories mimic cellular DNA damage foci, whereby a single DNA lesion results in a huge influx of factors to repair damage (Figure 4). Thus, by inducing and usurping the DDR pathways, HPVs can take advantage of major cellular pathways and resources

3.3. The Role of the DNA Damage Response during Initial Amplification of HPV

Difficulties in obtaining large numbers of virions have greatly hampered the study of the early events of HPV infection. Viral DNA (cleaved from plasmids propagated in bacteria and recircularized) can be transfected into keratinocytes or other cells as a surrogate for early infection. Such studies may not completely mimic delivery of a viral genome in a virion particle, but they can provide some insight into the early events required for infection. On the other hand, replication obtained with viral genomes deficient in E8^E2 repressor expression, or when viral genomes are co-transfected with E1 and E2 expression vectors, most likely represent the runaway replication observed in vegetative amplification.

It has been shown that PVs enter the nucleus and initiate their replication and transcription program adjacent to ND10 bodies, like many other viruses [20]. ND10 bodies are important for anti-viral defense and one of the components, Sp100, represses transcription and replication of incoming virions [84].

ND10 bodies are associated with regions of DNA damage in uninfected cells and may provide a link between early events in HPV entry and the initial rounds of unscheduled viral DNA synthesis required to initiate infection [85]. As HPV enters the cell it is likely that this unscheduled viral DNA synthesis will activate or use components of the DDR for limited amplification of the viral genome. A recent study from our laboratory demonstrated that the HPV E2 proteins bind to host chromatin in complex with BRD4 at regions of the genome undergoing replication stress [43], and we proposed that these interactions are important for both genome tethering during maintenance replication as well as nucleation of replication foci in vegetative amplification. We predict that the interaction of viral genomes with host chromatin becomes established at very early stages of infection and involves the DNA damage response.

Although it has been shown in some studies that transient replication of HPV16 is not inhibited by DNA damage signaling or by p53 induction [86,87], it is likely that these responses have to be tempered for the infected cell to transition into the maintenance phase. A quantitative colony-forming assay is a useful measure of genome establishment [84,88], but it indicates that this is a rare event. This is very similar to findings that establishment of Epstein-Barr virus derived replicons is infrequent [89]. Thus, the virus must evade intrinsic immune responses, modulate DDR responses, and tether to beneficial regions of host chromatin to ensure a long-term, persistent infection.

3.4. The Role of the DNA Damage Response during Maintenance Replication.

During the maintenance phase of replication, HPV genomes are replicated in S-phase in synchrony with host DNA replication. Cells containing HPV genomes have increased markers of ATM and ATR signaling, but pharmacological inhibition of the ATM pathway does not affect genome maintenance [69]. However, it has been reported that siRNA-mediated reduction of ATM, ATR or several other proteins in the DDR pathway, as well as Chk1 inhibition results in 40%–50% reduction in HPV16 copy number in W12 cells [90,91].

Many DNA tumor viruses inactivate pRB and p21 and derepress expression of the E2F transcription factor family and for HMCV this is important for ATM-driven viral replication [92]. Furthermore, deregulation of E2F1 by E7 induces the expression of Chk2 [93], implying that this function of E7 could promote HPV replication. E7 deregulation of E2F, and subsequent nucleotide deficiency, further promotes replication stress and genomic instability [94]. In addition, E7 can promote mitotic entry in the presence of a DDR response by accelerating the degradation of the Chk1 binding protein, claspin [95]. Therefore, HPVs integrate DNA damage signaling with anti-apoptotic and proliferative functions to create a unique cellular environment that supports viral replication.

Activation of ATM and ATR signaling results in activation of p53 with a concomitant growth arrest that would be detrimental for viral replication in dividing cells. However, several studies have shown that the ability of E6 to degrade and/or inactivate p53 is crucial for long-term genome maintenance [14,96,97]. Furthermore, inactivation of p53 or expression of a dominant negative p53 protein can complement genomes defective for E6 expression [87,98].

3.5. The Role of the DNA Damage Response during Vegetative Amplification of Viral Genomes

Most of what we know about the role of the DDR in HPV biology has been elucidated from studies of late viral DNA replication. The E1 and E2 replication proteins are induced to high levels by a differentiation-dependent induction of the late promoter [99] and this coincides with activation of a DDR [69]. Many studies have also shown that E1 can specifically upregulate and contribute to the activation of the DDR in non-differentiated cells, and when coexpressed with E2, many DDR factors such as pATM, pATR, γH2AX, pChk2, pChk1, BRCA1, RAD51, TopBP1 and pNBS1 colocalize within nuclear foci that replicate viral DNA to high levels [63,77,78,80].

In the more natural condition of a stratified epithelium, E7 plays an important role in inducing the ATM arm of the DDR in differentiated cells [16] and ATM signaling is required for genome amplification [69]. E7 specifically interacts with NBS1 (which is also required for viral replication), and this association can be separated from activation of the ATM pathway [100]. Further, studies using inhibitors of signal transducer and transactivator 5 (STAT5), a member of the JAK-STAT pathway and an important regulator of the immune response, displayed that STAT5 positively regulates vegetative amplification of HPV31 via potentiation of the ATM pathway through activation of Chk2 [101]. STAT5 activity was dependent on E7 expression, further demonstrating the role of E7 during vegetative amplification. Although the extent of the landscape of E7-driven regulation of cellular protein expression and signaling pathways is not fully understood, E7-mediated upregulation and accumulation of MRN and HR factors as well as stimulation of ATM through the activity of STAT5 is required to properly engage the DDR machinery to facilitate differentiation-dependent genome amplification, bridging the nexus of innate immunity and DNA repair.

The dysregulation of p53 via E6 during vegetative amplification is also necessary to provide an environment conducive for viral DNA amplification. Viruses that are unable to degrade or inactivate p53 are unable to amplify viral DNA in a stratified epithelium [102]. Separate from its role in checkpoint control, p53 can directly inhibit amplification replication in several PVs [103–105], perhaps by directly binding to the E2 protein [106]. Therefore, like other viruses, HPVs take advantage of some aspects of the DDR, but inactivate others.

The presence of several HR factors within HPV replication foci indicates that the transition from maintenance to amplification might also involve a switch to a distinct replication mechanism, such as recombination-dependent replication [67,68,82,107,108]. This has several advantages such as enabling replication in the G2 phase of the cell cycle, as well as generating large amounts of viral DNA without the need for replication initiator proteins to reinitiate DNA synthesis [109].

3.6. The Role of the DNA Damage Response in HPV Integration and Carcinogenesis

As described above, E7 and E6 have important roles in promoting the DDR to support viral DNA replication and render cells resistant to the consequences of checkpoint activation. However, this inadvertently leaves cells highly susceptible to mutation and genetic instability. This has been well studied for the oncogenic alpha-HPVs, but there is also evidence that the cutaneous beta-HPVs might manipulate the host DDR pathways to promote viral replication. Indeed, expression of beta-HPV E6 interferes with DDR signaling at many levels, rendering cellular genomes vulnerable to UV damage and carcinogenic genetic instability [110–116].

In many HPV associated cancers, the viral genome has become integrated into the host genome [117] often in regions of genetic instability called common fragile sites [118,119]. Could this be related to the reliance of the virus on the DDR for replication? We have shown recently that HPV E2 proteins associate with genetically unstable regions of the host chromosomes and also that late replication foci form adjacent to these sites [43]. It could be beneficial to the virus to associate with regions of host chromatin that are highly susceptible to replication stress and prone to late replication. However, the close association of viral and host replication (especially regions undergoing recombination-directed repair) could inadvertently lead to integration of the viral genome. Notably, common fragile sites and extrachromosomal HPV genomes have similar susceptibilities to ATR inhibitors, and to the replication inhibitor aphidicolin [90]. Recent studies have shown that HPV integration sites are highly unstable and involve many rearrangements and duplications of virus and host sequences [120]. It is generally thought that the E1 and E2 replication proteins are not expressed from integrated genomes but expression of these proteins from co-replicating, extrachromosomal HPV genomes induces recruitment of DDR proteins to the integration loci, resulting in onion skin replication and promoting genetic instability [121,122]. In the absence of the viral replication proteins, genetic instability can be further increased by homologous recombination-related looping mechanisms [120]. Any modification that results in increased expression of the E6 and E7 oncoproteins will further stimulate genetic instability and promote carcinogenesis.

4. Conclusions

DDR signaling upon infection is a common strategy utilized by many DNA viruses to recruit factors necessary for replication [74], and, as described here, activation of the DDR plays an important role in the HPV life cycle. As a small virus with limited coding capacity and few replication proteins, HPV needs to utilize the host DNA synthesis machinery to amplify itself. However, it must also reprogram and coordinate multiple cellular signaling pathways to establish an environment conducive to viral replication. Manipulation of the DDR provides a means to efficientlymodulate cell cycle checkpoints as well as recruit and usurp replication factors, especially in differentiated cells. The rapid expansion of the genome copy number during the amplification phase of the viral life cycle requires a replication mechanism with high fidelity and there is evidence that homologous recombination repair pathways may provide a means to both initiate replication and resolve DNA intermediates that occur during this phase of rapid DNA synthesis. Ongoing research in many laboratories should provide further mechanistic insight into the pathways and events that result in successful HPV propagation.

Acknowledgments

The authors' research is funded by the Intramural Research Program of the National Institute of Allergy and Infectious Disease of the National Institutes of Health.

Author Contributions

C.M., K.H., and A.M. wrote the manuscript.

References

1. Cubie, H.A. Diseases associated with human papillomavirus infection. *Virology* **2013**, *445*, 21–34.
2. McLaughlin-Drubin, M.E.; Meyers, J.; Munger, K. Cancer associated human papillomaviruses.

Curr. Opin. Virol. **2012**, *2*, 459–466. [CrossRef] [PubMed]

3. Zur Hausen, H. Papillomavirus infections—A major cause of human cancers. *Biochim. Biophys. Acta* **1996**, *1288*, F55–F78. [PubMed]
4. HPV-Associated Cancers Statistics. Available online: http://www.cdc.gov/cancer/hpv/statistics/ (accessed on 13 March 2015).
5. NIAID The Papillomavirus Episteme. Available online: http://pave.niaid.nih.gov/ (accessed on 13 March 2015).
6. McBride, A.A. Replication and partitioning of papillomavirus genomes. *Adv. Virus Res.* **2008**, *72*, 155–205. [PubMed]
7. Mohr, I.J.; Clark, R.; Sun, S.; Androphy, E.J.; MacPherson, P.; Botchan, M.R. Targeting the E1 replication protein to the papillomavirus origin of replication by complex formation with the E2 transactivator. *Science* **1990**, *250*, 1694–1699. [CrossRef] [PubMed]
8. Ustav, M.; Stenlund, A. Transient replication of BPV-1 requires two viral polypeptides encoded by the E1 and E2 open reading frames. *EMBO J.* **1991**, *10*, 449–457. [PubMed]
9. Ustav, M.; Ustav, E.; Szymanski, P.; Stenlund, A. Identification of the origin of replication of bovine papillomavirus and characterization of the viral origin recognition factor E1. *EMBO J.* **1991**, *10*, 4321–4329. [PubMed]
10. Sanders, C.M.; Stenlund, A. Recruitment and loading of the E1 initiator protein: An ATP-dependent process catalysed by a transcription factor. *EMBO J.* **1998**, *17*, 7044–7055.
11. Egawa, N.; Nakahara, T.; Ohno, S.; Narisawa-Saito, M.; Yugawa, T.; Fujita, M.; Yamato, K.; Natori, Y.; Kiyono, T. The E1 protein of human papillomavirus type 16 is dispensable for maintenance replication of the viral genome. *J. Virol.* **2012**, *86*, 3276–3283. [CrossRef] [PubMed]
12. Kim, K.; Lambert, P.F. E1 protein of bovine papillomavirus 1 is not required for the maintenance of viral plasmid DNA replication. *Virology* **2002**, *293*, 10–14. [CrossRef] [PubMed]
13. McLaughlin-Drubin, M.E.; Bromberg-White, J.L.; Meyers, C. The role of the human papillomavirus type 18 E7 oncoprotein during the complete viral life cycle. *Virology* **2005**, *338*, 61–68. [CrossRef] [PubMed]
14. Flores, E.R.; Allen-Hoffmann, B.L.; Lee, D.; Lambert, P.F. The human papillomavirus type 16 E7 oncogene is required for the productive stage of the viral life cycle. *J. Virol.* **2000**, *74*, 6622–6631.
15. Chow, L.T.; Duffy, A.A.; Wang, H.K.; Broker, T.R. A highly efficient system to produce infectious human papillomavirus: Elucidation of natural virus-host interactions. *Cell Cycle* **2009**, *8*, 1319–1323. [CrossRef] [PubMed]
16. Banerjee, N.S.; Wang, H.K.; Broker, T.R.; Chow, L.T. Human papillomavirus (HPV) E7 induces prolonged G2 following S phase reentry in differentiated human keratinocytes. *J. Biol. Chem.* **2011**, *286*, 15473–15482. [CrossRef] [PubMed]
17. Nakahara, T.; Peh, W.L.; Doorbar, J.; Lee, D.; Lambert, P.F. Human papillomavirus type 16 E1^E4 contributes to multiple facets of the papillomavirus life cycle. *J. Virol.* **2005**, *79*, 13150–13165.
18. Day, P.M.; Schelhaas, M. Concepts of papillomavirus entry into host cells. *Curr. Opin. Virol.* **2014**, *4*, 24–31. [CrossRef] [PubMed]
19. Culp, T.D.; Budgeon, L.R.; Christensen, N.D. Human papillomaviruses bind a basal extracellular

matrix component secreted by keratinocytes which is distinct from a membrane-associated receptor. *Virology* **2006**, *347*, 147–159. [CrossRef] [PubMed]

20. Day, P.M.; Baker, C.C.; Lowy, D.R.; Schiller, J.T. Establishment of papillomavirus infection is enhanced by promyelocytic leukemia protein (PML) expression. *Proc. Natl. Acad. Sci. USA* **2004**, *101*, 14252–14257. [CrossRef] [PubMed]
21. Pyeon, D.; Pearce, S.M.; Lank, S.M.; Ahlquist, P.; Lambert, P.F. Establishment of human papillomavirus infection requires cell cycle progression. *PLoS Pathog.* **2009**, *5*, e1000318.
22. Aydin, I.; Weber, S.; Snijder, B.; Samperio Ventayol, P.; Kuhbacher, A.; Becker, M.; Day, P.M.; Schiller, J.T.; Kann, M.; Pelkmans, L.; *et al.* Large scale RNAi reveals the requirement of nuclear envelope breakdown for nuclear import of human papillomaviruses. *PLoS Pathog.* **2014**, *10*, e1004162. [CrossRef] [PubMed]
23. Evans, M.F.; Aliesky, H.A.; Cooper, K. Optimization of biotinyl-tyramide-based *in situ* hybridization for sensitive background-free applications on formalin-fixed, paraffin-embedded tissue specimens. *BMC Clin. Pathol.* **2003**, *3*, e2. [CrossRef]
24. Peh, W.L.; Middleton, K.; Christensen, N.; Nicholls, P.; Egawa, K.; Sotlar, K.; Brandsma, J.; Percival, A.; Lewis, J.; Liu, W.J.; *et al.* Life cycle heterogeneity in animal models of human papillomavirus-associated disease. *J. Virol.* **2002**, *76*, 10401–10416. [CrossRef] [PubMed]
25. Ozbun, M.A. Human papillomavirus type 31b infection of human keratinocytes and the onset of early transcription. *J. Virol.* **2002**, *76*, 11291–11300. [CrossRef] [PubMed]
26. Stubenrauch, F.; Hummel, M.; Iftner, T.; Laimins, L.A. The E8E2C protein, a negative regulator of viral transcription and replication, is required for extrachromosomal maintenance of human papillomavirus type 31 in keratinocytes. *J. Virol.* **2000**, *74*, 1178–1186. [CrossRef] [PubMed]
27. Botchan, M.; Berg, L.; Reynolds, J.; Lusky, M. The bovine papillomavirus replicon. In *Papillomaviruses*; John Wiley & Sons: New York, NY, USA, 1986; pp. 53–67.
28. Roberts, J.M.; Weintraub, H. *Cis*-acting negative control of DNA replication in eukaryotic cells. *Cell* **1988**, *52*, 397–404. [CrossRef] [PubMed]
29. Gilbert, D.M.; Cohen, S.N. Bovine papilloma virus plasmids replicate randomly in mouse fibroblasts throughout S phase of the cell cycle. *Cell* **1987**, *50*, 59–68. [CrossRef] [PubMed]
30. Ravnan, J.-B.; Gilbert, D.M.; Ten Hagen, K.G.; Cohen, S.N. Random-choice replication of extrachromosomal bovine papillomavirus (BPV) molecules in heterogeneous, clonally derived BPV-infected cell lines. *J. Virol.* **1992**, *66*, 6946–6952. [PubMed]
31. Hoffmann, R.; Hirt, B.; Bechtold, V.; Beard, P.; Raj, K. Different modes of human papillomavirus DNA replication during maintenance. *J. Virol.* **2006**, *80*, 4431–4439. [CrossRef] [PubMed]
32. Fradet-Turcotte, A.; Moody, C.; Laimins, L.A.; Archambault, J. Nuclear export of human papillomavirus type 31 E1 is regulated by Cdk2 phosphorylation and required for viral genome maintenance. *J. Virol.* **2010**, *84*, 11747–11760. [CrossRef] [PubMed]
33. Yu, J.H.; Lin, B.Y.; Deng, W.; Broker, T.R.; Chow, L.T. Mitogen-activated protein kinases activate the nuclear localization sequence of human papillomavirus type 11 E1 DNA helicase to promote efficient nuclear import. *J. Virol.* **2007**, *81*, 5066–5078. [CrossRef] [PubMed]
34. Straub, E.; Dreer, M.; Fertey, J.; Iftner, T.; Stubenrauch, F. The viral E8^E2C repressor limits productive replication of human papillomavirus 16. *J. Virol.* **2014**, *88*, 937–947.

35. Gunasekharan, V.; Laimins, L.A. Human papillomaviruses modulate microRNA 145 expression to directly control genome amplification. *J. Virol.* **2013**, *87*, 6037–6043. [CrossRef] [PubMed]
36. Penrose, K.J.; McBride, A.A. Proteasome-mediated degradation of the papillomavirus E2-TA protein is regulated by phosphorylation and can modulate viral genome copy number. *J. Virol.* **2000**, *74*, 6031–6038. [CrossRef] [PubMed]
37. Skiadopoulos, M.H.; McBride, A.A. Bovine papillomavirus type 1 genomes and the E2 transactivator protein are closely associated with mitotic chromatin. *J. Virol.* **1998**, *72*, 2079–2088. [PubMed]
38. Ilves, I.; Kivi, S.; Ustav, M. Long-term episomal maintenance of bovine papillomavirus type 1 plasmids is determined by attachment to host chromosomes, which is mediated by the viral E2 protein and its binding sites. *J. Virol.* **1999**, *73*, 4404–4412. [PubMed]
39. Bastien, N.; McBride, A.A. Interaction of the papillomavirus E2 protein with mitotic chromosomes. *Virology* **2000**, *270*, 124–134. [CrossRef] [PubMed]
40. McBride, A.A.; Oliveira, J.G.; McPhillips, M.G. Partitioning viral genomes in mitosis: Same idea, different targets. *Cell Cycle* **2006**, *5*, 1499–1502. [CrossRef] [PubMed]
41. Oliveira, J.G.; Colf, L.A.; McBride, A.A. Variations in the association of papillomavirus E2 proteins with mitotic chromosomes. *Proc. Natl. Acad. Sci. USA* **2006**, *103*, 1047–1052. [CrossRef] [PubMed]
42. Jang, M.K.; Kwon, D.; McBride, A.A. Papillomavirus E2 proteins and the host BRD4 protein associate with transcriptionally active cellular chromatin. *J. Virol.* **2009**, *83*, 2592–2600.
43. Jang, M.K.; Shen, K.; McBride, A.A. Papillomavirus genomes associate with BRD4 to replicate at fragile sites in the host genome. *PLoS Pathog.* **2014**, *10*, e1004117. [CrossRef] [PubMed]
44. Helfer, C.M.; Yan, J.; You, J. The cellular bromodomain protein Brd4 has multiple functions in E2-mediated papillomavirus transcription activation. *Viruses* **2014**, *6*, 3228–3249.
45. Jang, M.K.; Anderson, D.E.; van Doorslaer, K.; McBride, A.A. A Proteomic approach to discover and compare interacting partners of Papillomavirus E2 proteins from diverse phylogenetic groups. *Proteomics* **2015**. [CrossRef]
46. McBride, A.A. The Papillomavirus E2 proteins. *Virology* **2013**, *445*, 57–79. [CrossRef] [PubMed]
47. Devaiah, B.N.; Singer, D.S. Two faces of brd4: Mitotic bookmark and transcriptional lynchpin. *Transcription* **2013**, *4*, 13–17. [CrossRef] [PubMed]
48. McBride, A.A.; Jang, M.K. Current understanding of the role of the Brd4 protein in the papillomavirus lifecycle. *Viruses* **2013** *5*, 1374–1394. [CrossRef] [PubMed]
49. You, J.; Croyle, J.L.; Nishimura, A.; Ozato, K.; Howley, P.M. Interaction of the bovine papillomavirus E2 protein with Brd4 tethers the viral DNA to host mitotic chromosomes. *Cell* **2004**, *117*, 349–360. [CrossRef] [PubMed]
50. Baxter, M.K.; McPhillips, M.G.; Ozato, K.; McBride, A.A. The mitotic chromosome binding activity of the papillomavirus E2 protein correlates with interaction with the cellular chromosomal protein, Brd4. *J. Virol.* **2005**, *79*, 4806–4818. [CrossRef] [PubMed]
51. McPhillips, M.G.; Ozato, K.; McBride, A.A. Interaction of bovine papillomavirus E2 protein with Brd4 stabilizes its association with chromatin. *J. Virol.* **2005**, *79*, 8920–8932.

52. McPhillips, M.G.; Oliveira, J.G.; Spindler, J.E.; Mitra, R.; McBride, A.A. Brd4 is required for e2-mediated transcriptional activation but not genome partitioning of all papillomaviruses. *J. Virol.* **2006**, *80*, 9530–9543. [CrossRef] [PubMed]
53. Rahman, S.; Sowa, M.E.; Ottinger, M.; Smith, J.A.; Shi, Y.; Harper, J.W.; Howley, P.M. The Brd4 extraterminal domain confers transcription activation independent of pTEFb by recruiting multiple proteins, including NSD3. *Mol. Cell. Biol.* **2011**, *31*, 2641–2652. [CrossRef] [PubMed]
54. Smith, J.A.; White, E.A.; Sowa, M.E.; Powell, M.L.; Ottinger, M.; Harper, J.W.; Howley, P.M. Genome-wide siRNA screen identifies SMCX, EP400, and Brd4 as E2-dependent regulators of human papillomavirus oncogene expression. *Proc. Natl. Acad. Sci. USA* **2010**, *107*, 3752–3757.
55. Schweiger, M.R.; Ottinger, M.; You, J.; Howley, P.M. Brd4 independent transcriptional repression function of the papillomavirus E2 proteins. *J. Virol.* **2007**, *81*, 9612–9622. [CrossRef] [PubMed]
56. Wu, S.Y.; Lee, A.Y.; Hou, S.Y.; Kemper, J.K.; Erdjument-Bromage, H.; Tempst, P.; Chiang, C.M. Brd4 links chromatin targeting to HPV transcriptional silencing. *Genes Dev.* **2006**, *20*, 2383–2396. [CrossRef] [PubMed]
57. Helfer, C.M.; Wang, R.; You, J. Analysis of the papillomavirus E2 and bromodomain protein Brd4 interaction using bimolecular fluorescence complementation. *PLoS ONE* **2013**, *8*, e77994.
58. Chang, S.-W.; Liu, W.-C.; Liao, K.-Y.; Tsao, Y.-P.; Hsu, P.-H.; Chen, S.-L. Phosphorylation of HPV-16 E2 at Serine 243 Enables Binding to Brd4 and Mitotic Chromosomes. *PLoS ONE* **2014**, *9*, e110882. [CrossRef] [PubMed]
59. Stubenrauch, F.; Colbert, A.M.; Laimins, L.A. Transactivation by the E2 protein of oncogenic human papillomavirus type 31 is not essential for early and late viral functions. *J. Virol.* **1998**, *72*, 8115–8123. [PubMed]
60. Senechal, H.; Poirier, G.G.; Coulombe, B.; Laimins, L.A.; Archambault, J. Amino acid substitutions that specifically impair the transcriptional activity of papillomavirus E2 affect binding to the long isoform of Brd4. *Virology* **2007**, *358*, 10–17. [CrossRef] [PubMed]
61. Sakakibara, N.; Chen, D.; Jang, M.K.; Kang, D.W.; Luecke, H.F.; Wu, S.Y.; Chiang, C.M.; McBride, A.A. Brd4 Is Displaced from HPV Replication Factories as They Expand and Amplify Viral DNA. *PLoS Pathog.* **2013**, *9*, e1003777. [CrossRef] [PubMed]
62. Wang, X.; Helfer, C.M.; Pancholi, N.; Bradner, J.E.; You, J. Recruitment of brd4 to the human papillomavirus type 16 DNA replication complex is essential for replication of viral DNA. *J. Virol.* **2013**, *87*, 3871–3884. [CrossRef] [PubMed]
63. Gauson, E.J.; Donaldson, M.M.; Dornan, E.S.; Wang, X.; Bristol, M.; Bodily, J.M.; Morgan, I.M. Evidence supporting a role for TopBP1 and Brd4 in the initiation but not continuation of human papillomavirus 16 E1/E2 mediated DNA replication. *J. Virol.* **2015**, *89*, 4980–4991.
64. Floyd, S.R.; Pacold, M.E.; Huang, Q.; Clarke, S.M.; Lam, F.C.; Cannell, I.G.; Bryson, B.D.; Rameseder, J.; Lee, M.J.; Blake, E.J.; *et al.* The bromodomain protein Brd4 insulates chromatin from DNA damage signalling. *Nature* **2013**, *498*, 246–250. [CrossRef] [PubMed]
65. Bedell, M.A.; Hudson, J.B.; Golub, T.R.; Turyk, M.E.; Hosken, M.; Wilbanks, G.D.; Laimins, L.A. Amplification of human papillomavirus genomes *in vitro* is dependent on epithelial differentiation. *J. Virol.* **1991**, *65*, 2254–2260. [PubMed]

66. Maglennon, G.A.; McIntosh, P.; Doorbar, J. Persistence of viral DNA in the epithelial basal layer suggests a model for papillomavirus latency following immune regression. *Virology* **2011**, *414*, 153–163. [CrossRef] [PubMed]
67. Flores, E.R.; Lambert, P.F. Evidence for a switch in the mode of human papillomavirus type 16 DNA replication during the viral life cycle. *J. Virol.* **1997**, *71*, 7167–7179. [PubMed]
68. Burnett, S.; Zabielski, J.; Moreno-Lopez, J.; Pettersson, U. Evidence for multiple vegetative DNA replication origins and alternative replication mechanisms of bovine papillomavirus type 1. *J. Mol. Biol.* **1989**, *206*, 239–244. [CrossRef] [PubMed]
69. Moody, C.A.; Laimins, L.A. Human Papillomaviruses Activate the ATM DNA Damage Pathway for Viral Genome Amplification upon Differentiation. *PLoS Pathog.* **2009**, *5*, e1000605.
70. Nakamura, J.; Mutlu, E.; Sharma, V.; Collins, L.; Bodnar, W.; Yu, R.; Lai, Y.; Moeller, B.; Lu, K.; Swenberg, J. The endogenous exposome. *DNA Repair* **2014**, *19*, 3–13. [CrossRef] [PubMed]
71. Jackson, S.P.; Bartek, J. The DNA-damage response in human biology and disease. *Nature* **2009**, *461*, 1071–1078. [CrossRef] [PubMed]
72. Stracker, T.H.; Usui, T.; Petrini, J.H. Taking the time to make important decisions: The checkpoint effector kinases Chk1 and Chk2 and the DNA damage response. *DNA Repair* **2009**, *8*, 1047–1054.
73. Chaurushiya, M.S.; Weitzman, M.D. Viral manipulation of DNA repair and cell cycle checkpoints. *DNA Repair* **2009**, *8*, 1166–1176. [CrossRef] [PubMed]
74. Luftig, M.A. Viruses and the DNA Damage Response: Activation and Antagonism. *Annu. Rev. Virol.* **2014**, *1*, 605–625. [CrossRef]
75. Sowd, G.A.; Li, N.Y.; Fanning, E. ATM and ATR activities maintain replication fork integrity during SV40 chromatin replication. *PLoS Pathog.* **2013**, *9*, e1003283. [CrossRef] [PubMed]
76. Sowd, G.A.; Mody, D.; Eggold, J.; Cortez, D.; Friedman, K.L.; Fanning, E. SV40 utilizes ATM kinase activity to prevent non-homologous end joining of broken viral DNA replication products. *PLoS Pathog.* **2014**, *10*, e1004536. [CrossRef] [PubMed]
77. Sakakibara, N.; Mitra, R.; McBride, A.A. The papillomavirus E1 helicase activates a cellular DNA damage response in viral replication foci. *J. Virol.* **2011**, *85*, 8981–8995. [CrossRef] [PubMed]
78. Fradet-Turcotte, A.; Bergeron-Labrecque, F.; Moody, C.A.; Lehoux, M.; Laimins, L.A.; Archambault, J. Nuclear accumulation of the papillomavirus E1 helicase blocks S-phase progression and triggers an ATM-dependent DNA damage response. *J. Virol.* **2011**, *85*, 8996–9012. [CrossRef] [PubMed]
79. Gillespie, K.A.; Mehta, K.P.; Laimins, L.A.; Moody, C.A. Human papillomaviruses recruit cellular DNA repair and homologous recombination factors to viral replication centers. *J. Virol.* **2012**, *86*, 9520–9526. [CrossRef] [PubMed]
80. Reinson, T.; Toots, M.; Kadaja, M.; Pipitch, R.; Allik, M.; Ustav, E.; Ustav, M. Engagement of the ATR-Dependent DNA Damage Response at the Human Papillomavirus 18 Replication Centers during the Initial Amplification. *J. Virol.* **2013**, *87*, 951–964. [CrossRef] [PubMed]
81. Kanginakudru, S.; DeSmet, M.; Thomas, Y.; Morgan, I.M.; Androphy, E.J. Levels of the E2 interacting protein TopBP1 modulate papillomavirus maintenance stage replication. *Virology* **2015**, *478*, 135–142. [CrossRef] [PubMed]
82. Sakakibara, N.; Chen, D.; McBride, A.A. Papillomaviruses use recombination-dependent

replication to vegetatively amplify their genomes in differentiated cells. *PLoS Pathog.* **2013**, *9*, e1003321. [CrossRef] [PubMed]

83. Swindle, C.S.; Zou, N.; van Tine, B.A.; Shaw, G.M.; Engler, J.A.; Chow, L.T. Human papillomavirus DNA replication compartments in a transient DNA replication system. *J. Virol.* **1999**, *73*, 1001–1009. [PubMed]
84. Stepp, W.H.; Meyers, J.M.; McBride, A.A. Sp100 provides intrinsic immunity against human papillomavirus infection. *MBio* **2013**, *4*, e00845–13. [CrossRef] [PubMed]
85. Everett, R.D. Interactions between DNA viruses, ND10 and the DNA damage response. *Cell. Microbiol.* **2006**, *8*, 365–374. [CrossRef] [PubMed]
86. King, L.E.; Fisk, J.C.; Dornan, E.S.; Donaldson, M.M.; Melendy, T.; Morgan, I.M. Human papillomavirus E1 and E2 mediated DNA replication is not arrested by DNA damage signalling. *Virology* **2010**, *406*, 95–102. [CrossRef] [PubMed]
87. Lorenz, L.D.; Rivera Cardona, J.; Lambert, P.F. Inactivation of p53 rescues the maintenance of high risk HPV DNA genomes deficient in expression of E6. *PLoS Pathog.* **2013**, *9*, e1003717.
88. Lace, M.J.; Turek, L.P.; Anson, J.R.; Haugen, T.H. Analyzing the Human Papillomavirus (HPV) Life Cycle in Primary Keratinocytes with a Quantitative Colony-Forming Assay. *Curr. Protoc. Microbiol.* **2014**, *33*, 14b.2.1–14b.2.13. [PubMed]
89. Leight, E.R.; Sugden, B. Establishment of an oriP replicon is dependent upon an infrequent, epigenetic event. *Mol. Cell. Biol.* **2001**, *21*, 4149–4161. [CrossRef] [PubMed]
90. Edwards, T.G.; Helmus, M.J.; Koeller, K.; Bashkin, J.K.; Fisher, C. Human papillomavirus episome stability is reduced by aphidicolin and controlled by DNA damage response pathways. *J. Virol.* **2013**, *87*, 3979–3989. [CrossRef] [PubMed]
91. Edwards, T.G.; Vidmar, T.J.; Koeller, K.; Bashkin, J.K.; Fisher, C. DNA damage repair genes controlling human papillomavirus (HPV) episome levels under conditions of stability and extreme instability. *PLoS ONE* **2013**, *8*, e75406. [CrossRef] [PubMed]
92. E, X.; Pickering, M.T.; Debatis, M.; Castillo, J.; Lagadinos, A.; Wang, S.; Lu, S.; Kowalik, T.F. An E2F1-mediated DNA damage response contributes to the replication of human cytomegalovirus. *PLoS Pathog.* **2011**, *7*, e1001342. [CrossRef] [PubMed]
93. Rogoff, H.A.; Pickering, M.T.; Frame, F.M.; Debatis, M.E.; Sanchez, Y.; Jones, S.; Kowalik, T.F. Apoptosis associated with deregulated E2F activity is dependent on E2F1 and Atm/Nbs1/Chk2. *Mol. Cell. Biol.* **2004**, *24*, 2968–2977. [CrossRef] [PubMed]
94. Bester, A.C.; Roniger, M.; Oren, Y.S.; Im, M.M.; Sarni, D.; Chaoat, M.; Bensimon, A.; Zamir, G.; Shewach, D.S.; Kerem, B. Nucleotide deficiency promotes genomic instability in early stages of cancer development. *Cell* **2011**, *145*, 435–446. [CrossRef] [PubMed]
95. Spardy, N.; Covella, K.; Cha, E.; Hoskins, E.E.; Wells, S.I.; Duensing, A.; Duensing, S. Human papillomavirus 16 E7 oncoprotein attenuates DNA damage checkpoint control by increasing the proteolytic turnover of claspin. *Cancer Res.* **2009**, *69*, 7022–7029. [CrossRef] [PubMed]
96. Thomas, J.T.; Hubert, W.G.; Ruesch, M.N.; Laimins, L.A. Human papillomavirus type 31 oncoproteins E6 and E7 are required for the maintenance of episomes during the viral life cycle in normal human keratinocytes. *Proc. Natl. Acad. Sci. USA* **1999**, *96*, 8449–8454.
97. Park, R.B.; Androphy, E.J. Genetic analysis of high-risk e6 in episomal maintenance of human papillomavirus genomes in primary human keratinocytes. *J. Virol.* **2002** *76*, 11359–11364.

98. Brimer, N.; Vande Pol, S.B. Papillomavirus E6 PDZ interactions can be replaced by repression of p53 to promote episomal human papillomavirus genome maintenance. *J. Virol.* **2014**, *88*, 3027–3030. [CrossRef] [PubMed]

99. Klumpp, D.J.; Laimins, L.A. Differentiation-induced changes in promoter usage for transcripts encoding the human papillomavirus type 31 replication protein E1. *Virology* **1999**, *257*, 239–246.

100. Anacker, D.C.; Gautam, D.; Gillespie, K.A.; Chappell, W.H.; Moody, C.A. Productive replication of human papillomavirus 31 requires DNA repair factor Nbs1. *J. Virol.* **2014**, *88*, 8528–8544.

101. Hong, S.; Laimins, L.A. The JAK-STAT Transcriptional Regulator, STAT-5, Activates the ATM DNA Damage Pathway to Induce HPV 31 Genome Amplification upon Epithelial Differentiation. *PLoS Pathog.* **2013**, *9*, e1003295. [CrossRef] [PubMed]

102. Kho, E.Y.; Wang, H.K.; Banerjee, N.S.; Broker, T.R.; Chow, L.T. HPV-18 E6 mutants reveal p53 modulation of viral DNA amplification in organotypic cultures. *Proc. Natl. Acad. Sci. USA* **2013**, *110*, 7542–7549. [CrossRef] [PubMed]

103. Lepik, D.; Ilves, I.; Kristjuhan, A.; Maimets, T.; Ustav, M. p53 protein is a suppressor of papillomavirus DNA amplificational replication. *J. Virol.* **1998**, *72*, 6822–6831.

104. Ilves, I.; Kadaja, M.; Ustav, M. Two separate replication modes of the bovine papillomavirus BPV1 origin of replication that have different sensitivity to p53. *Virus Res.* **2003**, *96*, 75–84.

105. Akgul, B.; Karle, P.; Adam, M.; Fuchs, P.G.; Pfister, H.J. Dual role of tumor suppressor p53 in regulation of DNA replication and oncogene E6-promoter activity of epidermodysplasia verruciformis-associated human papillomavirus type 8. *Virology* **2003**, *308*, 279–290.

106. Brown, C.; Kowalczyk, A.M.; Taylor, E.R.; Morgan, I.M.; Gaston, K. P53 represses human papillomavirus type 16 DNA replication via the viral E2 protein. *Virol. J.* **2008**, *5*, e5. [CrossRef]

107. Dasgupta, S.; Zabielski, J.; Simonsson, M.; Burnett, S. Rolling-circle replication of a high-copy BPV-1 plasmid. *J. Mol. Biol.* **1992**, *228*, 1–6. [CrossRef] [PubMed]

108. Auborn, K.J.; Little, R.D.; Platt, T.H.; Vaccariello, M.A.; Schildkraut, C.L. Replicative intermediates of human papillomavirus type 11 in laryngeal papillomas: Site of replication initiation and direction of replication. *Proc. Natl. Acad. Sci. USA* **1994**, *91*, 7340–7344.

109. Lydeard, J.R.; Lipkin-Moore, Z.; Sheu, Y.J.; Stillman, B.; Burgers, P.M.; Haber, J.E. Break-induced replication requires all essential DNA replication factors except those specific for pre-RC assembly. *Genes Dev.* **2010**, *24*, 1133–1144. [CrossRef] [PubMed]

110. Wallace, N.A.; Robinson, K.; Howie, H.L.; Galloway, D.A. HPV 5 and 8 E6 abrogate ATR activity resulting in increased persistence of UVB induced DNA damage. *PLoS Pathog.* **2012**, *8*, e1002807. [CrossRef] [PubMed]

111. Wallace, N.A.; Galloway, D.A. Manipulation of cellular DNA damage repair machinery facilitates propagation of human papillomaviruses. *Semin. Cancer Biol.* **2014**, *26*, 30–42.

112. Wallace, N.A.; Robinson, K.; Galloway, D.A. Beta human papillomavirus E6 expression inhibits stabilization of p53 and increases tolerance of genomic instability. *J. Virol.* **2014**, *88*, 6112–6127.

113. Wallace, N.A.; Robinson, K.; Howie, H.L.; Galloway, D.A. beta-HPV 5 and 8 E6 Disrupt Homology Dependent Double Strand Break Repair by Attenuating BRCA1 and BRCA2 Expression and Foci Formation. *PLoS Pathog.* **2015**, *11*, e1004687. [CrossRef] [PubMed]

114. Jackson, S.; Storey, A. E6 proteins from diverse cutaneous HPV types inhibit apoptosis in

response to UV damage. *Oncogene* **2000**, *19*, 592–598. [CrossRef] [PubMed]

115. Giampieri, S.; Storey, A. Repair of UV-induced thymine dimers is compromised in cells expressing the E6 protein from human papillomaviruses types 5 and 18. *Br. J. Cancer* **2004**, *90*, 2203–2209. [PubMed]
116. Holloway, A.; Simmonds, M.; Azad, A.; Fox, J.L.; Storey, A. Resistance to UV-induced apoptosis by beta-HPV5 E6 involves targeting of activated BAK for proteolysis by recruitment of the HERC1 ubiquitin ligase. *Int. J. Cancer J. Int. Cancer* **2015**, *136*, 2831–2843. [CrossRef]
117. Durst, M.; Gissmann, L.; Ikenberg, H.; zur Hausen, H. A papillomavirus DNA from a cervical carcinoma and its prevalence in cancer biopsy samples from different geographic regions. *Proc. Natl. Acad. Sci. USA* **1983**, *80*, 3812–3815. [CrossRef] [PubMed]
118. Thorland, E.C.; Myers, S.L.; Gostout, B.S.; Smith, D.I. Common fragile sites are preferential targets for HPV16 integrations in cervical tumors. *Oncogene* **2003**, *22*, 1225–1237.
119. Smith, P.P.; Friedman, C.L.; Bryant, E.M.; McDougall, J.K. Viral integration and fragile sites in human papillomavirus-immortalized human keratinocyte cell lines. *Genes Chromosomes Cancer* **1992**, *5*, 150–157. [CrossRef] [PubMed]
120. Akagi, K.; Li, J.; Broutian, T.R.; Padilla-Nash, H.; Xiao, W.; Jiang, B.; Rocco, J.W.; Teknos, T.N.; Kumar, B.; Wangsa, D.; *et al.* Genome-wide analysis of HPV integration in human cancers reveals recurrent, focal genomic instability. *Genome Res.* **2013**. [CrossRef]
121. Kadaja, M.; Sumerina, A.; Verst, T.; Ojarand, M.; Ustav, E.; Ustav, M. Genomic instability of the host cell induced by the human papillomavirus replication machinery. *EMBO J.* **2007**, *26*, 2180–2191. [CrossRef] [PubMed]
122. Kadaja, M.; Isok-Paas, H.; Laos, T.; Ustav, E.; Ustav, M. Mechanism of genomic instability in cells infected with the high-risk human papillomaviruses. *PLoS Pathog.* **2009**, *5*, e1000397.

Permissions

All chapters in this book were first published by MDPI; hereby published with permission under the Creative Commons Attribution License or equivalent. Every chapter published in this book has been scrutinized by our experts. Their significance has been extensively debated. The topics covered herein carry significant findings which will fuel the growth of the discipline. They may even be implemented as practical applications or may be referred to as a beginning point for another development.

The contributors of this book come from diverse backgrounds, making this book a truly international effort. This book will bring forth new frontiers with its revolutionizing research information and detailed analysis of the nascent developments around the world.

We would like to thank all the contributing authors for lending their expertise to make the book truly unique. They have played a crucial role in the development of this book. Without their invaluable contributions this book wouldn't have been possible. They have made vital efforts to compile up to date information on the varied aspects of this subject to make this book a valuable addition to the collection of many professionals and students.

This book was conceptualized with the vision of imparting up-to-date information and advanced data in this field. To ensure the same, a matchless editorial board was set up. Every individual on the board went through rigorous rounds of assessment to prove their worth. After which they invested a large part of their time researching and compiling the most relevant data for our readers.

The editorial board has been involved in producing this book since its inception. They have spent rigorous hours researching and exploring the diverse topics which have resulted in the successful publishing of this book. They have passed on their knowledge of decades through this book. To expedite this challenging task, the publisher supported the team at every step. A small team of assistant editors was also appointed to further simplify the editing procedure and attain best results for the readers.

Apart from the editorial board, the designing team has also invested a significant amount of their time in understanding the subject and creating the most relevant covers. They scrutinized every image to scout for the most suitable representation of the subject and create an appropriate cover for the book.

The publishing team has been an ardent support to the editorial, designing and production team. Their endless efforts to recruit the best for this project, has resulted in the accomplishment of this book. They are a veteran in the field of academics and their pool of knowledge is as vast as their experience in printing. Their expertise and guidance has proved useful at every step. Their uncompromising quality standards have made this book an exceptional effort. Their encouragement from time to time has been an inspiration for everyone.

The publisher and the editorial board hope that this book will prove to be a valuable piece of knowledge for researchers, students, practitioners and scholars across the globe.

List of Contributors

Gabrielė Stakaitytė, Jennifer J. Wood, Laura M. Knight, Hussein Abdul-Sada, Noor Suhana Adzahar, Nnenna Nwogu, Andrew Macdonald and Adrian Whitehouse
School of Molecular and Cellular Biology and Astbury Centre of Structural Molecular Biology, University of Leeds, Leeds, LS2 9JT, UK

Zachary L. Pratt
Department of Bacteriology and Food Research Institute, Microbial Sciences Building, University of Wisconsin- Madison, Madison, WI 53706, USA

Bill Sugden
Department of Oncology, McArdle Laboratory for Cancer Research, Madison, WI 53706, USA

Nagayasu Egawa, Heather Griffin and John Doorbar
Division of Virology, Department of Pathology, University of Cambridge, Tennis Court Road, Cambridge CB2 1QP, UK
The Francis Crick Institute Mill Hill Laboratory, the Ridgeway, Mill Hill, London NW7 1AA, UK

Kiyofumi Egawa
Department of Dermatology, The Jikei University School of Medicine, 3-25-8 Nishi shinbashi, Minato-ku, Tokyo 105-0003, Japan
Department of Microbiology, Kitasato University School of Allied Health and Sciences,
1-15-1 Kitasato, Sagamihara, Kanagawa 252-0373, Japan

Robert Hollingworth, George L. Skalka, Grant S. Stewart, Andrew D. Hislop and Roger J. Grand
School of Cancer Sciences, the College of Medicine and Dentistry, University of Birmingham, Birmingham B15 2TT, UK

David J. Blackbourn
School of Biosciences and Medicine, University of Surrey, Surrey GU2 7XH, UK

Özlem Cesur, Clare Nicol, Helen Groves, Jamel Mankouri, George Eric Blair and Nicola J. Stonehouse
School of Molecular and Cellular Biology, Faculty of Biological Sciences and Astbury Centre for Structural Molecular Biology, University of Leeds, Leeds LS2 9JT, UK

Jennifer Biryukov and Craig Meyers
Department of Microbiology and Immunology, The Pennsylvania State University, 500 University Drive, Hershey, PA 17033, USA

Abigail Morales-Sánchez
Unidad de Investigación en Virología y Cáncer, Hospital Infantil de México Federico Gómez. Dr. Márquez 162, Col. Doctores, C.P. 06720. México D.F., Mexico
Programa de Doctorado en Ciencias Biomédicas, Facultad de Medicina, Universidad Nacional Autónoma de Mexico. Av. Universidad 3000, Col. Universidad Nacional Autónoma de México, C.U., C.P. 04510 México D.F., México

Ezequiel M. Fuentes-Pananá
Unidad de Investigación en Virología y Cáncer, Hospital Infantil de México Federico Gómez. Dr. Márquez 162, Col. Doctores, C.P. 06720. México D.F., Mexico

Caleb C. McKinney, Katherine L. Hussmann and Alison A. McBride
Laboratory of Viral Diseases, National Institute of Allergy and Infectious Diseases, National Institutes of Health, Bethesda, MD 20892, USA

Index